Complications During and After Cataract Surgery

Ulrich Spandau · Gabor B. Scharioth

Complications During and After Cataract Surgery

From Phacoemulsification Over Secondary IOL Implantation to Dropped Nucleus

Second Edition

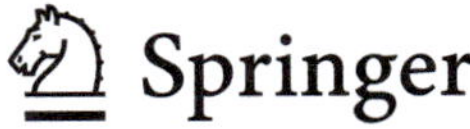 Springer

Ulrich Spandau
St. Eriks hospital
University of Stockholm
Stockholm, Sweden

Gabor B. Scharioth
Aurelios Augenzentrum
Recklinghausen, Germany

ISBN 978-3-030-93533-7   ISBN 978-3-030-93531-3   (eBook)
https://doi.org/10.1007/978-3-030-93531-3

This Springer imprint is published by the registered company Springer Nature Switzerland AG
The registered company address is: Gewerbestrasse 11, 6330 Cham, Switzerland

Introduction

How to manage a posterior capsule rupture or a zonular lysis? How to operate a dropped nucleus? What to do with a subluxated IOL? If you are seeking answers to these questions, then you found the right book. In this book, these questions and many, many more will be answered.

What is new in this second edition? The complete book is updated. We included several new techniques such as IOL rolling, Yamane technique, IOL fixation to the iris with suture and many more. Not last but least, the posterior segment section is completely redone. An exciting new technique for surgical management of dropped nucleus with a phacoemulsification handpiece is demonstrated. In addition, we demonstrate a trocar cannula technique which increases the surgical spectrum of a cataract surgeon immensely. For all operations, only a phacoemulsification machine was used.

The operations are described like in a cookbook. First, the ingredients and then the step-by-step preparations. These steps are illustrated with many pictures and drawings, followed by several surgical videos.

In my opinion, there are three parameters that make a good surgeon. They are surgical skill, experience and mastery of different surgical techniques.

Every surgeon is afraid of complications. This book takes the cataract surgeon's fear of complications by giving him a clear scheme in his hand after which he must proceed. Complications cannot be avoided, but you can learn to master them. And at the same time, you will also become a better surgeon.

All videos can be found in a playlist of my YouTube channel:
https://www.youtube.com/playlist?list=PL0dKYclPD7yMJRuQAIt9Dr7pOtuI0
Seex

I wish you much fun in the OR!

Stockholm, Sweden
Recklinghausen, Germany

Ulrich Spandau
Gabor B. Scharioth

Contents

Abbreviations

ECCE	Extracapsular cataract extraction
G	Gauge
I/A	Irrigation and aspiration
ICCE	Intracapsular cataract extraction
IOL	Intraocular lens
IOL in-the-bag	Intraocular lens is located inside the lens capsule
PCO	Posterior capsular opacification
PFCL	Perfluorocarbon liquid
PPV	Pars plana vitrectomy
PVD	Posterior vitreous detachment
SICS	Small incision cataract surgery (=modified ECCE)

Part I
Fundamentals for Complication Management

Basics

1

Contents

Abstract

In this chapter the basics of cataract surgery are explained; the difficulty of cataract surgery in relation to the density of the nucleus, the examination of pseudophakic eyes at the slit lamp and all you need to know about the intraocular lens.

Keywords

Basics · Cataract surgery · Intraocular lens · IOL

1.1 Difficulty of Cataract Surgery in Relation to Density of Nucleus

The difficulty of a cataract surgery depends on several factors. One important factor is the density of the nucleus.

A soft nucleus (Fig. 1.1) consists of an almost homogeneous soft nucleus and epinucleus. The age of the patient is approximately 50 years. A typical indication is a refractive lens exchange. The surgery is rather difficult. The nucleus is difficult to crack because it is so soft.

© The Author(s), under exclusive license to Springer Nature Switzerland AG 2022

3

U. Spandau and G. B. Scharioth, *Complications During and After Cataract Surgery*,
https://doi.org/10.1007/978-3-030-93531-3_1

Fig. 1.1 A soft nucleus. Nucleus and epinucleus are homogeneously soft. Not too easy to operate

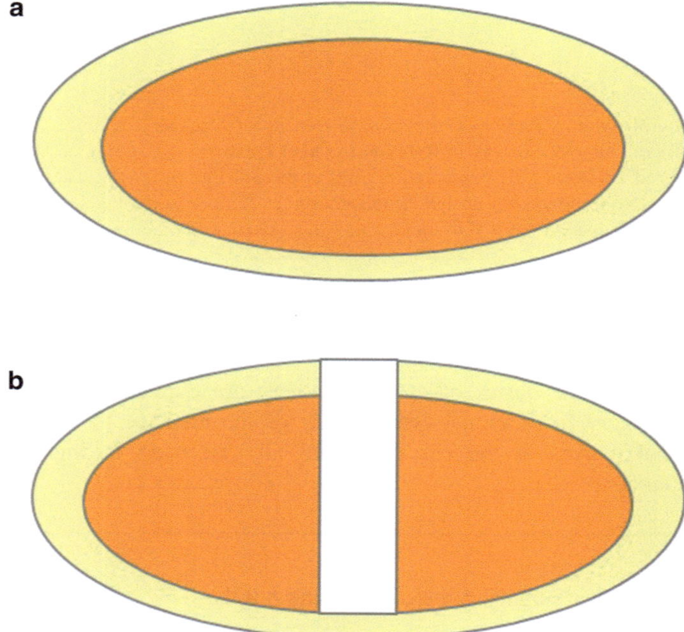

Fig. 1.2 Medium hard nucleus. **a** The nucleus is hard but the epinucleus is soft. **b** After cracking of the hard nucleus, the soft epinucleus remains as a scaffold for the posterior capsule. Good eye for a beginner

A medium hard nucleus (Fig. 1.2) consists of a hard nucleus and a soft epinucleus. The age of the patient is approximately 70 years. This cataract is rather easy to operate because the nucleus is easy to crack, and the soft epinucleus serves as a scaffold for the posterior capsule.

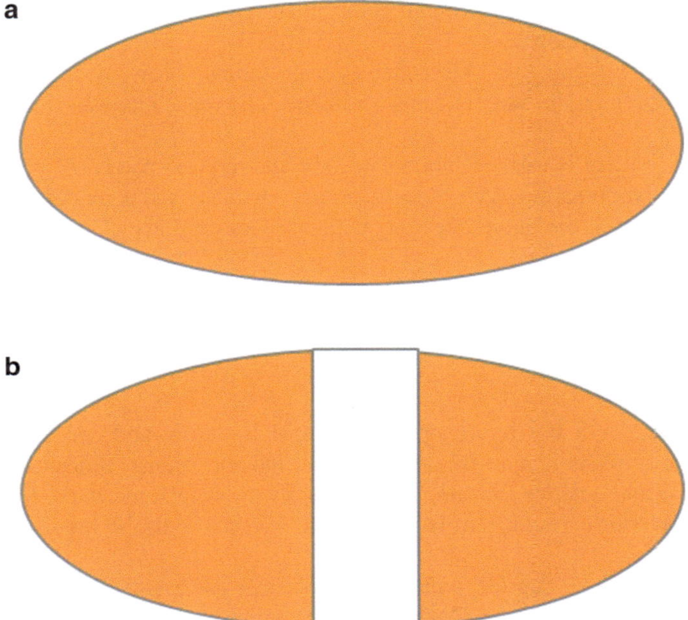

Fig. 1.3 Hard nucleus. **a** Nucleus and epinucleus are homogeneously hard. An epinucleus is practically not existent. **b** After cracking of the nucleus and epinucleus, the risk to damage the posterior capsule is high. There is no epinucleus left to protect the posterior capsule. Difficult to operate

A rock-hard nucleus (Fig. 1.3) consists of a hard nucleus and hard epinucleus. The lens is completely mature, i.e. nucleus and epinucleus are one hard mass and cannot be separated from each other. The patient is approximately 90 years old. The difficulty of this surgery is very high. The hard nucleus requires a high phacoemulsification energy, which may cause damage to the endothelium. Grooving is difficult because the red reflex is weak and because the epinucleus is as hard as the nucleus. Cracking is difficult because you need to crack the nucleus and the epinucleus. Removal of the quadrants is difficult because the soft epinucleus as scaffold is missing. In addition, the floppy posterior capsule may easily be aspirated into the phaco tip and be damaged.

1.2   Difficulty of Cataract Surgery in Relation to Other Factors

Patient selection: There are difficult patients with easy eyes, and there are easy patients with difficult eyes. It is impossible to say, which is worse.

What is a <u>difficult patient</u>? Spinal deformities, mental and motor restlessness and especially claustrophobia.

What is a <u>difficult eye</u>? Deep set eye, prominent brow, nystagmus, corneal opacities, small pupil, hard nucleus and especially phacodonesis due to zonular lysis.

An <u>easy patient</u> is relaxed, normal weight and approximately 70 <u>years</u> old. An <u>easy eye</u> is exophthalmic with a deep anterior chamber and a moderate cataract.

Try to select in the beginning <u>easy patients with easy eyes</u>.

1.3   Anatomy of Different IOL Implantation Sites at the Slit Lamp

It is difficult for a beginning ophthalmologist to know and see the difference between an implantation in the lens capsule and the sulcus. Sulcus is the space between iris and anterior capsule. The IOL is always implanted in the lens capsule. But if a posterior capsular rent is present, the IOL can only be implanted into the sulcus.

The anterior lens capsule undergoes a fibrosis and phimosis reaction after a cataract operation (Fig. 1.4). During the contractive reaction of the phimosis, the IOL optic may move before the edge of the rhexis. The reason for this is the rhexis size. If the rhexis has a regular size, then the optic will not move out of the rhexis. If the rhexis is too large, then the optic can flip before the rhexis. In most cases, only one part of the optic flips before the rhexis. The haptics however do not flip out of the capsular bag.

Examine an operated eye for these features. Observe the capsular fibrosis of the rhexis and check if it is located anterior or posterior to the optic edge (Fig. 1.4). The anterior capsular fibrosis may be completely (360°) located before the IOL (Fig. 1.4) or only partially (Fig. 1.5). The latter can be often seen. In this case, the

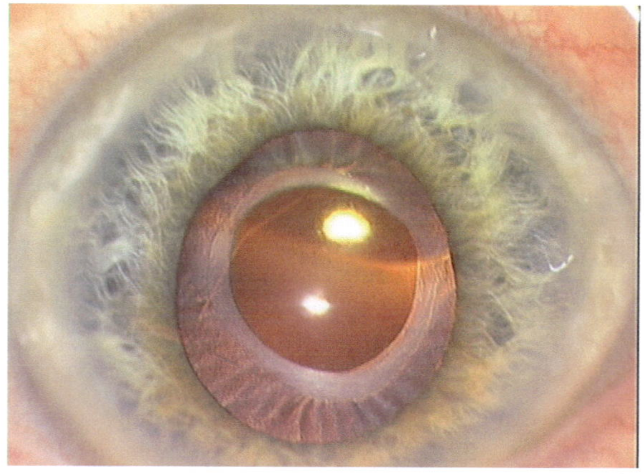

Fig. 1.4 A regular in the bag implantation. The anterior capsule underwent a fibrosis and a phimosis. The anterior capsule is 360° located anterior to the IOL

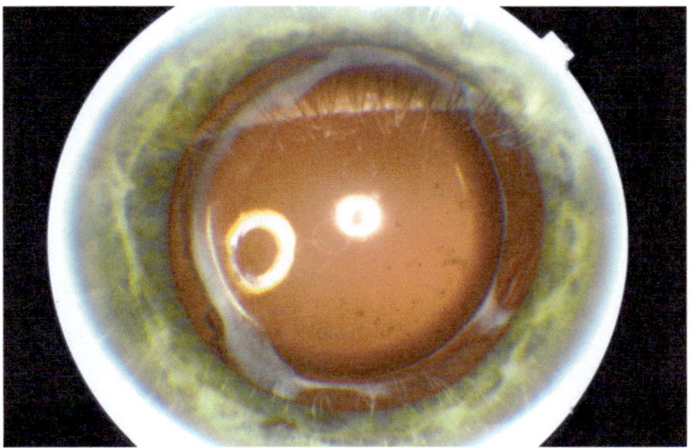

Fig. 1.5 Right eye: A regular in the bag implantation. The left part of the rhexis is located behind the IOL, the haptics at 1 o'clock and 7 o'clock are behind the rhexis, but the right part of the rhexis is located behind the IOL. The reason for this is that the right part of the rhexis flipped behind the IOL during the phimosis reaction

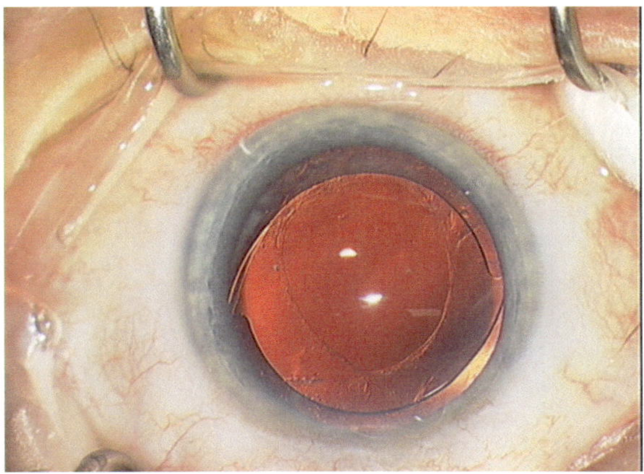

Fig. 1.6 This IOL is located in the sulcus. The sulcus is the space between iris and anterior capsule. The anterior capsule is located behind the IOL. Both, the haptics and the optic, are located before the anterior capsule. The lens and the posterior capsule were damaged due to a trauma, and a sulcus implantation was performed

right side of the rhexis flipped behind the IOL under the phimosis reaction of the anterior capsule. In case of a posterior capsule rupture, the lens is implanted in the sulcus. In this case, the anterior capsule is located behind the IOL (Fig. 1.6). If the IOL is implanted in the sulcus, it is possible to flip or buttonhole the optic behind the rhexis edge (lens capture) (Fig. 1.7). The lens is now centred, and a stable IOL-lens capsule diaphragm is obtained.

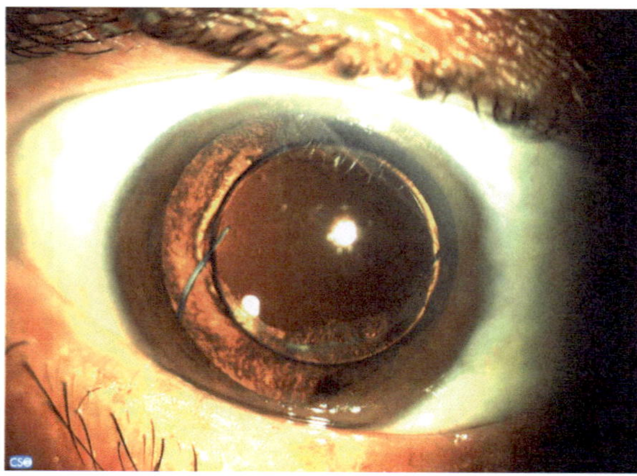

Fig. 1.7 This is a special case of a sulcus IOL: An IOL with lens capture. The optic is located behind the anterior capsule (behind the rhexis), but the haptics are located before the anterior capsule (sulcus). Typical is an oval form of the anterior capsule. The posterior capsule is damaged, and the IOL was fixated inside the rhexis in order to centre the IOL

Fig. 1.8 Subluxated IOL. Only the IOL is subluxated, the anterior lens capsule is intact and centred. The IOL can be repositioned in the sulcus

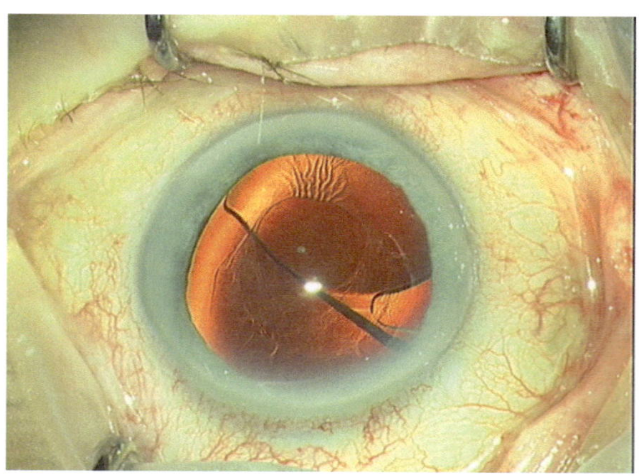

If the IOL is dislocated (subluxated), then observe if the lens capsule is also subluxated or not (Figs. 1.8 and 1.9). If the IOL was implanted into the sulcus, then it may happen that the IOL is dislocated and the (anterior) lens capsule is intact (Fig. 1.8). If the IOL was implanted into the lens capsule, it may occur that the in-the-bag-IOL subluxates man years later due to zonular lysis (Fig. 1.7).

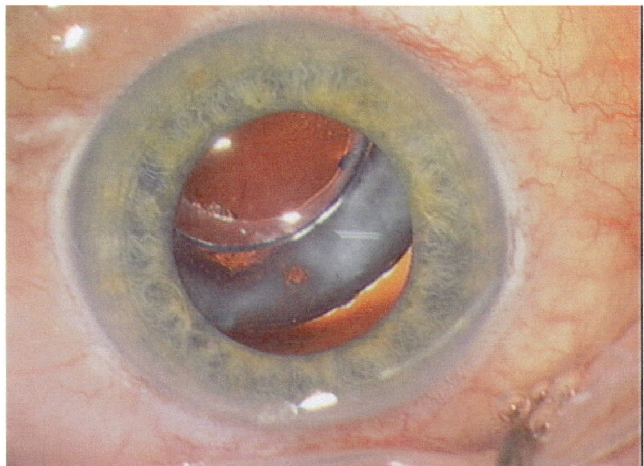

Fig. 1.9 Subluxated bag-IOL complex. The lens capsule with the IOL is subluxated due to zonular lysis. The IOL cannot be repositioned in the sulcus. A scleral or iris fixation is necessary.

1.4   Anatomic Requirements for an IOL Implantation

The best location for an IOL is the lens capsule (Fig. 1.10) because this is the natural place and because the lens capsule and IOL form a diaphragm separating the anterior from the posterior chamber. A rift in the anterior capsule is no hinder for an implantation in the lens capsule. A rift in the posterior capsule, however, is not acceptable. A round rhexis in the posterior capsule, however, is no problem. An alternative to the in-the-bag implantation is the sulcus implantation (Fig. 1.11). The sulcus is located between the iris and the anterior capsule. The requirement is an intact <u>anterior</u> lens capsule. A rift in the anterior capsule is not acceptable (with a few exceptions).

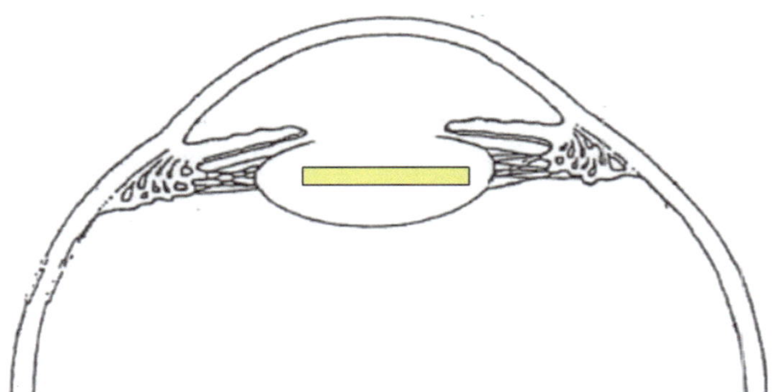

Fig. 1.10 Drawing of the anatomy of a regular in the bag implantation

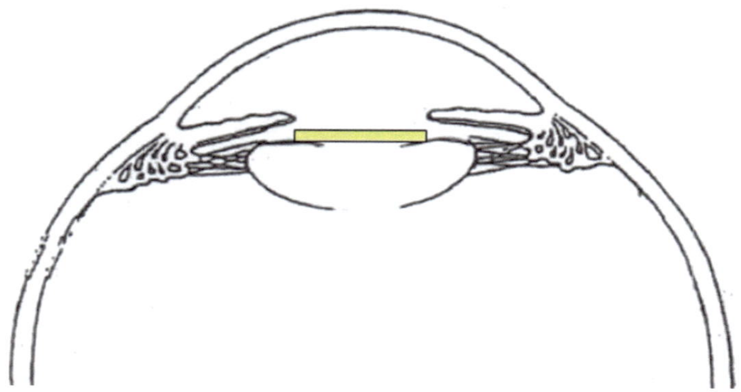

Fig. 1.11 Drawing of the anatomy of a sulcus-fixated IOL. The IOL is located between the iris and the anterior capsule

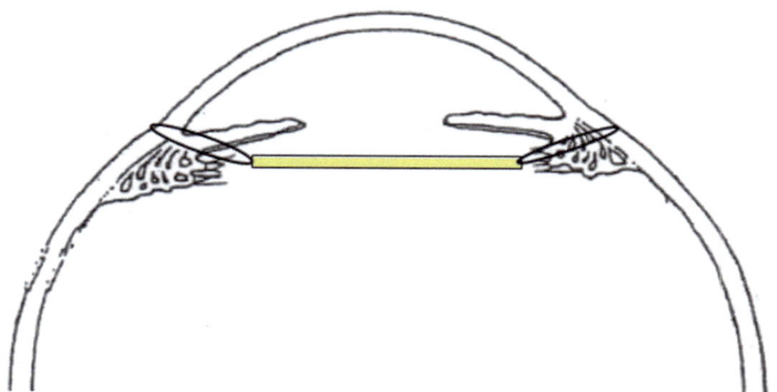

Fig. 1.12 Drawing of the anatomy of a scleral-fixated IOL. The lens capsule is absent

If the lens capsule is completely absent, then IOL implantation gets more difficult. The most popular method today is the intrascleral fixation of an IOL (Fig. 1.12). The haptics are inserted into the sclera (*intrascleral fixation*). No sutures are required. Alternatively, the haptics are sutured against the posterior iris (*iris suturing*). Another alternative is an iris fixation. A special iris-claw IOL is enclavated into the iris tissue (*Artisan IOL*) (Fig. 1.13).

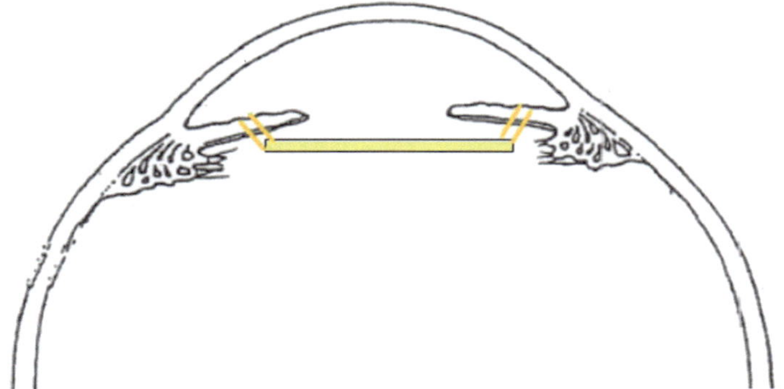

Fig. 1.13 Drawing of the anatomy of an iris-fixated IOL (retropupillar). The lens capsule is absent

1.5   1-piece IOL Versus 3-piece IOL

Intraocular lenses have an optic and two haptics. The most IOLs have also a sharp edge at the posterior side of the optic. This sharp edge functions as a barrier for ingrowing cells from the equator of the lens capsule preventing a posterior capsular opacification. Depending on the haptic design, there are two IOL designs on the market: 1-piece IOL which is made of one piece (Fig. 1.14) and a 3-piece IOL (Fig. 1.15) which is made of one optic and two haptics. A 1-piece IOL can only be implanted into the lens capsule but not in the sulcus because the thick haptics cause iris chafing with glaucoma–uveitis–hyphaema (GUH) (Fig. 1.16). The 3-piece IOL has thin haptics and can be implanted into the lens capsule as well into the sulcus.

Fig. 1.14 1-piece IOL. The IOL is made of one piece

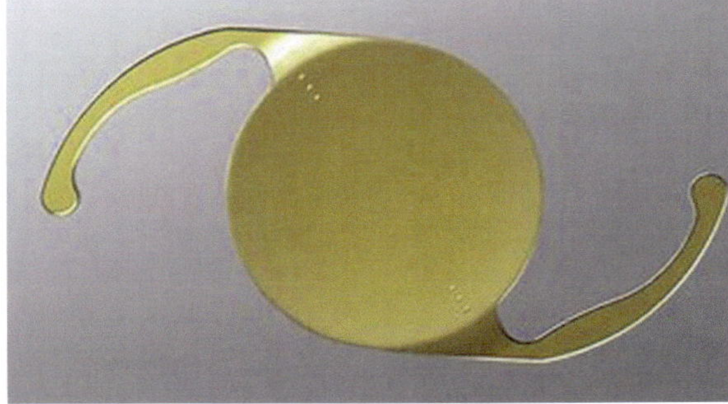

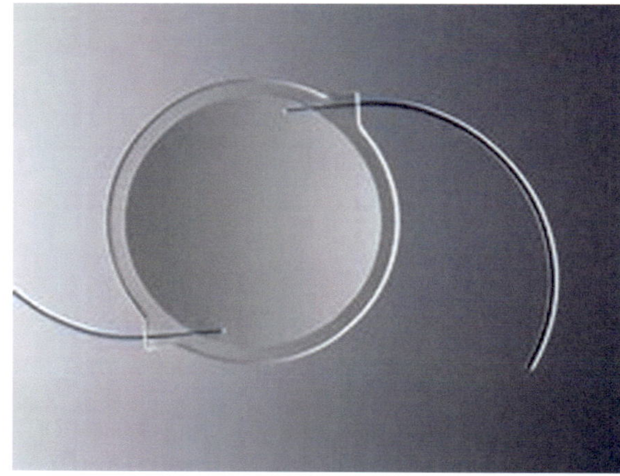

Fig. 1.15 3-piece IOL. The IOL is made of three pieces, one optic and two haptics

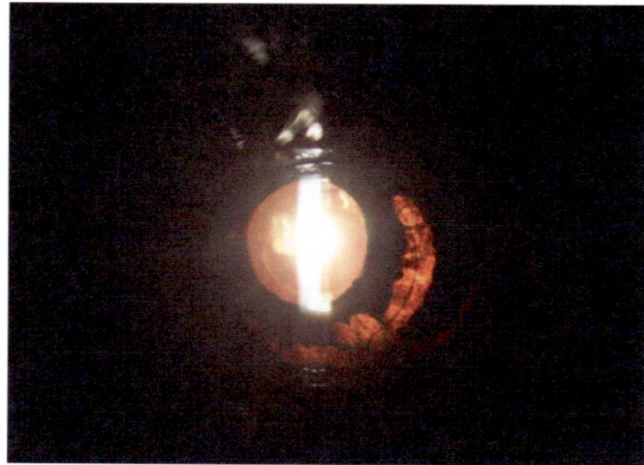

Fig. 1.16 Iris depigmentation secondary to implantation of a 1-piece IOL into the sulcus (iris chaffing)

1.6 Correct IOL Choice

If the IOL is not located in the bag, calculations for the IOL should take into consideration the effective lens position of the optic within the eye. The general rule is: The more anterior the IOL the less dioptre. An anterior chamber lens has less dioptre than an in-the-bag IOL. If the IOL is completely in the sulcus, the optic will be more anterior and the power should be decreased by 0.5D. Intrascleral-fixated IOLs end up having the same power calculations as in-the-bag placement. Retropupillar-fixated iris claw IOLs have approximately 2D less than in the bag IOLs. (Figs. 1.17, 1.18 and 1.19).

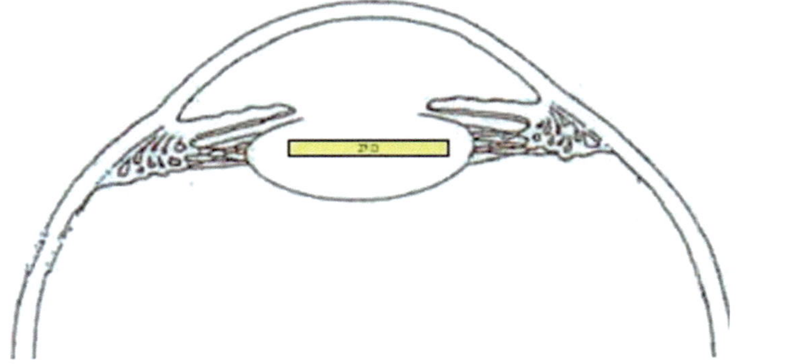

Fig. 1.17 Drawings for the surgical planning of IOL power in case of a complication. The normal case is an in-the-bag location with a +23.0D IOL

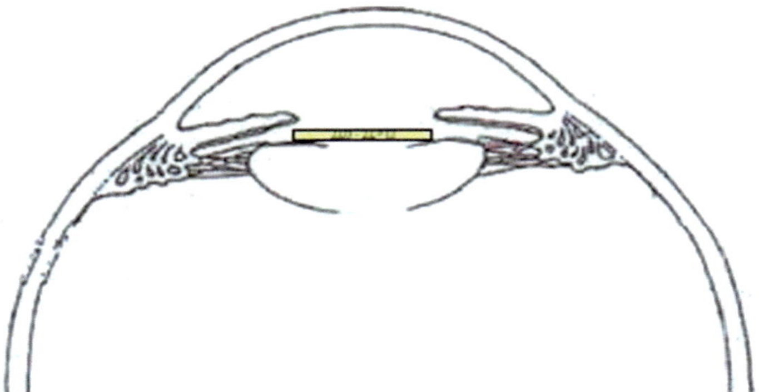

Fig. 1.18 Sulcus implantation. The IOL power is between 22.0 and 22.5D

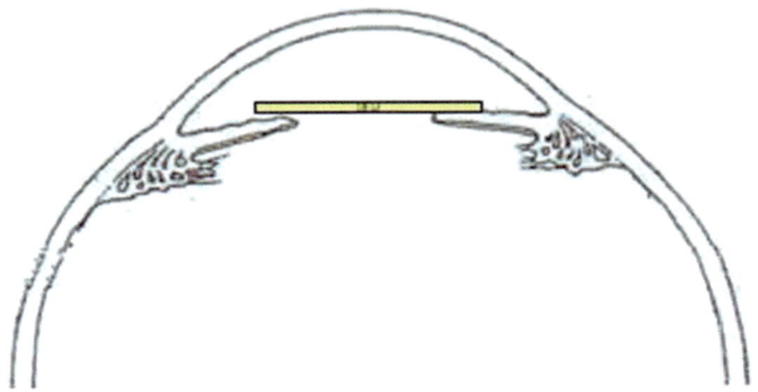

Fig. 1.19 Antepupillar iris-fixated IOL. The IOL power is approximately 18.0D

Essential Surgical Techniques for Complication Management

2

Contents

Abstract

Complication management requires the knowledge of special surgical techniques. In this chapter the techniques SICS and trocar surgery are introduced.

Keywords

SICS · Trocar surgery · Trocar

If you want to be able to operate all cataracts, also the difficult cases, you must be ready to learn more techniques than only phacoemulsification. A cataract with advanced zonular lysis cannot be operated with phacoemulsification. For this difficult case, you must learn the SICS technique. A subluxated IOL, a posterior capsular opacification in a child, a positive vitreous pressure during phacoemulsification can only be solved with a trocar surgery from pars plana.

2.1 Surgical Technique: SICS, the Modified ECCE

The SICS technique is nowadays the standard surgical technique for cataract surgery in Africa and rural parts of Asia. If the nucleus is too hard for phacoemulsification, you can remove the nucleus easier and with less trauma with the SICS

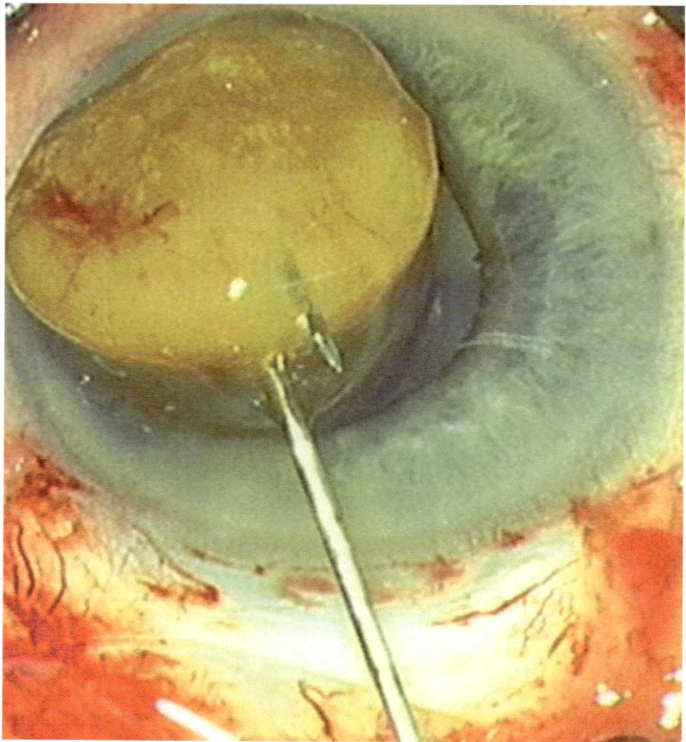

Fig. 2.1 SICS technique: The rock-hard nucleus is removed with a "fish hook". At 12 o'clock, an 8 mm broad frown incision was performed

technique. The SICS technique (small incision cataract surgery) is an evolution of ECCE. The main characteristic of a SICS technique is a self-sealing scleral tunnel wound (frown incision) where the entire nucleus is extracted. The "small" in the abbreviation relates to the "small" scleral incision being relatively smaller than an ECCE, although it is still markedly larger than a phaco tunnel. This technique is very useful in case of a rock-hard nucleus or zonular lysis (Fig. 2.1).

2.2 Trocar Surgery for Cataract Surgeons

In this book, we will introduce you to trocar surgery from pars plana. Trocar surgery increases the surgical spectrum of a cataract surgeon immensely. A vitreous prolapse after a posterior capsular defect is usually removed with a vitreous cutter from the limbus. The disadvantage of this technique is that it is not possible to remove the complete anterior vitreous because the iris and the lens capsule are in

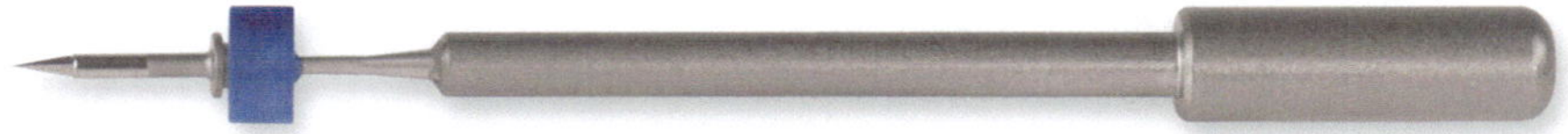

Fig. 2.2 A trocar with a blue valve and the inserter. The inserter is removed after insertion of the trocar in the sclera

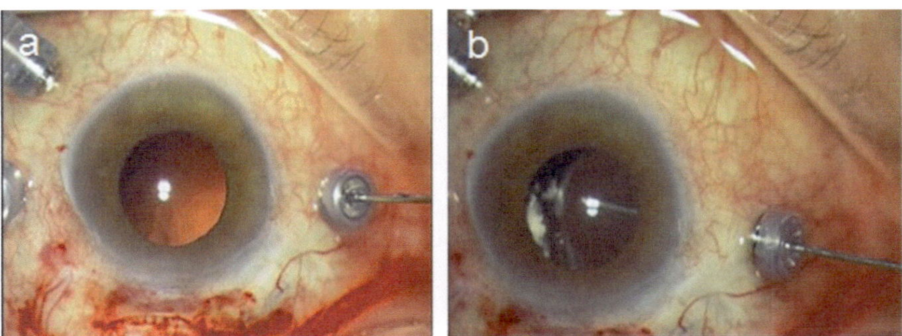

Fig. 2.3 **a** A dislocated IOL secondary to zonular lysis. The IOL cannot be elevated from the limbus into the anterior chamber. **b** After insertion of a trocar, the IOL can be easily elevated with the viscoelastic cannula or vitreous cutter into the anterior chamber

the way. We will describe an anterior vitrectomy from pars plana, which can be performed with a phaco machine. A trocar is inserted through the sclera, and then the anterior vitreous is removed from pars plana through the trocar. This method functions with a regular anterior cutter.

You can also elevate dislocated IOLs, remove a PCO from pars plana and much more. Trocar cannulas are easy to insert (Fig. 2.2); in the most cases, only one or two trocars are required (Fig. 2.3).

2.3 Get Acquainted with Your Surgical Equipment

Before you start surgery, get acquainted with your equipment. Test the surgical chair and get used to the surgical microscope. This can be done without a patient in the OR.

Instruments

It is essential to know about a broad variety of ophthalmic instruments. Especially if you operate outside the routine cataract procedure, you may need other instruments. Inform yourself what instruments are standard in the cataract set of your department and keep yourself updated regarding new instruments. You can visit the companies on surgical conferences or update yourself using the internet. The specific instruments for each surgery are listed in the chapter.

2.4 Summary

Master the following three techniques to become a complete cataract surgeon

The phacoemulsification technique, the small incision cataract surgery (SICS) technique and the trocar surgery from pars plana are necessary and sufficient to become a complete cataract surgeon. These three techniques make you independent from a posterior segment surgeon.

Planning for Surgical Complications

Contents

Abstract

The spectrum of surgical complications is high and every complication requires a specific planning and preparation. This chapter gives a short introduction how to approach a complication.

Keywords

Complication · Approach · Surgery

If a complication such as posterior capsular defect occurs, you should ask yourself the following questions:

What is the problem?
Can I solve the problem myself?
Have I solved the problem before, and do I have the required equipment sterile on site?
Do I have enough time to solve the complication now?

If you are uncertain whether you can solve the problem yourself, then you should remove the viscoelastic from the anterior chamber and send the patient to an experienced clinic. It is psychologically difficult to stop the surgery, but it is a laudable decision. It is much easier to continue with surgery than to stop. But if you do not master the complication, you are doing no service to the patient; on the

© The Author(s), under exclusive license to Springer Nature Switzerland AG 2022
U. Spandau and G. B. Scharioth, *Complications During and After Cataract Surgery*,
https://doi.org/10.1007/978-3-030-93531-3_3

contrary, you can make the situation worse. In addition, you might increase the surgical trauma, which makes the second operation more difficult.

3.1 Different Cases for Surgical Planning

First case: Anteriorly dislocated IOL-in-the-bag, Fig. 3.1

An IOL in-the-bag is a dislocated IOL with lens capsule. The IOL in-the-bag is spontaneously dislocated due to zonular lysis. It is possible to approach the IOL in-the-bag from the anterior chamber. Dissect a 6 mm broad frown-incision and extract the IOL with the lens capsule and continue with a secondary IOL implantation.

An elegant alternative are the Hoffmann technique and the iris suture technique. For details, see chapter "Secondary IOL implantation".

Second case: Dislocated IOL with partially defective capsular bag, Fig. 3.2

The surgical planning depends on the status of the anterior capsule. Examine the anterior capsule preoperatively. If the anterior capsule is intact you can implant an IOL into the sulcus. In this case, an inferior rift is present in the anterior capsule. A sulcus implantation is not possible.

Third case: Zonular lysis, Fig. 3.3

If the zonular lysis is limited (about 1–2 quadrants), insert four iris retractors and fixate them in the rhexis instead of the iris. You have to work very atraumatic, in order not to enlarge the zonular lysis. Implant after hydrodissection a capsular tension ring. If the zonular lysis includes 2–3 quadrants, remove the nucleus with the lens (ICCE or SICS). See chapter "Zonular lysis".

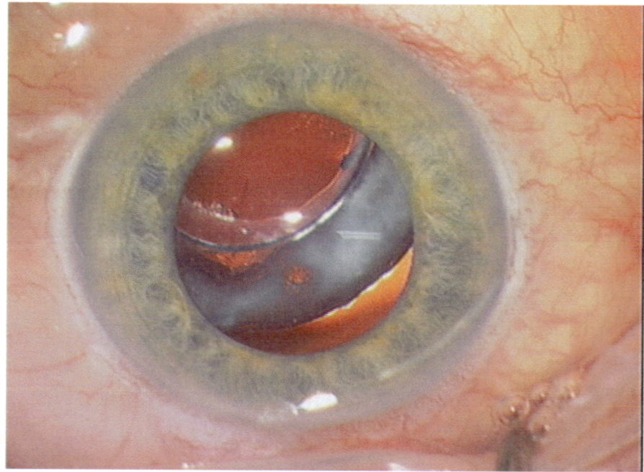

Fig. 3.1 Anterior dislocated bag-IOL complex due to zonular lysis

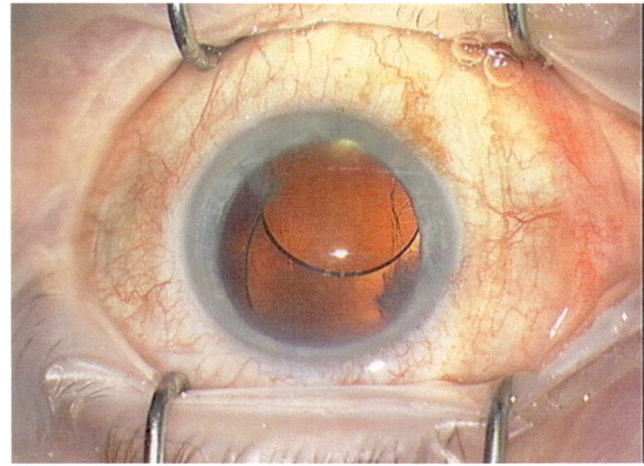

Fig. 3.2 Anterior dislocated IOL after a complicated cataract surgery. The posterior capsule is defective, and the anterior capsule is inferior defective

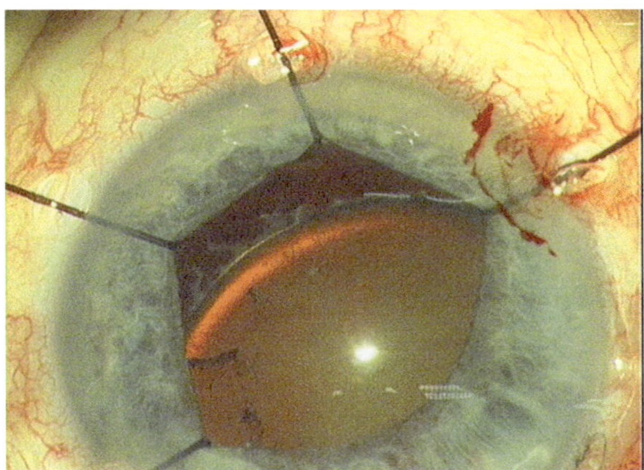

Fig. 3.3 An eye with a large zonular defect secondary to pseudoexfoliation syndrome

Fourth case: Posteriorly dislocated (dropped) nucleus, Fig. 3.4

A clear case. A vitreoretinal intervention is required. Why? The vitreous must be removed to access the nucleus: Then the nucleus is removed with the phaco handpiece. The complete surgery can be done with a cataract machine. See chapter "Surgical management of a dropping and dropped nucleus".

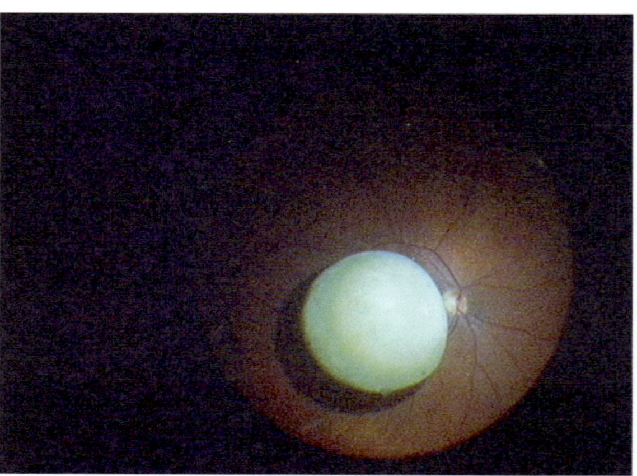

Fig. 3.4 Posterior dislocated nucleus after a trauma for 15 years ago. The patient had no symptoms. With courtesy of the Kaden Verlag

Part II

Easy and Difficult Phacoemulsification

All videos of this part be found in a playlist of my YouTube channel:
https://www.youtube.com/playlist?list=PL0dKYclPD7yMJRuQAIt9Dr7pOtuI0
Seex

Phacoemulsification of an Easy Cataract

4

Contents

Abstract

This chapter explains in detail the phacoemulsification of an easy cataract. All instruments are demonstrated and the surgery is described step-by-step.

Keywords

Phacoemulsification · Easy cataract · Cataract surgery

All videos can be found in a playlist of my YouTube channel:

https://www.youtube.com/playlist?list=PL0dKYclPD7yMJRuQAIt9Dr7pOtuI0Seex.

The emphasis in this chapter lies on the management of an easy cataract, the following chapter on the management of a difficult cataract. The surgery is performed in topical and intracameral anaesthesia.

4.1 Equipment

Phacoemulsification machine

Phacoemulsification was developed by Mr Kelman in the seventies and phacoemulsification surgery became standard in the nineties. The phacoemulsification handpiece emulsifies the nucleus with ultrasound. The phacoemulsification

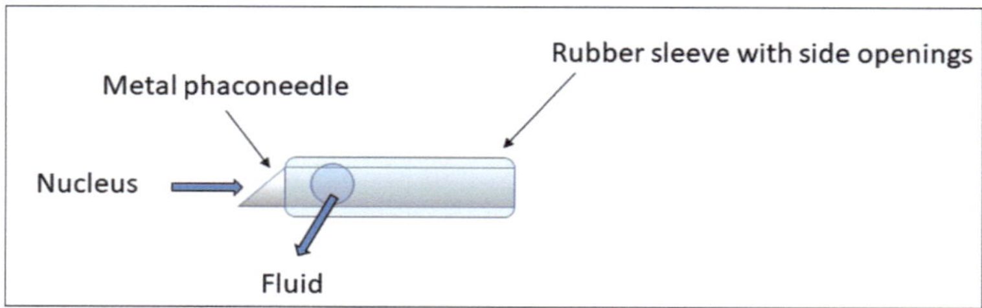

Fig. 4.1 Phaco needle with sleeve. The fluid flows through the side openings into the eye

handpiece includes aspiration and irrigation. The tip of the handpiece contains a needle for phacoemulsification and a sleeve for injection of fluid into the anterior chamber (Fig.4.1). The emulsified nucleus is aspirated, and at the same time, fluid is injected into the eye to avoid a collapse of the anterior chamber.

The modern phacoemulsification machines have an excellent phaco mode and a good vitrectomy mode. In most cases, the vitreous cutter is 23G with a cutting frequency of 2500–4000 cuts/min. The 23G vitreous cutter fits through a paracentesis, whereas an old 20G vitreous cutter only fits through the main incision.

Standard instruments for an easy phacoemulsification

What is the name of this forceps? What is the function of that instrument? The knowledge of all instruments on your phaco set is essential for a successful surgery and a clear communication in the OR. In addition, you need to know the name and function of those instruments, which are not in the regular set. Why? Because the scrub nurse has to fetch the specific instrument you requested. I also recommend looking at some instrument brochures, e.g. Geuder or Katena, to get an idea about the huge variety of instruments available.

Phaco set

Here you find all details of our phacoemulsification instrument set, which we use at the University Hospital of Uppsala (Fig. 4.2). The content of course varies from hospital to hospital.

1× forceps, capsulorhexis (Geuder 31299 or 31308).

1× forceps, Mc Pherson (Geuder 31623).

1× manipulator, chopper after Neuhann (Geuder 32162).

1× manipulator, push–pull after Dardenne (Geuder 16175).

1× handpiece, aspiration.

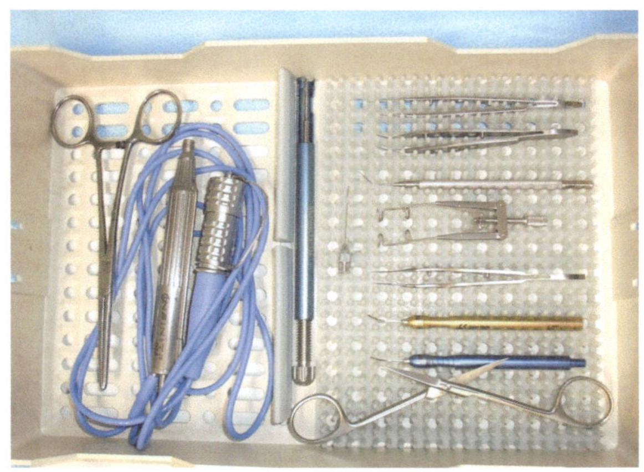

Fig. 4.2 A phacoemulsification set. It is important to know all instruments in the set

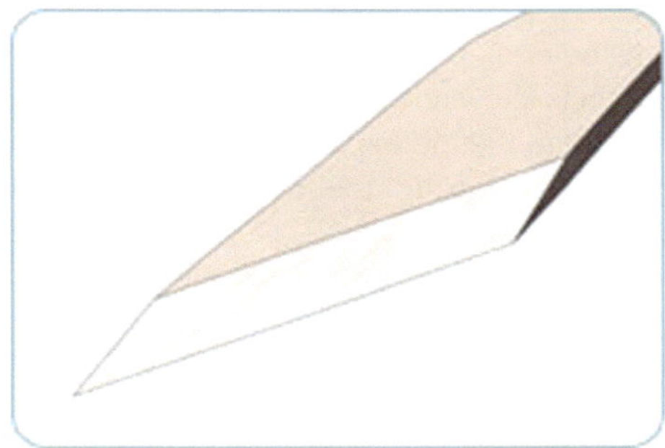

Fig. 4.3 A 15° knife. The main indication is a paracentesis. DORC. 51.4891

1× handpiece, irrigation.

1× phaco handpiece.

1× injector for IOL.

Incisions

Paracentesis knife, 1.3 mm

15° knife (1.3 mm). Indication: Paracentesis (Fig. 4.3). Many suppliers: DORC or Beaver-Visitec.

OR

Angled trapezoid knife, 1.2 mm. Alcon: 8065 921541.

Main incision knife, 2.4 mm

Indication: Main incision (Fig. 4.4). Slit knife. Many suppliers: DORC or Beaver-Visitec, 581129.

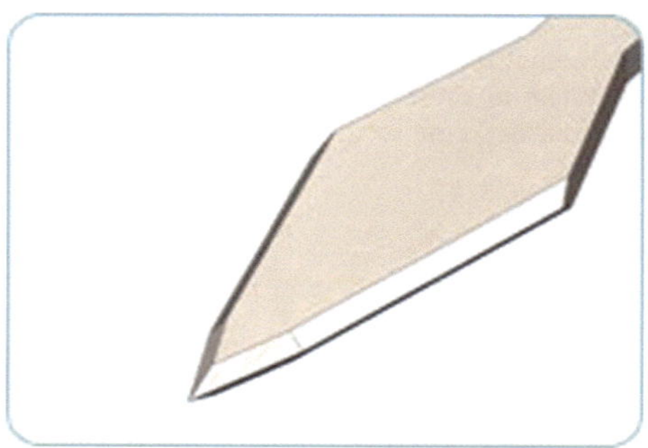

Fig. 4.4 Tunnel incision knife, 2.4 mm. Indication: Main section. Slit knife. DORC. 54.5725 or Alcon. 8065992445

Rhexis

Viscoelastics

There are two different types of viscoelastic available, the one being dispersive and the other being cohesive. The first type disperses in the anterior chamber and protects the endothelium during phacoemulsification. The second type "coheres" meaning that it expands and maintains the anterior chamber. The first type is important during the rhexis, and the latter type is required during the lens implantation.

An example of a dispersive viscoelastic is Viscoat (Alcon Laboratories, Inc, Fort Worth, Texas), and an example of a cohesive viscoelastic is Provisc (Alcon Laboratories, Inc, Fort Worth, Texas).

Cystotome

Indication: Designed for Capsulorhexis, highly recommended to start capsulotomy, for deep set eyes and small pupils. (Fig. 4.5) Many suppliers: Beaver-Visitec, Oasis.

Capsulorhexis forceps

Indication: Capsulorhexis (Fig. 4.6). Many vendors such as Geuder 31299 or 31308

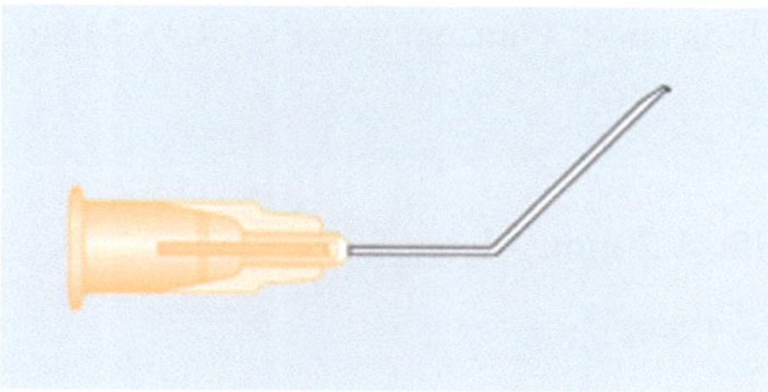

Fig. 4.5 Cystotome. Indication: Capsulorhexis. Several companies: Beaver-Visitec, Oasis. Alternatively, bend a grey 17G cannula to a cystotome

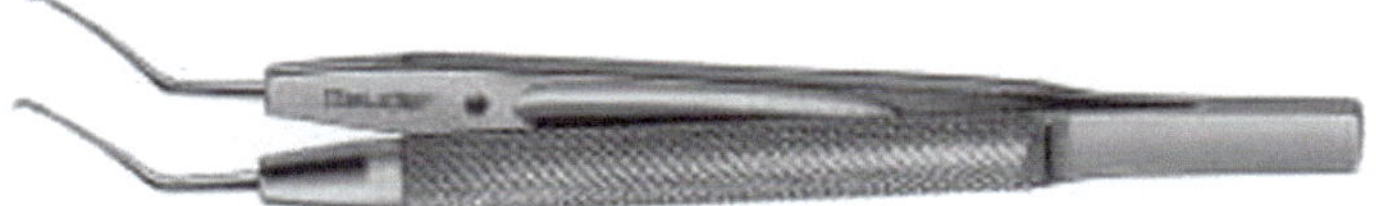

Fig. 4.6 Capsulorhexis forceps. Indication: Capsulorhexis. Many vendors such as Geuder 31299 or 31308

Phacoemulsification handpiece

During phacoemulsification, the dominant hand holds the phaco handpiece and the non-dominant hand a manipulator (e.g. Chopper, spatula or push–pull).

Push–Pull (=Sinskey hook)

The push–pull instrument is a very useful instrument for anterior segment surgery. Indication: Manipulation of the nucleus and rotation of IOL (Fig. 4.7). In addition, you can widen a small pupil with a push–pull instrument or examine the periphery of the capsular bag. Geuder: Iris hook Dardenne (push–pull), Geuder 16175.

Drysdale manipulator

This manipulator is very useful in manipulating the nucleus (Fig. 4.8). The round tip prevents a rupture of the lens capsule. Geuder 16185.

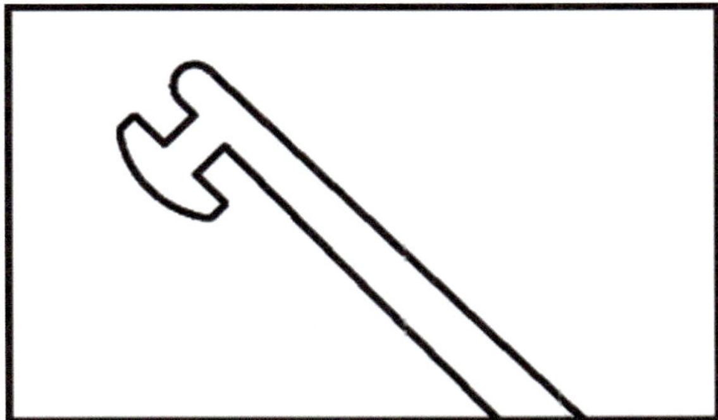

Fig. 4.7 Push–pull manipulator (Sinskey hook). Indication: Manipulation of the nucleus and the IOL. Geuder: Iris hook Dardenne (push–pull), Geuder 16175

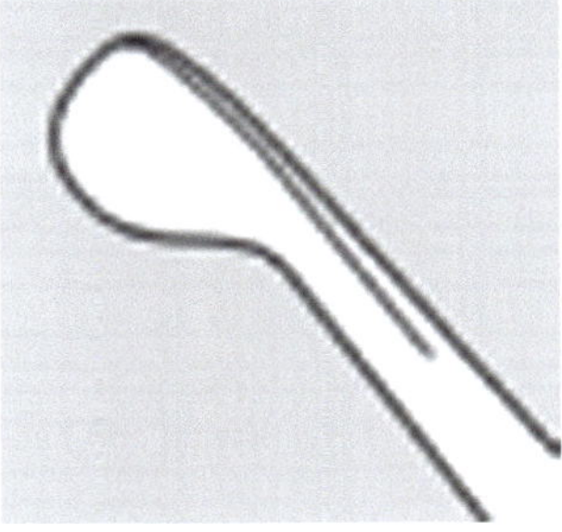

Fig. 4.8 A Drysdale nucleus manipulator. Geuder 16185

Chopper

(1) Combined instrument with push–pull and chopper. Indication: Chopping a hard nucleus with the chopper, manipulation of the nucleus and of the IOL with the push–pull. Chopper by Neuhann, Geuder 32162
(2) Chopper by Agarwal. Indication: Chopping of a hard nucleus. Geuder 32282

Irrigation and Aspiration (I/A)

I/A handpiece, bimanual

One handpiece is for aspiration (Fig. 4.10) and the other handpiece for irrigation (Fig. 4.11). You access the anterior chamber through two paracenteses. I recommend bimanual I/A because they are easier to use than the monomanual I/A. Geuder: Irrigating handpiece and aspirating handpiece.

I/A handpiece, monomanual

This monomanual or coaxial handpiece has both functions (irrigation and aspiration) integrated in one handpiece (Fig. 4.12). The handpiece is comparable in size to the phaco handpiece, and you enter the eye through the tunnel incision.

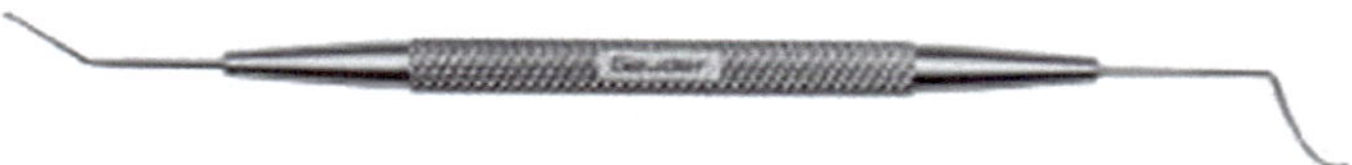

Fig. 4.9 Chopper. Combined instrument with push–pull and chopper. Indication: Chopping a hard nucleus with the chopper; manipulation of the nucleus and of the IOL with the push–pull. Chopper by Neuhann, Geuder 32162

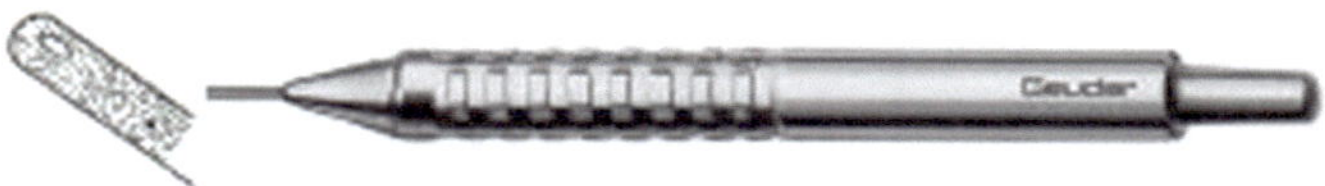

Fig. 4.10 Aspiration tip and handpiece for bimanual I/A. Useful is a rough tip for polishing. Geuder: Aspirating handpiece, 22101

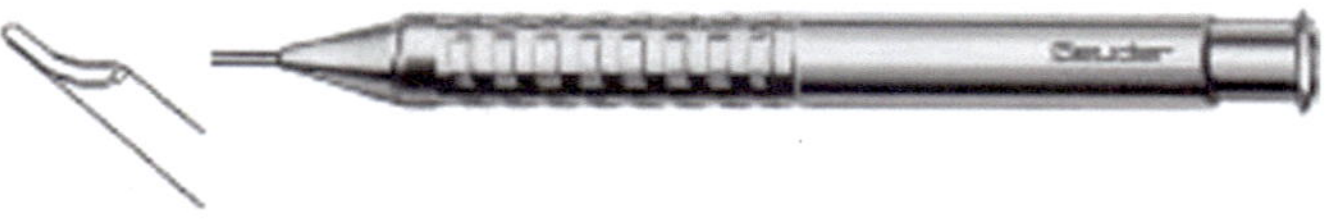

Fig. 4.11 Irrigation tip and handpiece. Geuder: Irrigating handpiece, Geuder 22100

4.2 Surgery of an Easy Cataract

Instruments

Phaco set

Individual steps

1. Paracentesis incisions at 10:30 o'clock and 1:30 o'clock
2. Intracameral lidocaine and viscoelastics
3. Corneal tunnel incision at 9 o'clock
4. Capsulorhexis
5. Hydrodissection and hydrodelineation
6. Phacoemulsification
7. Irrigation and Aspiration (I/A)
8. IOL implantation
9. Removal of viscoelastics
10. Hydration of corneal incisions
11. Intracameral cefuroxime.

The surgery step-by-step:

1. Paracentesis incisions at 10:30 o'clock and 1:30 o'clock
2. Intracameral lidocaine and viscoelastics
3. Corneal tunnel incision at 9 o'clock.

Instrumentation:

Paracentesis: Paracentesis knife, 1,3 mm.

Tunnel incision: Tunnel knife: 2.4 mm.

Intracameral anaesthesia: 1% lidocaine, several manufacturers.

Operation:

We recommend fixating the globe during these steps with a toothed forceps (e.g. Castroviejo) or even better with a cotton swab (does not cause conjunctival haemorrhage) (Fig. 4.13). The dominant hand performs a paracentesis at the grey/white (arcus senilis/limbus) border. One paracentesis is situated at 10:30 o'clock and the other at 1:30 o'clock (Fig. 4.14). Inject next 1% lidocaine into the anterior chamber (Fig. 4.15). Proceed with injection of viscoelastics into the anterior chamber (Fig. 4.16). The next step is the corneal tunnel incision at 9 o'clock. The tunnel is more difficult than it looks, it is important to have a drawing in mind when performing this procedure for the first times (Fig. 4.17). The corneal incision has 3–4 movements (see also drawing): (1) Parallel to the iris (Fig. 4.18),

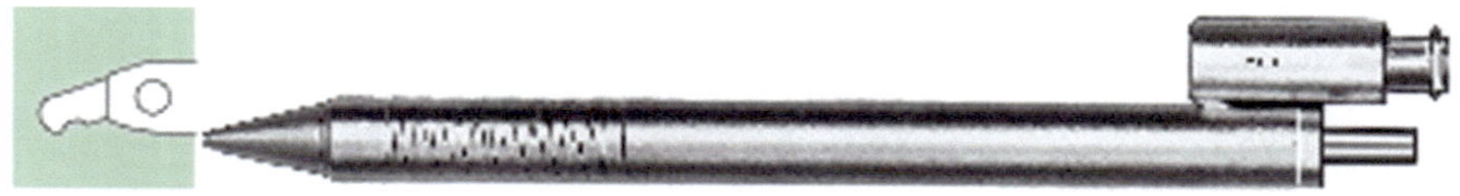

Fig. 4.12 I/A handpiece, monomanual. This monomanual or coaxial handpiece has both functions (irrigation and aspiration) integrated in one handpiece. The handpiece is comparable in size to the phaco handpiece, and you enter the eye through the tunnel incision. Geuder 22540

(2) up and parallel to the cornea (Fig. 4.19), (3) parallel to the iris (Fig. 4.20) and (4) point to the apex of the cornea for the residual part of the knife (Fig. 4.12).

The main incision at 9 o'clock is much more convenient than a main incision at 12 o'clock, because it is easier to hold the phaco handpiece sidewards like a pen than downward.

4. Capsulorhexis

Instrumentation:

Rhexis: Cystotome and capsulorhexis forceps

Viscoelastic

Operation:

The nucleus has a convex shape. The function of the viscoelastic is to maintain the anterior chamber while performing a rhexis and to flatten the nucleus (Fig. 4.21). Imagine you walk along a steep hill and your feet threaten to slip away. Exactly the same happens with the rhexis if the nucleus has a convex (steep) shape. This can be avoided by (re)injecting viscoelastics (Fig. 4.22).

The rhexis can be performed with a cystotome or with a capsulorhexis forceps. I recommend performing the first part of the rhexis with the cystotome until you created a flap, and then proceed with the forceps or even continue with the cannula. Insert the cystotome needle as depicted in Fig. 4.23 and <u>not</u> as in Fig. 4.24.

Then puncture the anterior capsule in the centre with the cystotome (Fig. 4.25) and draw the cystotome to the midperiphery (Fig. 4.24). Then pull the cystotome to create a flap (Fig. 4.27). This step is tricky because you need to control carefully the depth of the cystotome tip. If you come too deep you shovel up anterior cortex and obscure your view, if you are too high you lose the flap. Keep attention that the flap lies flat, then grasp the flap at the peripheral edge with the capsulorhexis forceps and make a circular rhexis (Figs. 4.28, 4.29, 4.30). While pulling, always keep attention that the flap is nicely folded over. In the beginning, you will make many interruptions but try with time to draw the flap for a longer and longer distance. When finishing the capsulorhexis pull the flap towards the centre of the pupil (Fig. 4.26).

Fig. 4.13 Fixate the globe with a cotton swab. Perform a paracentesis at 10:30 o'clock with the 15° knife

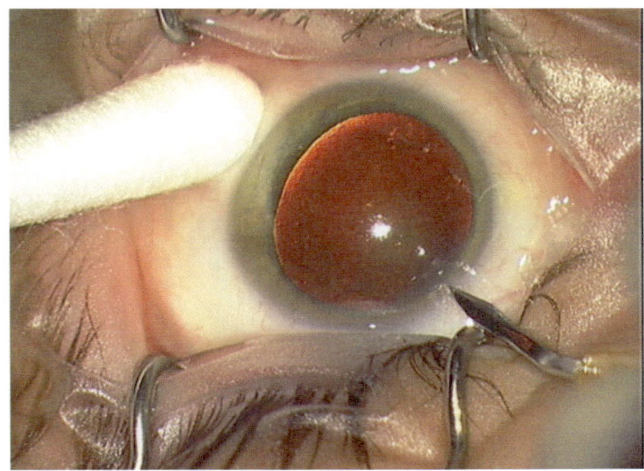

Fig. 4.14 Fixate the globe with a cotton swab. Perform a paracentesis at 1:30 o'clock with the 15° knife or this trapezoid knife (Alcon, ClearCut Sideport Angled; 1.2 mm 8065 921541)

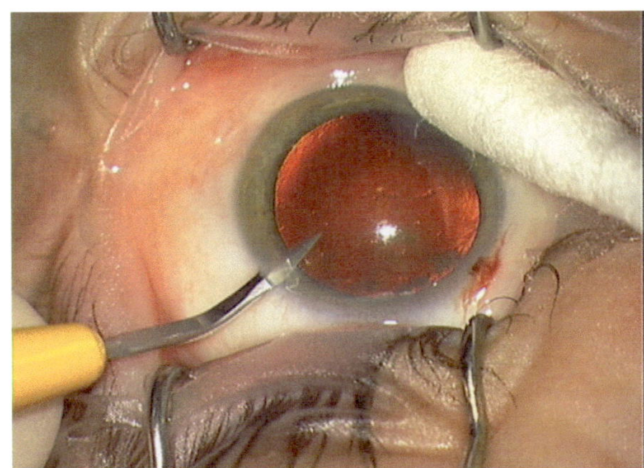

Fig. 4.15 Inject 1% lidocaine into the anterior chamber

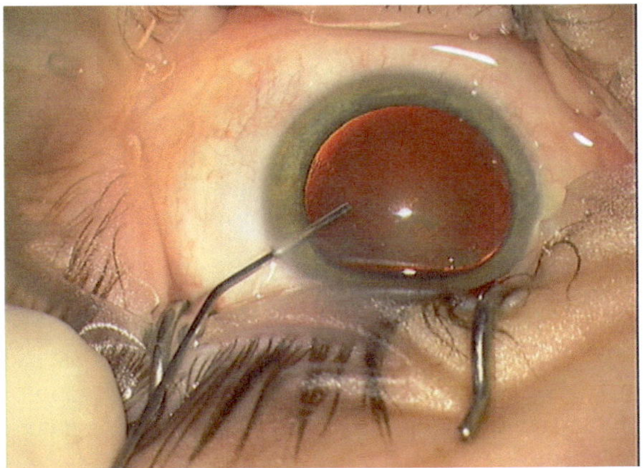

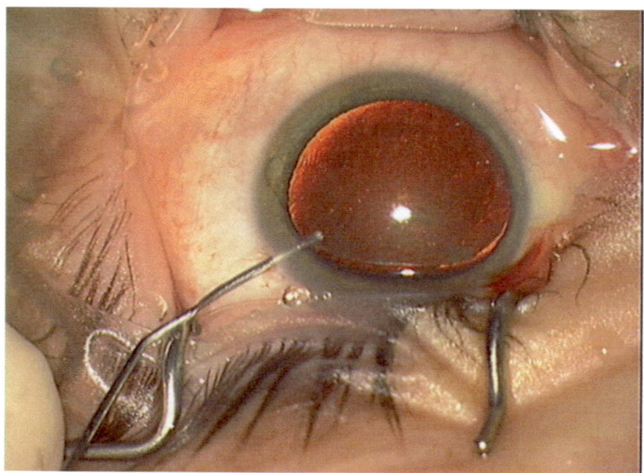

Fig. 4.16 Inject viscoelastics into the anterior chamber

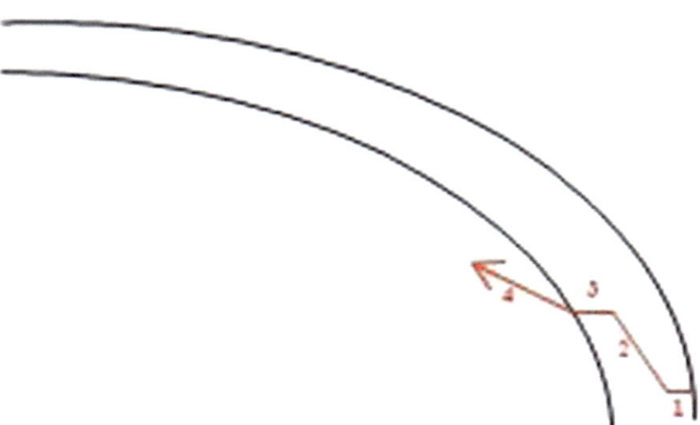

Fig. 4.17 Drawing of a tunnel incision. The incision is lamellar and therefore watertight and requires no suture. The first movement is horizontal (1), the second movement is upwards (2), the third movement is again horizontal (3) and the final movement points towards the apex of the cornea (4)

Important: Check if the rhexis is complete. If it remains incomplete you will aspirate the flap into the phaco probe and create a posterior capsular rupture.

Pits & Pearls no. 1

Two advices which makes life for the beginning cataract surgeon much easier. (1) Optics. A main problem of the beginner is bad optics. Use methylcellulose instead of BSS for the cornea. (2) Constant irrigation. Use constant irrigation during phaco and I/A. You will always have a stable anterior chamber.

Fig. 4.18 First movement is horizontal (see also Fig. 4.15)

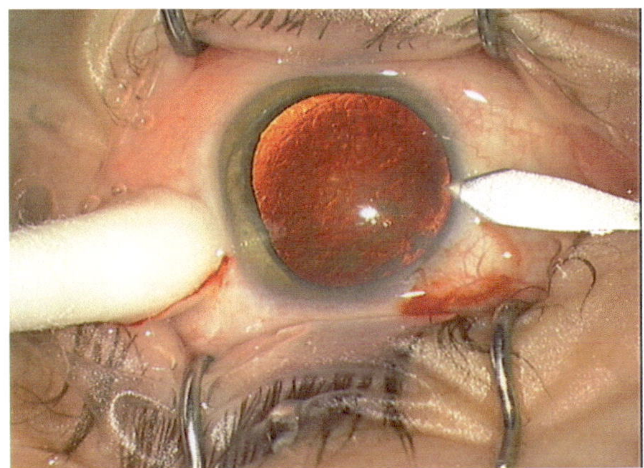

Fig. 4.19 Bend the knife downwards until it touches the conjunctiva and move it upwards parallel to the epithelium. Stop this movement if the marking on the knife reaches the entrance of the tunnel incision (see also Fig. 4.18)

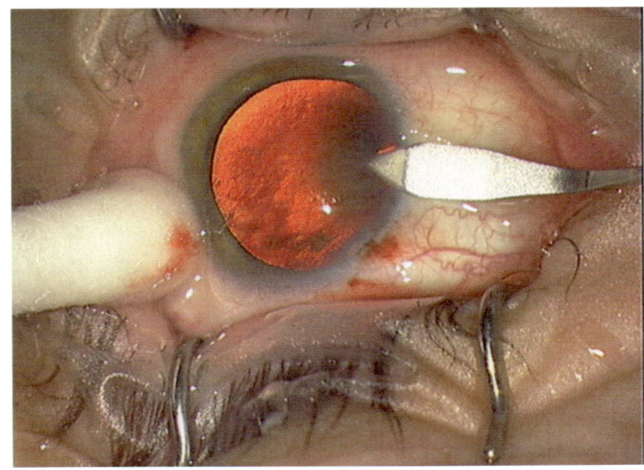

Fig. 4.20 Continue with a horizontal movement (see also Fig. 4.17). If you want to optimize the main incision, then point the knife to the apex of the cornea as soon as you enter the anterior chamber

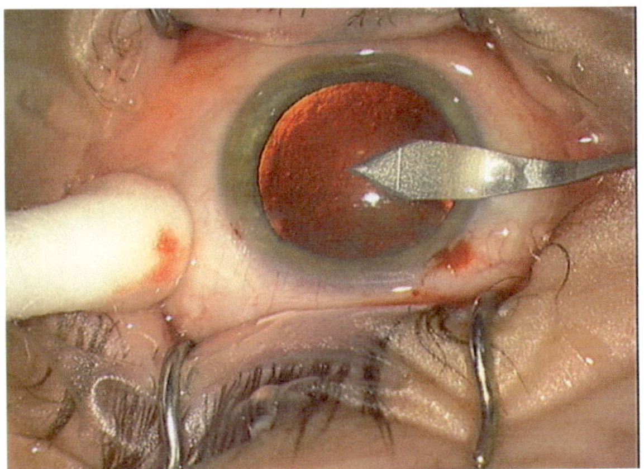

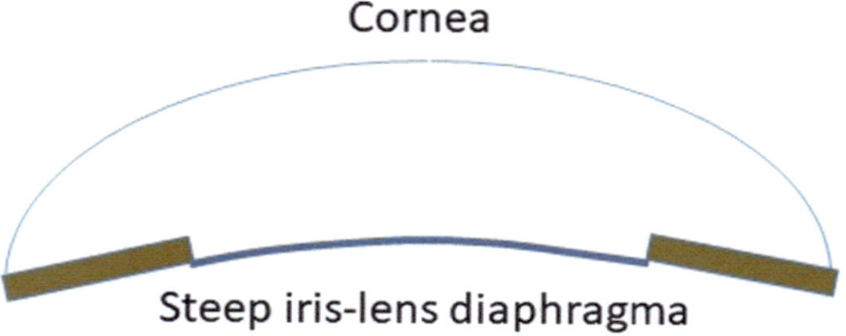

Fig. 4.21 Short eye with steep iris–lens diaphragma. The capsulorhexis is difficult

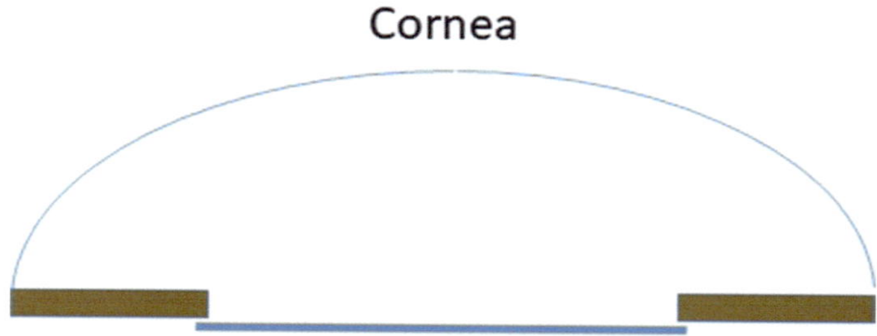

Fig. 4.22 After injection of sufficient viscoelastics, the iris–lens diaphragm is flat and the rhexis is easy

Fig. 4.23 Next step is the capsulorhexis with the cystotome. The insertion of the cystotome is difficult for the beginner. This is the correct way to insert the cystotome

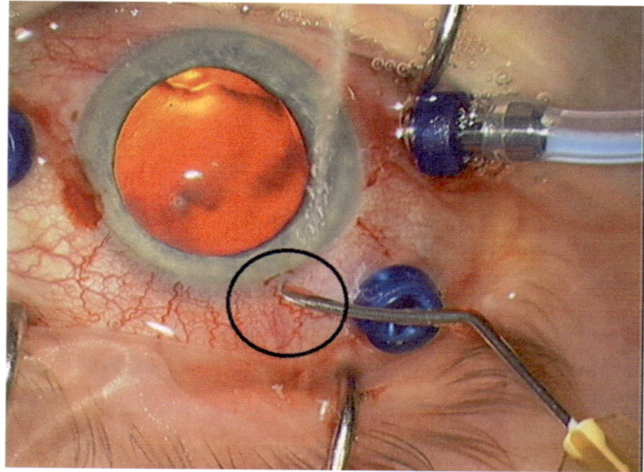

Fig. 4.24 This is the wrong way to insert the cystotome

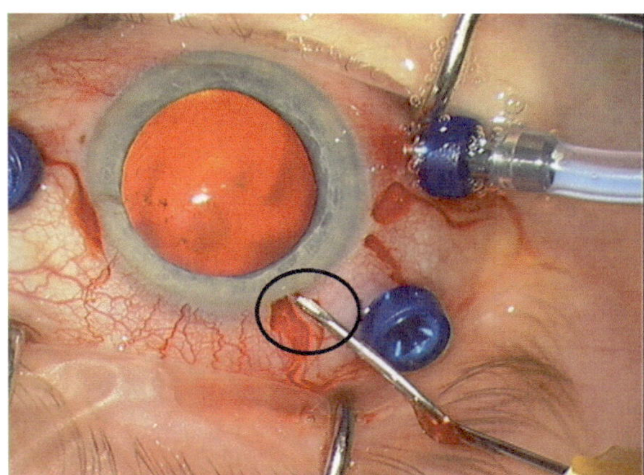

Fig. 4.25 Place the cystotome in the middle of the cornea and open/pinch the anterior capsule

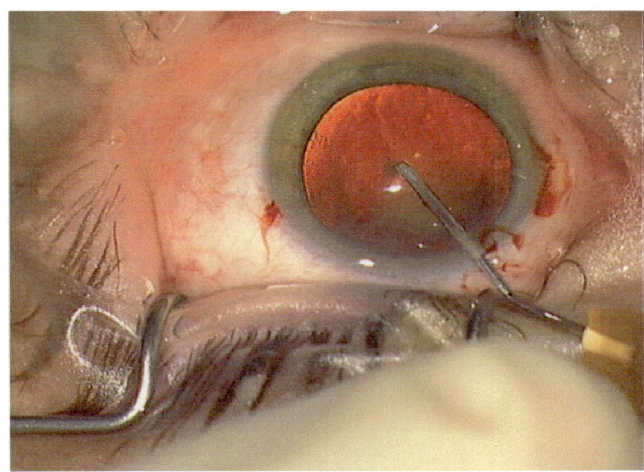

Fig. 4.26 Draw the cannula to the midperiphery approximately 2 mm away from the centre

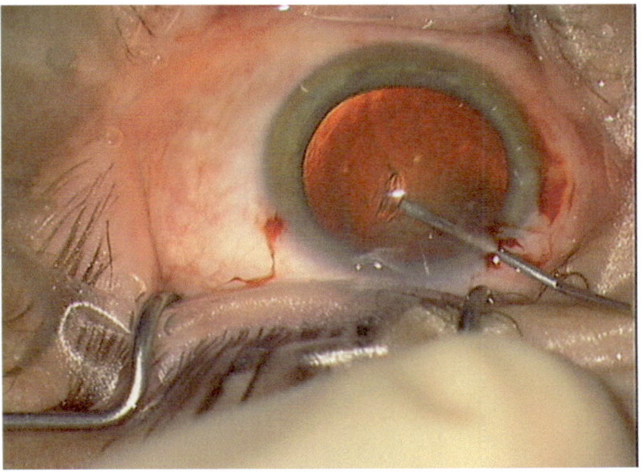

Fig. 4.27 Create a flap. This is a difficult manoeuvre. Hold the cannula superficial in order only to pull the anterior capsule; if you are too deep with the cannula then cortical material will obscure the view

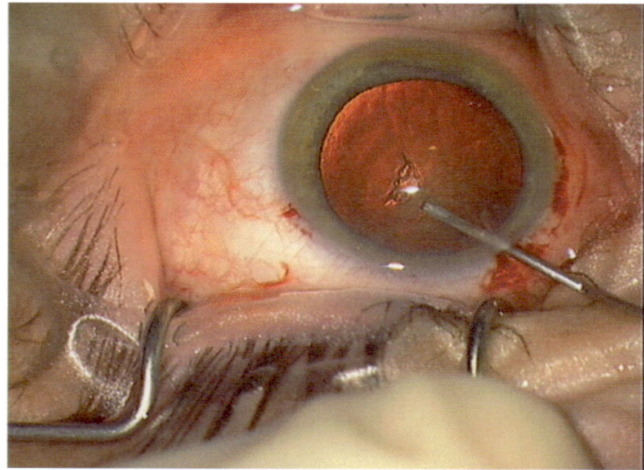

Fig. 4.28 Continue with the rhexis. Place the tip of the cystotome on the flap and draw a circular rhexis

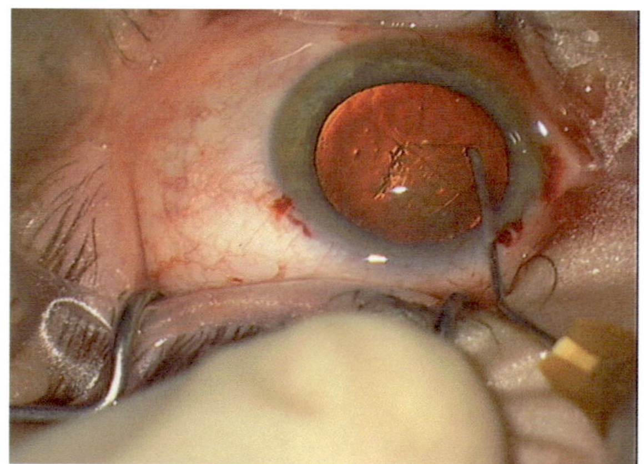

Fig. 4.29 Try to draw the flap a long stretch and do not interrupt the movement too much. The flap should always lie flat as depicted

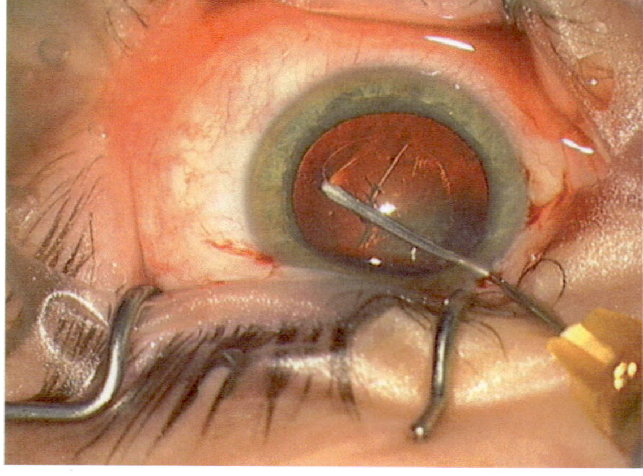

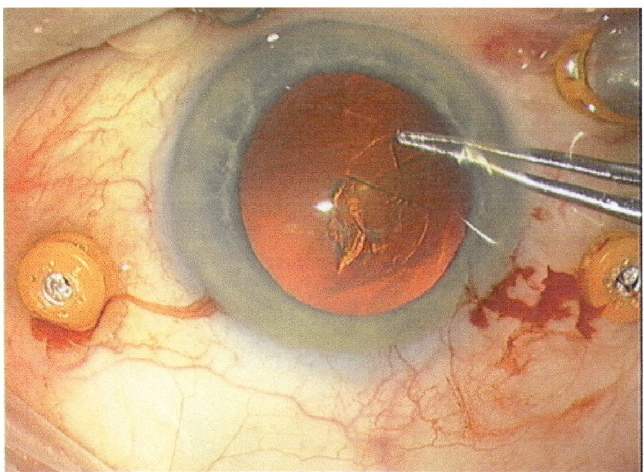

Fig. 4.30 Instead of using a cystotome, you can use a capsulorhexis forceps. Check at the end of the rhexis that the rhexis is really complete. An incomplete rhexis is dangerous because the remaining flap can be sucked in by the phaco tip resulting in an anterior rift or even in a posterior capsular defect

5. Hydrodissection and hydrodelineation

Instrumentation:

Syringe filled with BSS and anterior chamber maintainer cannula (Fig. 4.31).

Operation:

As a beginner, you underestimate the importance of this step. But it is actually a vital step for a successful and smooth going phacoemulsification. This step must be performed through the main incision and <u>not</u> through the paracentesis (Fig. 4.32). If

Fig. 4.31 An anterior chamber cannula attached to a 3 ml syringe filled with BSS. Indication: Injection of BSS into the anterior chamber

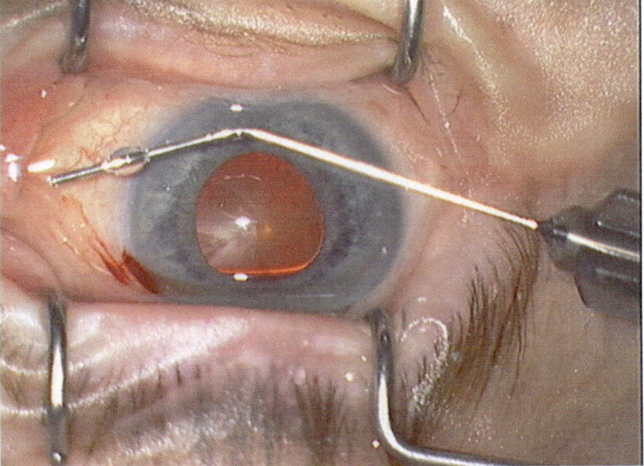

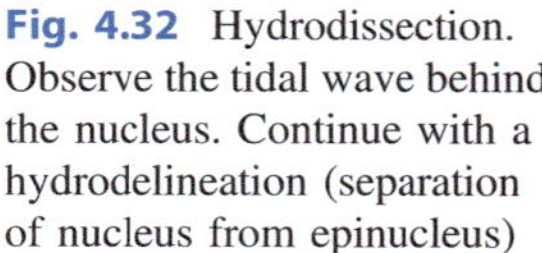

Fig. 4.32 Hydrodissection. Observe the tidal wave behind the nucleus. Continue with a hydrodelineation (separation of nucleus from epinucleus)

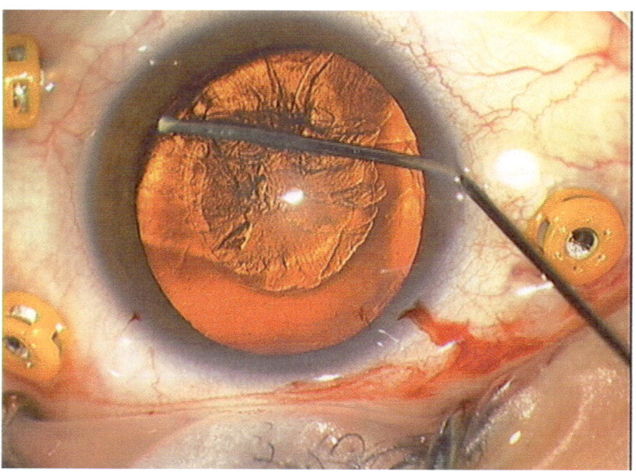

you inject through the paracentesis you will inflate the anterior chamber with subsequent iris prolapse and stress on the zonules. If you inject BSS through the main incision the fluid can also escape through the main incision without inflating the anterior chamber. When performing hydrodissection press, the cannula on the scleral part of the tunnel to facilitate fluid outflow when injecting fluid. This is especially important in a shallow anterior chamber.

Place the cannula under the anterior capsule directly across from the tunnel incision. Hold the cannula tip in position and provide forceful injection of fluid. A successful hydrodissection is visible through a propagating wave along the posterior capsule.

If no wave is evident after the first irrigation, then check first with your index finger how hard the globe is. If the globe is hard then wait before you continue with the next irrigation. Place the cannula at a different position and try again. The lens should be completely mobile before you continue with phacoemulsification. The next step is the hydrodelineation where the nucleus is separated from the epinucleus. Direct the cannula into the nucleus approximately at the edge of the rhexis. A successful hydrodissection is evident by a golden ring (Fig. 4.33).

Pits & Pearls no. 2

<u>Soft nucleus</u>: A soft nucleus is a difficult case. Do not operate a soft nucleus as a beginner. The problem is that the nucleus is difficult to remove. There are two tricks for a soft nucleus: (1) Luxate the nucleus with hydrodissection outside the lens capsule. The nucleus is now located in the anterior chamber. Remove the nucleus with the phaco handpiece in "epinucleus" mode. (2) Remove the nucleus inside the lens capsule with the phaco handpiece in "epinucleus" mode.

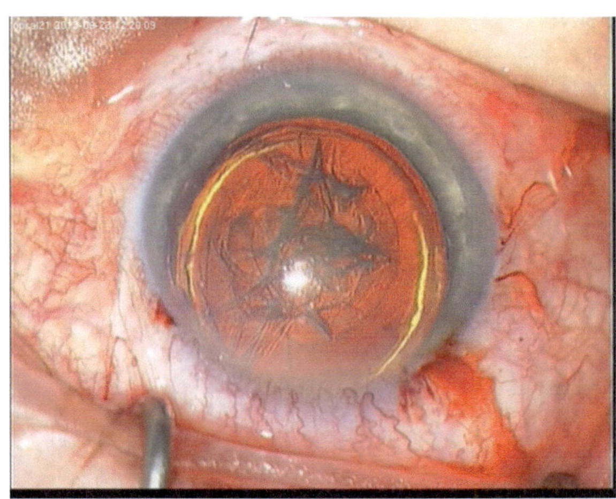

Fig. 4.33 A successful hydrodelineation is seen as a golden ring

6. Phacoemulsification

Instrumentation:

Dominant hand: Phacoemulsification handpiece

Non-dominant hand: Manipulator or chopper

Operation:

When you operate a phaco, you are working in different machine settings (modes). All modes depend on two parameters: (1) **Vacuum/aspiration** and (2) **phacoemulsification power**.

Phaco 1 mode (Sculpting or Grooving): Little aspiration, much phaco. Indication: To carve the groove. Grooving requires little aspiration but much phaco power.

Phaco 2 mode (Quadrant removal): Much aspiration, much phaco: Indication: To aspirate the quadrants and emulsify them. The aspiration of nuclear fragments requires much vacuum and emulsification of the nuclear fragments requires much phaco energy.

Phaco 3 Mode (Epinucleus): Much aspiration, little phaco. The epinucleus is soft, you need little phaco but much aspiration.

I/A 1 mode (Cortex): Much aspiration: It requires a lot of aspiration to remove the cortex.

I/A 2 mode (Polishing): Little aspiration: You may only work with little aspiration at the posterior capsule in order to remove cortical strands or fibrosis.

Fig. 4.34 Side openings of the sleeve must be located in the anterior chamber

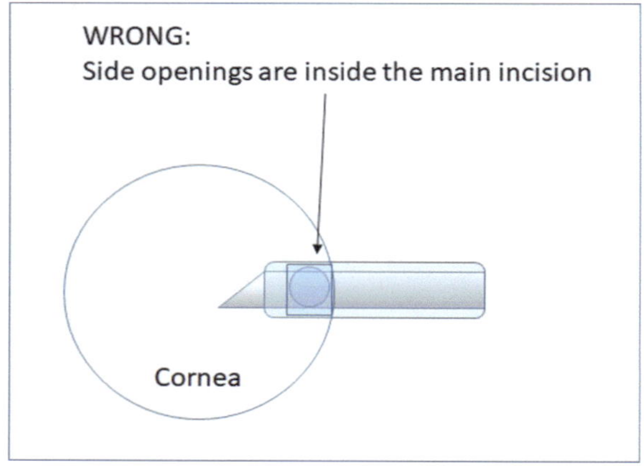

Fig. 4.35 Side openings may not be located in the main incision because the fluid cannot flow into the anterior chamber

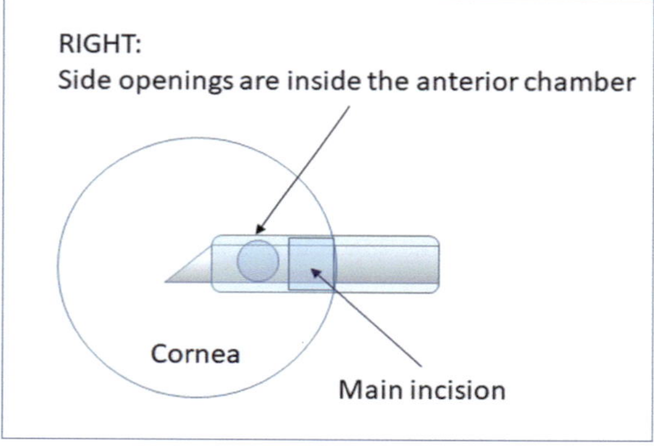

If you insert the phaco needle into the anterior chamber, check that the side openings of the sleeve are not located inside the main incision but inside the anterior chamber. If they are located inside the main incision, then the anterior chamber will collapse (Figs. 4.34 and 4.35).

Grooving & Cracking

Two remarks about the phaco handpiece: Firstly: The phaco handpiece has much power, be cautious when using it. It is possible to aspirate the complete iris or the complete capsular bag. If you aspirate once a part of the iris into the phaco tip, then you will inadvertently aspirate it again and again. Secondly: The phaco handpiece is coaxial which means that irrigation and emulsification are integrated in one instrument. The irrigation must always be switched on; otherwise, the anterior chamber will collapse. The problem is in order to have a continuous irrigation you need to press permanently on the foot pedal. As a beginner, you can take advantage of the continuous irrigation mode of the phaco machine. I recommend doing so for the first 100 cataracts.

Grooving: Begin by aspirating the cortex within the rhexis margins to improve the view onto the nucleus. Then sculpt the groove such as depicted in Fig. 4.36 and <u>not</u> as in Fig. 4.35. Point the phaco tip steep by moving the phaco tip downwards and then horizontally. The groove should not be too short and stretch from rhexis edge to rhexis edge (in a medium-sized rhexis). Focus the microscope on the middle of the groove, in order to detect the red reflex. The fundus reflex is a secure sign with the exception of a rock-hard nucleus. Here you may be working just above the lens capsule without seeing a red reflex.

Cracking: Hold the phaco tip (only irrigation, no phaco) at the left bottom edge of the groove and the manipulator at the right bottom edge of the groove (Fig. 4.38) and then move both instruments simultaneously to the side; in a slight horizontal and upward direction (Fig. 4.39). The cracking is easy if the groove is deep enough (Fig. 4.37).

Rotate

Begin by placing both instruments at the far periphery of the groove (Figs. 4.40, 4.41). Then push simultaneously both instruments so that the nucleus rotates. You can rotate clockwise or anticlockwise but adjust the instruments appropriately. The rotation manoeuvre requires some learning time. Rotate 90 degrees and sculpt the next groove. Crack the groove again and continue with the quadrant removal.

Quadrant removal (phaco or flip)

Do not move the phaco tip too much, stay more or less in the middle of the pupil. Use instead the manipulator to feed the phaco tip with nuclear fragments.

The first quadrant is always the most difficult to remove, the subsequent quadrants come easy. First check if the quadrant you want to remove is mobile. Have both edges been fully cracked? If not, then finish this job first before removing the quadrant. Otherwise, you will not succeed. Then change the machine settings to quadrant removal mode. You need more aspiration than in the sculpting mode in order to suck in the quadrant. Touch the quadrant with the phaco tip, increase aspiration and draw slowly the phaco handpiece backwards. Check if the quadrant follows or if it remains stuck. You can repeat this manoeuvre a few times but every

Fig. 4.36 Phacoemulsification. The groove must be steep at the edges and deep in the middle

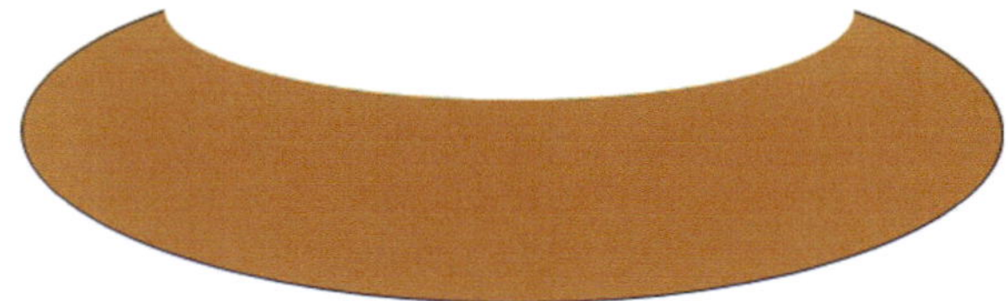

Fig. 4.37 This is a typical beginner groove. Flat at the edges and shallow in the middle. Do not perform your groove like this

Fig. 4.38 Cracking. Place the phaco tip and the manipulator at the very bottom of the groove. This manoeuvre is easier with a dense than with a soft nucleus

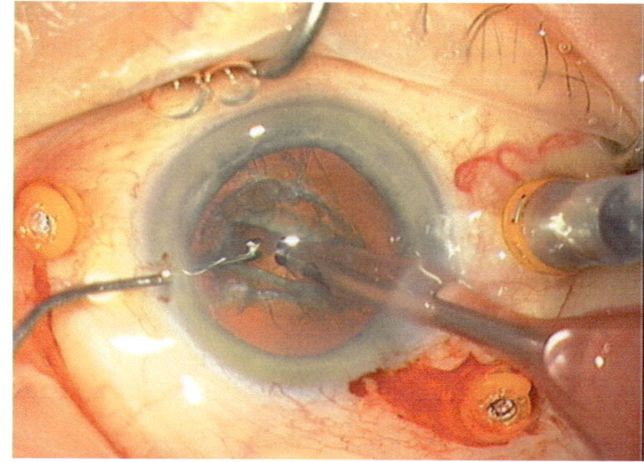

Fig. 4.39 Cracking. Move both instruments apart. The manoeuvre succeeds if the groove is deep enough. If not, then deepen the groove with phacoemulsification

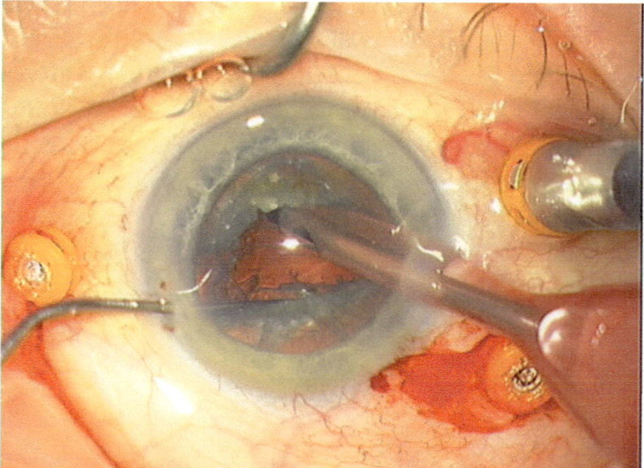

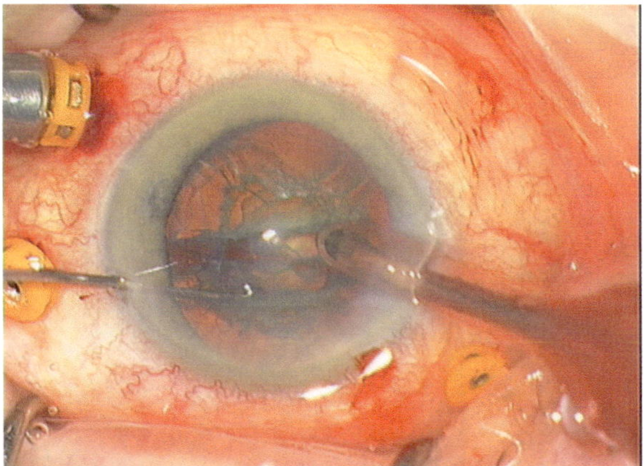

Fig. 4.40 Rotation of nucleus. A precondition of a successful rotation is a good hydrodissection. Place the manipulator at one peripheral end of the groove and the phaco tip at the opposite peripheral end of the groove and perform a rotational movement

Fig. 4.41 A successful rotation of the nucleus

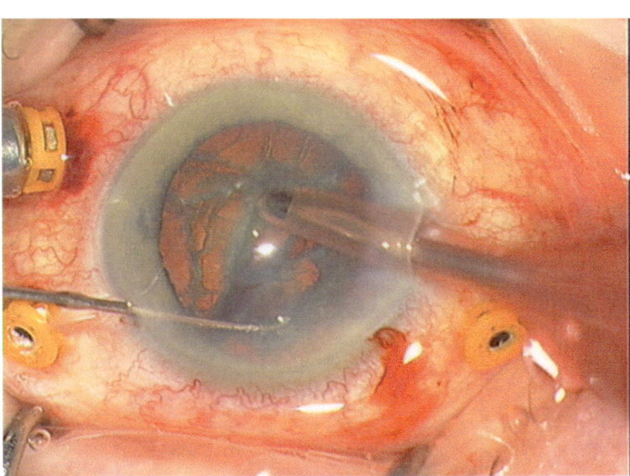

time you will remove some tissue from the quadrant until it gets difficult to aspirate the residual quadrant.

In this case a "flip" manoeuvre helps (Figs. 4.42, 4.43, 4.44). You need a blunt manipulator such as a push–pull manipulator. A good alternative is a Drysdale nucleus manipulator (see instruments) because there is no risk to damage the posterior capsule. Begin by rotating the quadrant you want to remove onto the opposite side of the paracentesis with the manipulator (see drawing). Direct the tip of the manipulator between the nucleus and the epinucleus. The risk to damage the posterior capsule is low. Then flip the nucleus up and move it in front of the phaco tip. After emulsification of the first quadrant, rotate the next quadrant in front of the

Fig. 4.42 Drawing of a flip manoeuvre. Place the manipulator below the fragment and elevate (flip) the fragment. The flip manoeuvre is a great help especially for the beginner. If you are not able to remove the first fragment with the phaco tip, then perform a flip manoeuvre

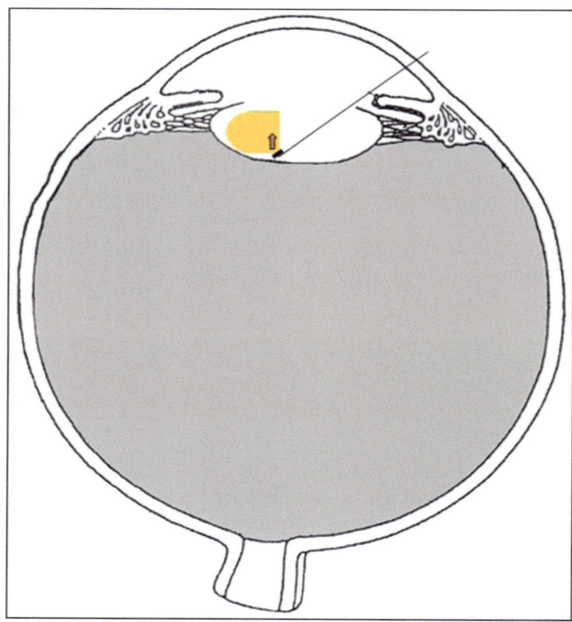

Fig. 4.43 Flip manoeuvre. The push–pull manipulator is placed below the fragment

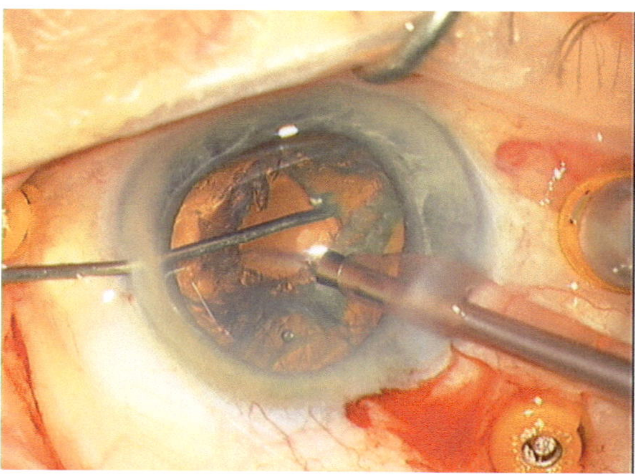

phaco tip. Aspirate it and emulsify it. The last half fragment can either be emulsified in to or - and what we recommend - be cracked first. Rotate the fragment in front of the tip (Fig. 4.45), change the machine setting to sculpting mode, make a groove in the nuclear fragment and crack it in two halves. Then change the machine setting to quadrant removal and emulsify the last two quadrants.

During removal of the nucleus, epinucleus sometimes comes in the way. Avoid removing it in this stage because it serves as a protection of the posterior capsule.

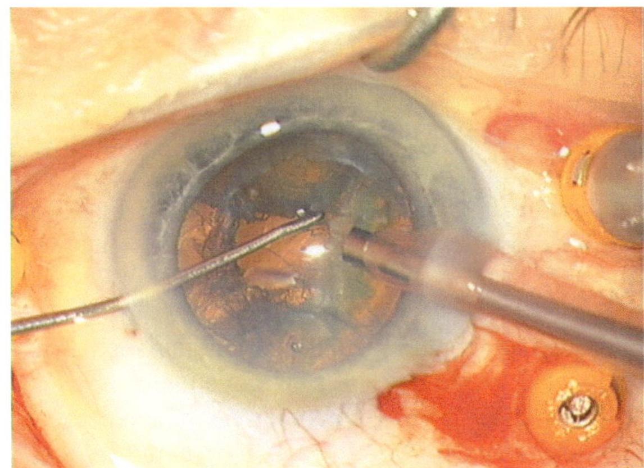

Fig. 4.44 Flip manoeuvre. The nuclear fragment is elevated and can now be easily removed with phacoemulsification

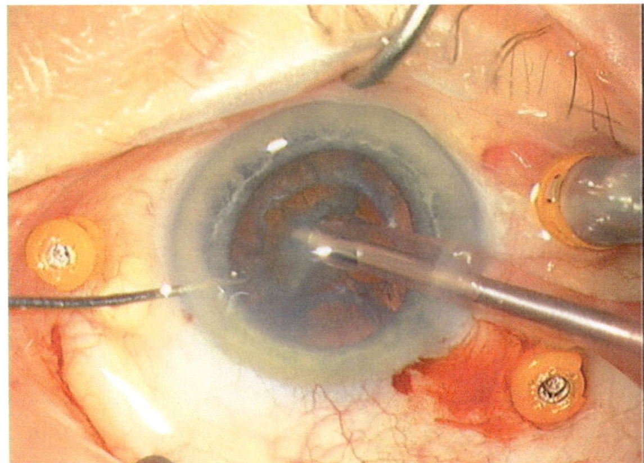

Fig. 4.45 Grooving of a half fragment. This manoeuvre must be performed in the "sculpting" mode, not in the "fragment removal" mode. After grooving the half fragment has to be cracked in two quarters

Pits & Pearls no. 3

<u>Epinucleus during phaco</u>. Do not remove the epinucleus during the removal of quadrants. Why? The epinucleus serves as a scaffold for the posterior capsule. The epinucleus prevents a floppy movement of the posterior capsule and consequently prevents that the posterior capsule is aspirated into the phaco tip.

Pits & Pearls no. 4

<u>Removal of phaco handpiece from anterior chamber</u>. Remove first the manipulator (e.g. chopper) and then the hand piece, NOT vice versa. Why? If you remove the phaco handpiece first, the anterior chamber will flatten, and you will struggle to remove the manipulator. The same applies for I/A with bi-manual handpieces. Remove irrigation last.

Pits & Pearls no. 5

<u>Unsuccessful quadrant removal</u>. Cause: Insufficient hydrodissection. Solution: Repeat hydrodissection. Take a syringe with BSS and place the cannula between the anterior capsule and the nucleus you want to remove. Inject BSS and press the cannula a bit down at the same time. If you succeed, the nuclear fragment will luxate up in the capsular bag. I recommend performing this step every time when you have problems removing or rotating a quadrant.

Epinucleus removal

The success of this step depends again on a successful hydrodissection. As a beginner, it might be wise to remove the epinucleus with bimanual I/A handpieces or even easier with a coaxial I /A handpiece. Change the machine settings to Epinucleus mode. Place the phaco tip at the epinucleus and aspirate the epinucleus. Don´t touch the rhexis edge! Aspirate slowly and try to remove adjacent epinucleus by moving the phaco tip horizontally. The epinucleus around the main tunnel incision is difficult to remove if hydrodissection was not complete. Remove it in the next step.

7. Irrigation and Aspiration (I/A)

<u>Instrumentation:</u>

I/A handpiece, bimanual. One handpiece is for irrigation and another handpiece for aspiration. You access the anterior chamber through two paracenteses.

<u>Operation:</u>

Change the machine settings to I/A mode. We recommend using bimanual I/A handpieces (Fig. 4.46). If you are a beginner, then use the continuous irrigation mode to avoid an anterior chamber collapse. Begin by placing the irrigation tip in

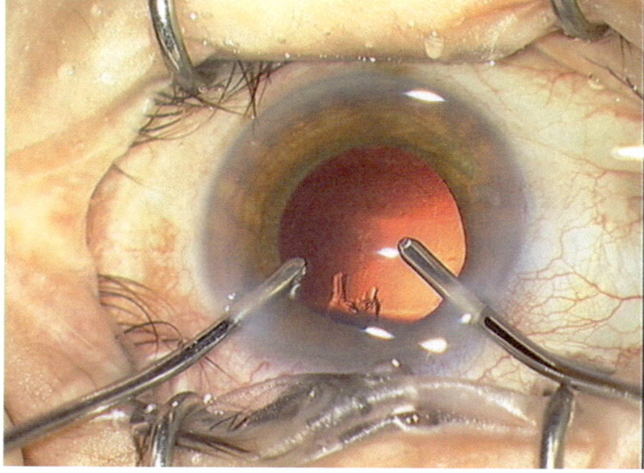

Fig. 4.46 Bimanual I/A. Sometimes a residual cortex remains at 12 o'clock, which is difficult to remove

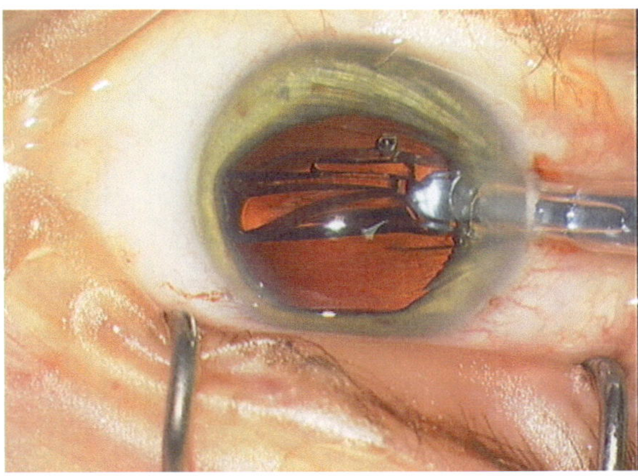

Fig. 4.47 IOL implantation. If the main incision is too small for the cartridge, then enlarge it with the main incision blade. The implantation of a 1-piece IOL is simple. The implantation of a 3-piece IOL requires some training

the anterior chamber and holding it still. Proceed by directing the aspiration tip under the anterior capsule approximately 1–2 mm beyond the rhexis edge. Aspirate and observe if cortex get aspirated. If so, draw the aspiration tip slowly towards the middle of the pupil. Make sure that the cortex follows with, if not increase aspiration. If you are finished with one side of the lens capsule, then change instruments and do the other side.

Caution: Cortical and nuclear fragments are often located at the side and main incisions. Don't miss to remove them because they cause an uveitis.

8. IOL implantation
9. Removal of viscoelastics

I recommend learning how to load an IOL in a cartridge and injector. Every skill you master on your own is worth it. Inflate the capsular bag with viscoelastic. Hold the injector like a pencil and rotate the tip into the tunnel incision (Fig. 4.47). If it does not fit, then do not insist but enlarge the tunnel with the 2.4 mm knife. Place the tip in the capsular bag and turn with the non-dominant hand the screw thread until the IOL is completely inside the anterior chamber. You can either press the IOL into the capsular bag or rotate it into the capsular bag. For the latter, place a push–pull instrument at a haptic and rotate the IOL into the capsular bag. Double-check that both haptics are located behind the anterior capsule. The easiest way to do so is by checking whether the anterior capsule lies above or below the haptics. It is a frequent beginner mistake to leave one haptic in the sulcus (Fig. 4.48). If one haptic remains in the sulcus, then the rhexis would be oval, not round; in addition, an IOL with both haptics in the bag lies more posterior and is not tilted.

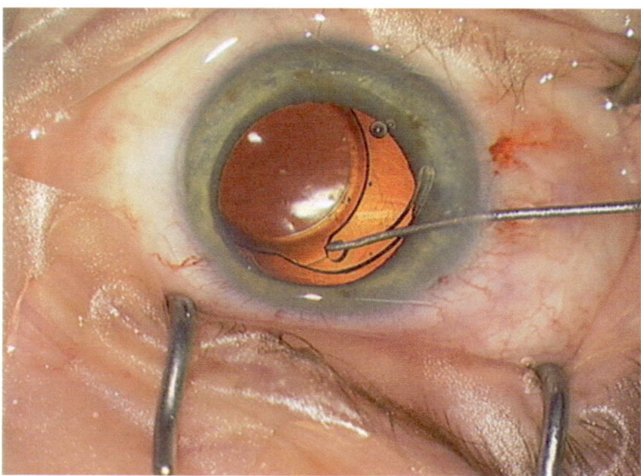

Fig. 4.48 The push–pull instrument facilitates the IOL implantation, especially in case of a 3-piece IOL. Place the tip of the instrument at the haptic and rotate the IOL into the lens capsule. Check after implantation that the IOL is completely implanted into the bag. Examine especially the haptics: Is the lens capsule at the haptic round (haptic in the bag) or oval (haptic in the sulcus)

Fig. 4.49 Hydration of paracentesis. Make the side incisions watertight by injecting BSS into the corneal stroma

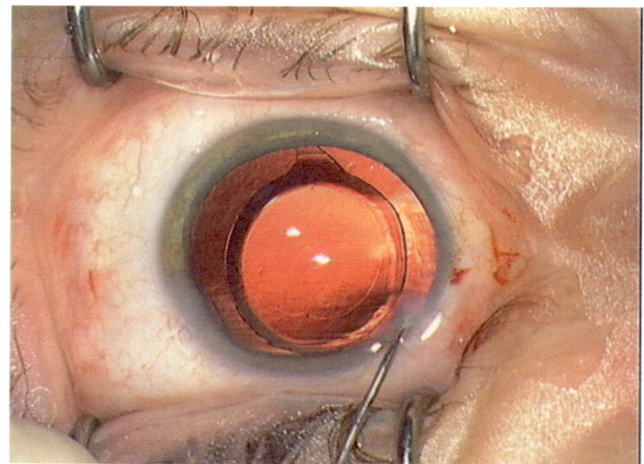

Pits & Pearls no. 6

Unstable anterior chamber. If you have an unstable anterior chamber, then inject air into the anterior chamber. Air has a higher surface tension than BSS. The anterior chamber is therefore more stable under air than under BSS.

10. Hydration of corneal incisions
11. Intracameral cefuroxime

Place the syringe filled with BSS almost parallel to the limbus into the paracentesis incision and inject a little BSS (Fig. 4.49). The manoeuvre is easier than it looks. Inject finally intracameral cefuroxime as endophthalmitis prophylaxis (cefuroxime, several providers such as GlaxoSmithKline and others).

Contents

Abstract

This chapter shows in detail the phacoemulsification of a difficult cataract. First the required instruments are demonstrated and then the surgery is explained step-by-step.

Keywords

Phacoemulsification · Difficult cataract

U. Spandau and G. B. Scharioth, *Complications During and After Cataract Surgery*,
https://doi.org/10.1007/978-3-030-93531-3_5

5.1 How to Approach a Difficult Cataract

The planning for a difficult eye starts at the slit lamp. The eye may be difficult, but the patient is "difficult". In contrast, the patient may be "difficult" but the eye is easy. The most difficult cases are a deep-set eye, short eye, flat anterior chamber, small pupil, hard nucleus and zonular lysis and a nervous and obese patient.

A complication may occur from the first to the final step. A complication in the first step influences the next steps. For example, a too short main incision may cause iris prolapse making all following steps difficult.

5.2 Anaesthesia

Ten years ago, peribulbar anaesthesia was standard for cataract surgery. Nowadays, a combined topical and intracameral anaesthesia is standard for phacoemulsification surgery. This anaesthesia is also sufficient for the most but not for all patients. In case of a nervous patient or a short eye, we recommend a peribulbar anaesthesia. In case of a complication, for example a posterior capsular rupture, we recommend also strongly a peribulbar anaesthesia. The latter can be added during surgery. I operated many patients with complicated phacoemulsifications. And all patients complained of terrible pain because the first surgeon continued with complication surgery using only a topical anaesthesia.

If you have a posterior capsular rupture you have two options: (1) Terminate surgery immediately and send the patient to an experienced surgeon. (2) Continue with complication management but add first an additional anaesthesia. If you choose the first option, you are a brave surgeon, and the patient will never be angry with you. If you choose the second option, you will make the patient unhappy unless you are an experienced surgeon and use additional anaesthesia.

I add often anaesthesia in case of a difficult cataract. The easiest way to add extra anaesthesia is to inject 3 ml Carbocaine into the caruncle. Wait one minute before you continue.

Remember: In case of blepharospasm, obese patient, nervous patient and short eye add peribulbar anaesthesia. The surgery will be much easier and the risk for complication much less. Add 3 ml Carbocaine through caruncle or 3–5 ml subtenonal.

5.3 Instruments for a Difficult Phacoemulsification

The number of instruments for a difficult phacoemulsification is much higher than for an easy phacoemulsification. In the following you will find a list of essential instruments for a difficult cataract surgery. **In my experience**, the most important items for difficult phacoemulsification are (1) additional (peribulbar) anaesthesia,

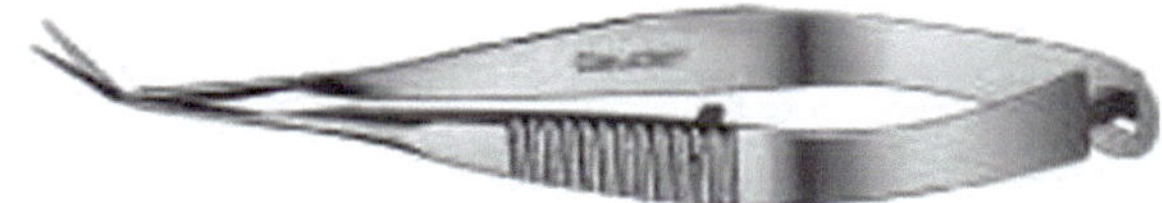

Fig. 5.1 Regular capsulotomy scissors. The instrument fits only through a main incision. Geuder 19,776

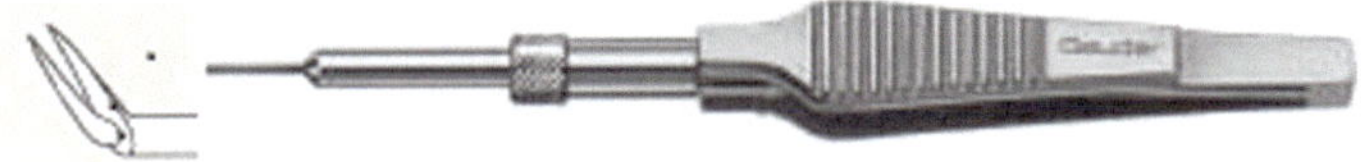

Fig. 5.2 Capsule scissors after Kampik. The instrument fits through a paracentesis. Indication: Cutting of capsule or iris. Geuder 38,215

(2) vision blue, (3) lens capsule scissors (Figs. 5.1 and 5.2), (4) iris hooks (Fig. 5.3) and (5) cystotome.

Scissors:

See Fig. 5.1.

OR

See Fig. 5.2.

Miscellaneous:

In the following, you will find the surgical management of possible complications step-by-step from the beginning to the end (Fig. 5.3).

5.4   Problems During Side Incisions

A conjunctival chemosis may occur at the paracenteses and especially at the tunnel incision and may be disturbing. The cause for the chemosis is a too posterior incision. Take the tunnel knife and make a small incision in the conjunctiva to the left or the right from the tunnel (Fig. 5.4).

5.5   Problems During Main Incision

If the main incision is too short, then an iris prolapse may occur during surgery. If the iris prolapse is small, I recommend to continue. If the iris prolapse is, however, big, then I recommend closing the main incision with an Ethilon 10-0 X-stitch and create a new main incision.

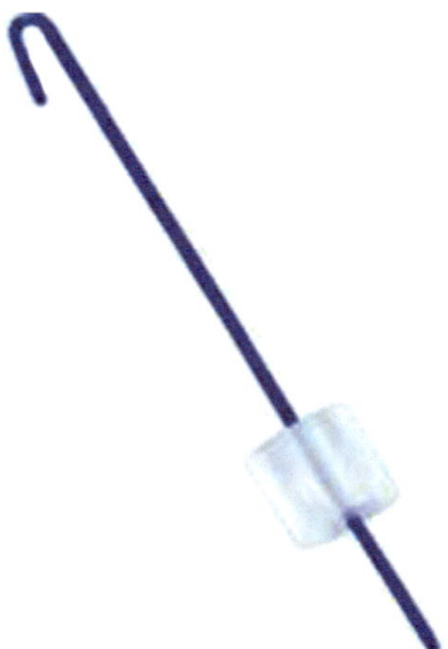

Fig. 5.3 Iris retractors:
Alcon/Grieshaber: Flexible
Iris Retractors REF 611.75

Fig. 5.4 Conjunctival
chemosis. The cause is a too
posterior (scleral) main or side
incision. Cut the conjunctiva
(3–4 mm limbal incision) at
the left and right side of the
main incision

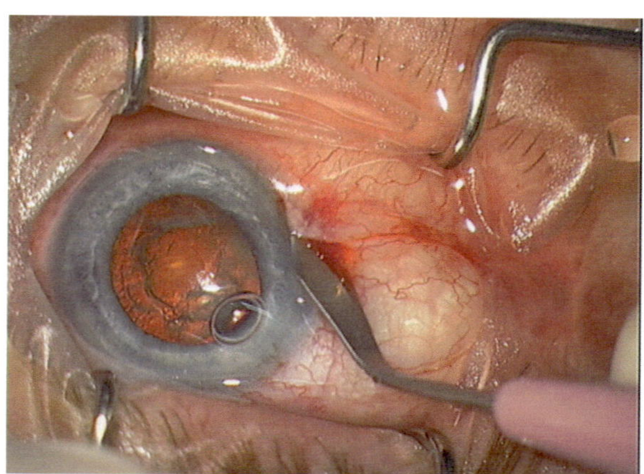

5.6   Problems During Capsulorhexis

(1) <u>**Posterior synechiae**</u> do not cause a surgical problem in most cases; inject
     viscoelastic into the anterior chamber and remove the synechiae with the
     viscoelastic cannula (Figs. 5.5, 5.7 and 5.8). If you have circular posterior
     synechiae, you have to work from both paracenteses. If the pupil is not suf-
     ficiently dilated after removal of the synechiae, you should use iris retractors. If
     the nucleus is mature and you want to stain with Vision Blue then you must
     first remove the synechiae and then inject the dye; otherwise you will only
     stain the small pupil (Figs. 5.6, 5.7 and 5.8).

Fig. 5.5 Posterior synechiae do not present a surgical problem

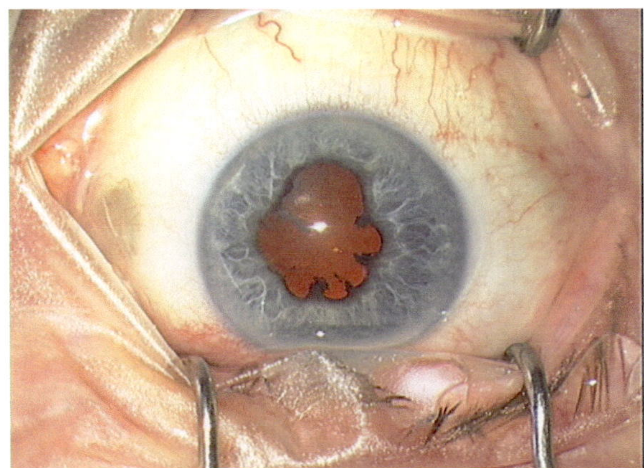

Fig. 5.6 Posterior synechiae. Inject viscoelastics

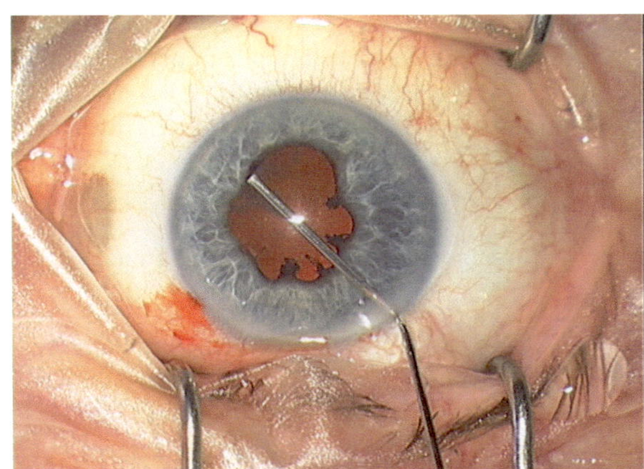

Fig. 5.7 Posterior synechiae. Remove the synechiae with the viscoelastics cannula

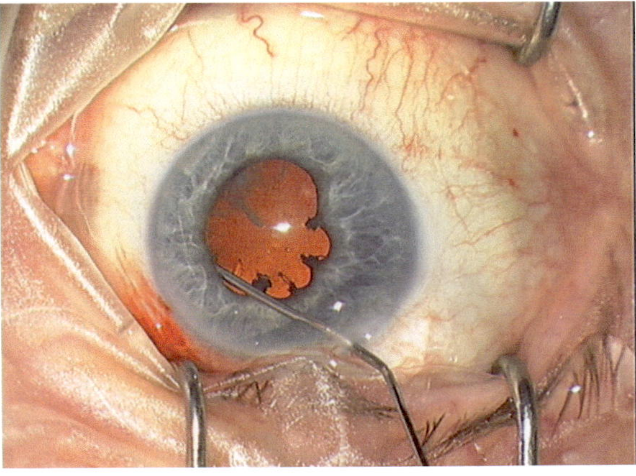

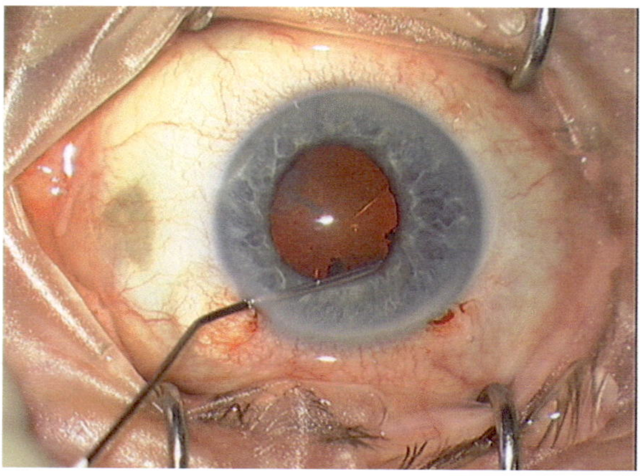

Fig. 5.8 Posterior synechiae. If necessary, work from both side incisions

(2) **Small pupil.** Especially as a beginner you should always work with a wide pupil. Do not perform a cataract operation if the pupil is small. You will regret it. There are several possibilities to widen the pupil: (A) With 2 push–pull instruments, (B) with iris hooks, (C) with Malyugin ring. And in case of a small fibrosed pupil you can perform (D) a sphincterectomy.

(A)   Instrumentation for widening with push–pull instruments:

Two push–pull instruments (Geuder, Germany)
  Insert both push–pull instruments simultaneously through both side incisions. Place the instrument at the opposite side at the pupillary edge and widen the pupil horizontally (Fig. 5.9). Then perform the same manoeuvre vertically. Inject again viscoelastics. If you are not satisfied with the pupil's size, then you have to continue with insertion of iris retractors.

(B)   Instrumentation and material for iris retractors insertion:

  The following videos demonstrate the surgery:

(1) Iris retractors
(2) Toothed forceps. Indication: Manipulation of suture or iris retractor. Castroviejo suturing forceps, Geuder, 19,023 (Fig. 5.10)
(3) Tying (anatomic) forceps. Indication: Manipulation of suture or iris retractor. Tying forceps, Geuder, 19,032 (Fig. 5.11)
(4) A grey 27G cannula attached to a 3 cc syringe (Fig. 5.12).

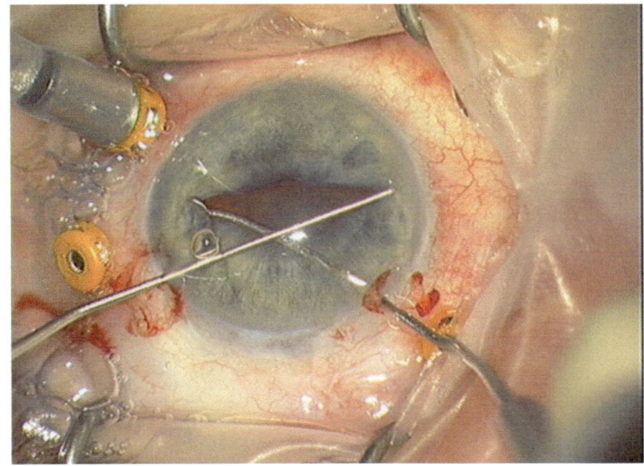

Fig. 5.9 Pupil stretching: Insert two push–pull instruments through the side incisions, place them at the pupillary edge at the opposite side and dilate the pupil. Perform the same manoeuvre at 6 o'clock and 12 o'clock, then reinject viscoelastics and perform the rhexis

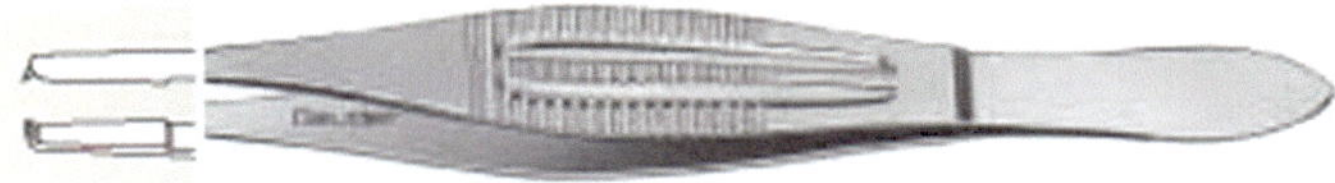

Fig. 5.10   Toothed forceps

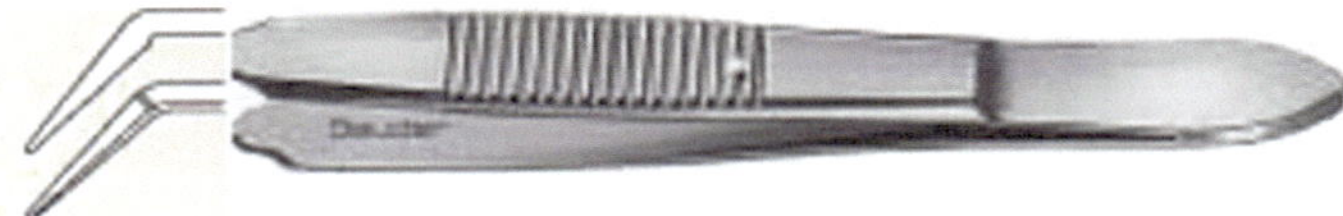

Fig. 5.11   Tying forceps

Place a grey cannula (27G) on a 3 ml syringe and bend the cannula rectangularly (Fig. 5.12). Make a paracentesis with the grey cannula at the limbus (Fig. 5.13). Grasp an iris hook with an anatomic tying forceps and insert the iris hook in the anterior chamber (Fig. 5.14). You can fixate it at once or after insertion of all iris retractors. Then introduce the remaining three iris retractors. For fixation of the iris hook grasp, the silicone stopper with the toothed forceps and turn the iris hook around its axis until the hook lies correctly behind the pupillary edge (tricky manoeuvre). Take the anatomic suturing forceps in the other hand, grasp the end of the iris hook and push the silicone stopper towards the limbus (Figs. 5 14, 5.15 and 5.16). If you do not get the hook under the iris, then inject viscoelastics behind the

Fig. 5.12 A grey 27G cannula attached to a 3 cc syringe

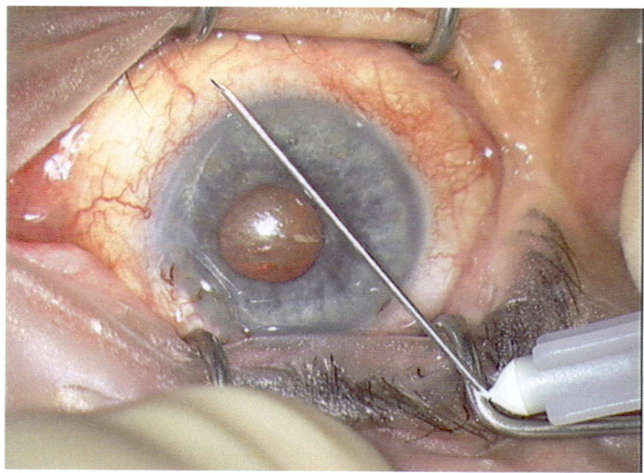

Fig. 5.13 Insertion of iris retractors: Perform a scleral incision with the grey cannula attached to a syringe

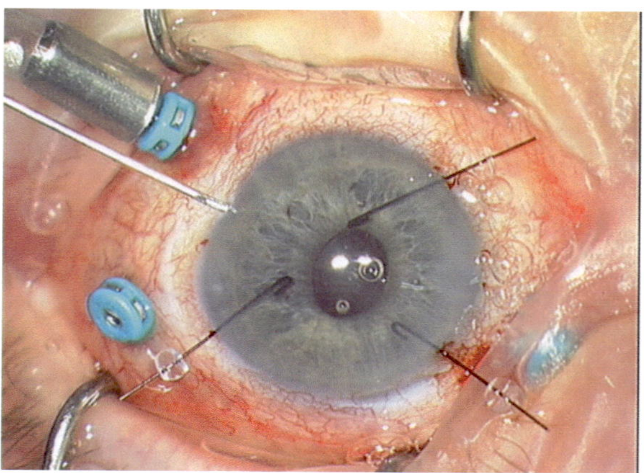

Fig. 5.14 Insertion of iris retractors: Hold an iris retractor with the tying forceps and insert the iris retractor

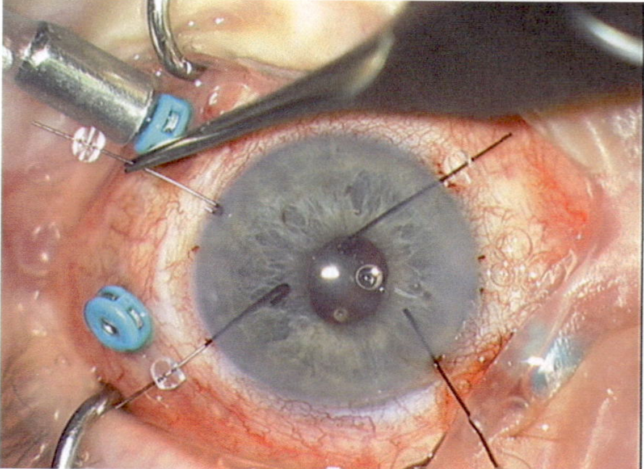

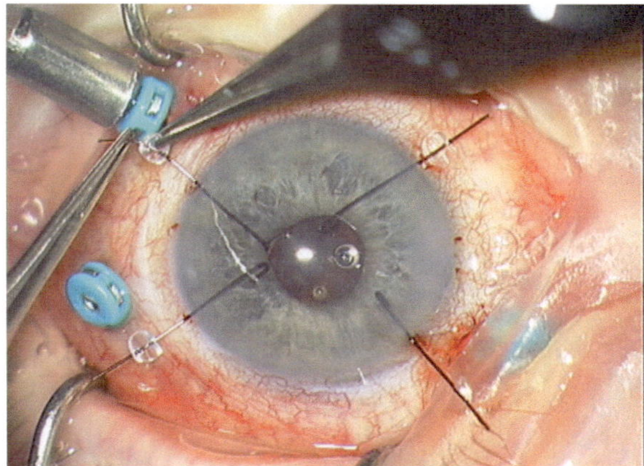

Fig. 5.15 Insertion of iris retractors: Hold the iris retractor with the tying forceps and pull the silicone stopper with the suturing forceps towards the limbus

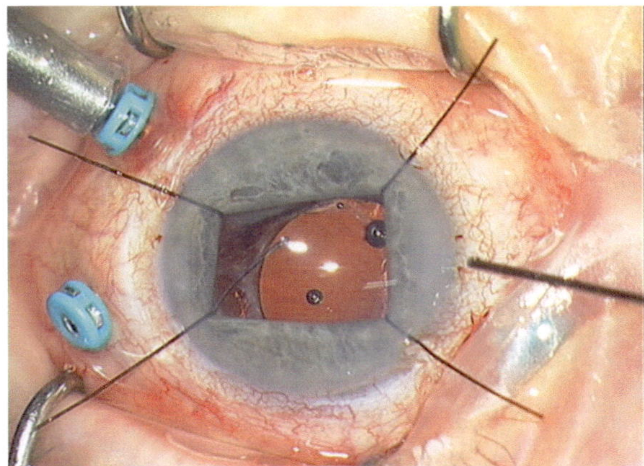

Fig. 5.16 Insertion of iris retractors: The insertion of four iris hooks is usually sufficient. Here the iris hooks were inserted to visualize the lens capsule

iris so that the iris is elevated. If necessary, you can ever insert a fifth iris hook (Fig. 5.17).

For removal, grasp the hook at the limbus with the tying forceps and the silicone stopper with the suturing forceps (Fig. 5.18). Pull the silicone stopper upwards while fixating the iris hook with the tying forceps. Loosen the hook at the pupillary edge and pull the hook slowly and obliquely outside.

(C)   <u>Insertion of a Malyugin ring (Video available):</u>

The Malyugin ring creates a round enlarged pupil (Fig. 5.19) compared to iris retractors which create a rectangle. The Malyugin ring is easy to implant and explant but more traumatic to the iris tissue than iris retractors. Damage to the iris sphincter is less common if you use the 6.25 mm Malyugin ring.

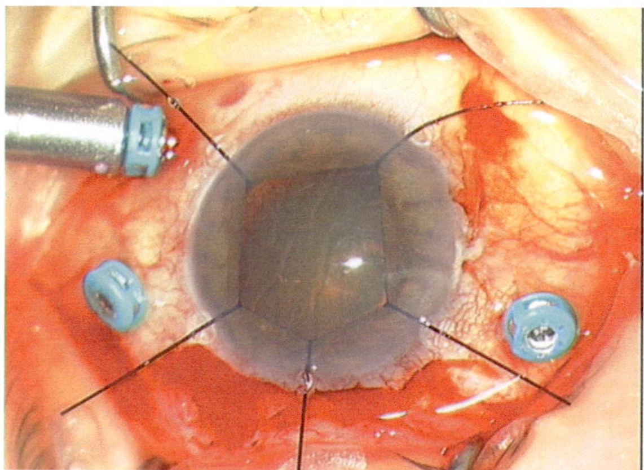

Fig. 5.17 Insertion of iris retractors: If necessary, insert five iris retractors

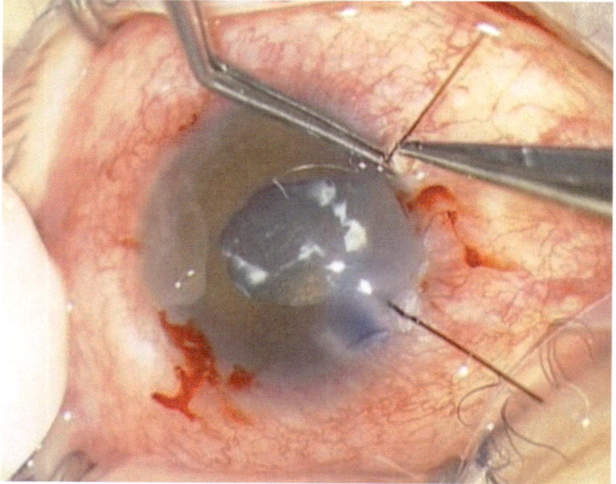

Fig. 5.18 Removal of iris retractors: Hold the iris retractor with the tying forceps between limbus and silicone stopper (left instrument). Then grasp the silicone stopper with the suturing forceps and retract the silicone stopper (right instrument). Then remove the iris hook cautiously with the tying forceps

<u>Instrumentation and material for Malyugin ring:</u>

(1) Malyugin ring with injector (MST, USA)
(2) Implantation: Kuglen hook or push–pull manipulator
(3) Explantation: Intravitreal forceps or toothed forceps

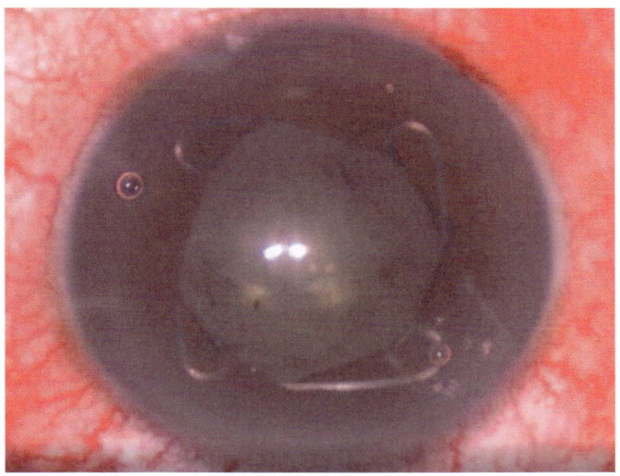

Fig. 5.19 A Malyugin ring achieves a round dilatation of the pupil. Photo courtesy V.O. Ponomarev

A Malyugin ring has four scrolls. Main incision at 12 o'clock. Inject the ring, place the distal scroll in the pupillary edge at 6 o'clock. Remove the injector. Position the proximal scroll at 12 o'clock with a manipulator and then finally position the lateral scrolls.

For removal, disengage the distal scroll, then the proximal scroll and finally the lateral scrolls. Place the ring on top of the iris. Grab the scroll at 12 o'clock with the forceps from the main incision and extract the complete ring.

(D) <u>Sphincterotomy in small fibrosed pupil (video available):</u>

In case of very small pupil and fibrosed sphincter (Fig. 5.20) or fibrosed membranous pupillary ring, a very effective method to increase pupil size is mechanical removal of the membrane and cutting the sphincter muscle (sphincterectomy). This usually results in moderate pupil dilatation sufficient for phacoemulsification.

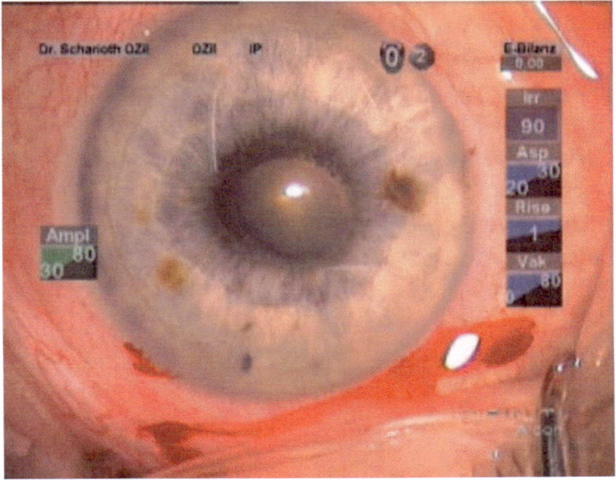

Fig. 5.20 Very small pupil with fibrosed pupillary margin prior to any manipulation

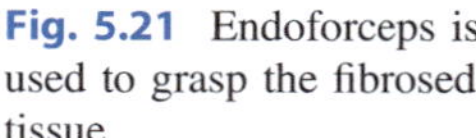

Fig. 5.21 Endoforceps is used to grasp the fibrosed tissue

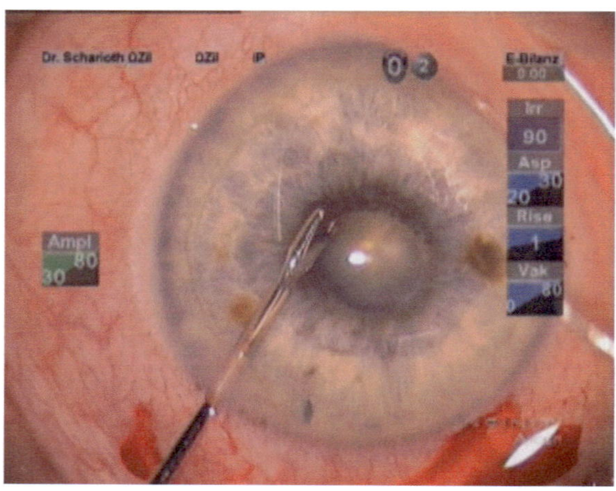

Instruments

Endoforceps (e.g. Scharioth IOL fixation forceps set 1286.SFD, DORC Int., The Netherlands).

Individual steps

1. Insertion of permanent infusion or injection of more OVD
2. Releasing of posterior synechiae
3. Removal of fibrosed tissue from pupillary margin
4. Refill with OVD (e.g. Healon5) to increase pupil size.

Standard main incision and side ports are prepared. Anterior chamber is filled with OVD. Posterior synechiae are released with blunt instrument (e.g. spatula). Through side port incision, an endoforceps is introduced and the fibrosed tissue at pupillary margin is grasped (Fig. 5.21). Then this tissue is pulled to release contraction (Fig. 5.22). Sometimes second instrument is used to counterpressure the tissue and to facilitate separation (Fig. 5.23). This procedure is repeated 360° all around. Occasionally the tissue cannot be removed just by pulling; in this case, dense tissue could be cut with endoscissors. After complete removal of the fibrosed tissue, the anterior chamber is refilled with OVD. The use of viscoadaptive OVD (e.g. Healon5, AMO, USA) could lead to additional increase in pupil size. These manipulations should result in moderate pupil dilatation sufficient for phacoemulsification (Fig. 5.24). Otherwise, additional techniques and/or devices are needed.

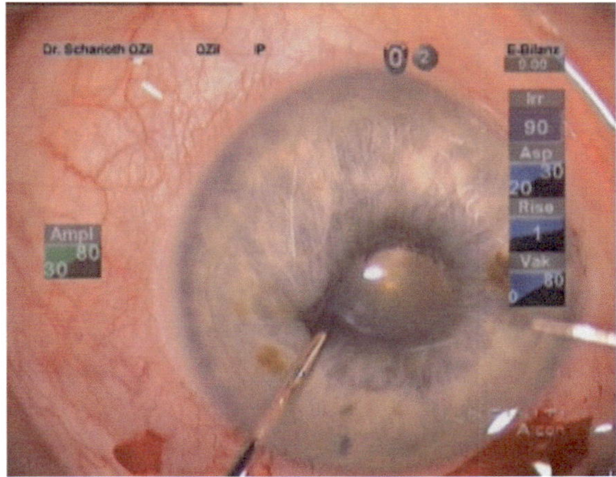

Fig. 5.22 With the endoforceps the fibrosed tissue is pulled from iris tissue

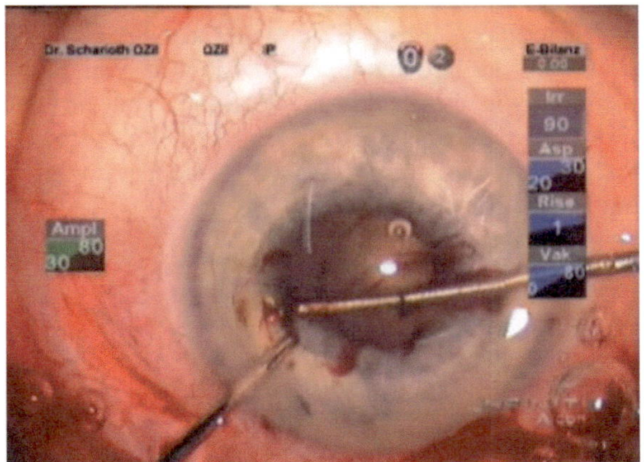

Fig. 5.23 In case of very strong adhesion of the fibrosed tissue to iris a second instrument could be used to help separation

5.7   Problems DURING Capsulorhexis

(1)   Flat anterior chamber (Video available)

In case of a flat anterior chamber, inject Healon GV. It facilitates the capsulorhexis very much. In addition, perform a long main incision in order to prevent iris prolapse.

Tips: In case of a flat anterior chamber, use a cystotome or alternatively a rhexis forceps through the SIDE incision.

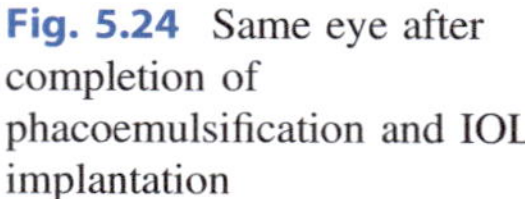

Fig. 5.24 Same eye after completion of phacoemulsification and IOL implantation

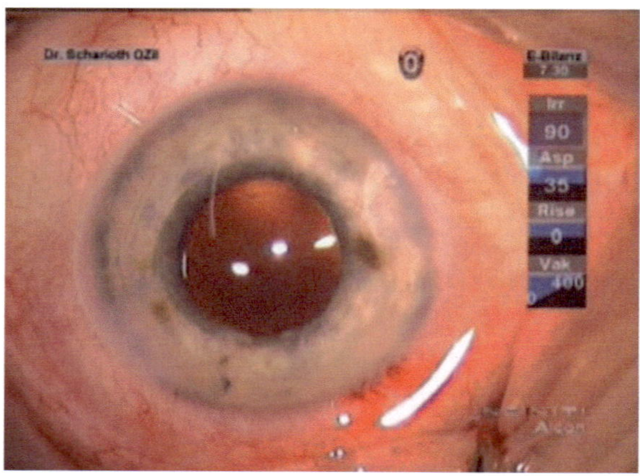

Pits & Pearls no. 7

Flat anterior chamber. When using a regular capsulorhexis forceps, you lose viscoelastics through the main incision. If you perform the rhexis from the side incision, you do not lose viscoelastics and the anterior chamber remains stable. From the side incision, you can use (1) a cystotome, (2) a special capsulorhexis forceps. These instruments enable a rhexis through the side incision and prevent an outflow of viscoelastics.

(2) **Peripheral extension of the rhexis**

Instrumentation:

(1) Capsulotomy scissors (Fig. 5.1)

Halt the rhexis, reinject viscoelastic to flatten the nucleus until the anterior segment deepens. If the rhexis extended peripherally to the zonules, do not use force to retrieve it because the rift may continue to the posterior capsule (Fig. 5.25a).

You have two options (Fig. 5.25b). You can (a) place back the flap of the lens capsule, (b) grasp the peripheral edge with the forceps and pull the capsule towards the centre (Figs. 5.26, 5.27). If the manoeuvre succeeds, the rhexis continues from the zonules inwards, then fold the capsular flap back and continue with the rhexis. Alternatively, you can cut the lens capsule with a capsulotomy scissors (Fig. 5.28) and complete the rhexis. For the beginner, I recommend the second method, because it is technically easier.

Important: A rhexis, which extends peripherally to the zonules, is stable and does not continue to the posterior capsule. It may, however, continue to the posterior capsule if you use too much force.

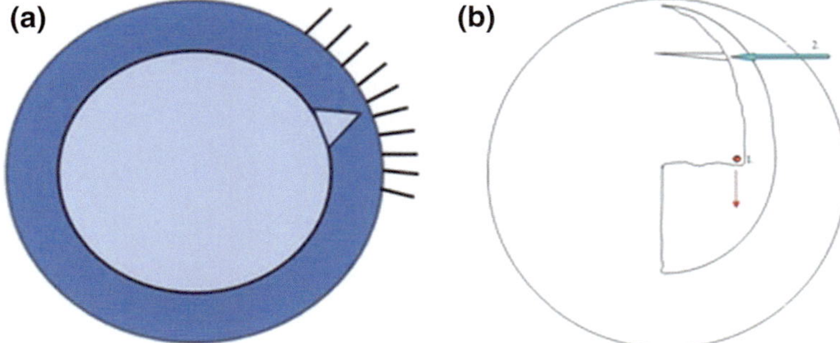

Fig. 5.25 **a** Peripheral extension of capsulorhexis. **b** Two solutions: (1) Place the flap back. Grasp the edge of the flap with the capsulorhexis forceps and pull the flap in the direction of the arrow. The peripheral rhexis will continue centrally. (2) Cut the anterior capsule with the capsulorhexis forceps and continue with the rhexis

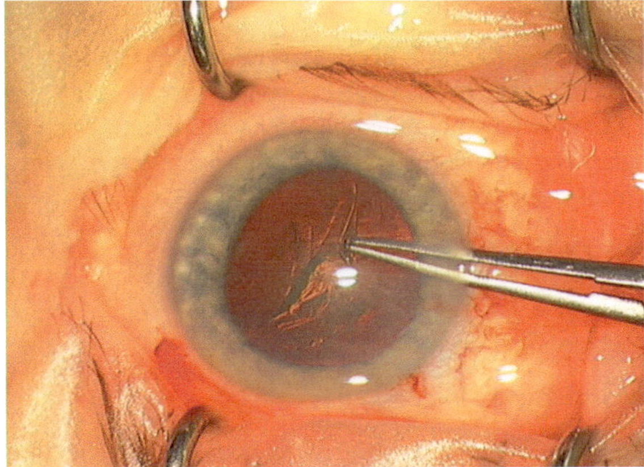

Fig. 5.26 Peripheral extended rhexis with first solution. Place the flap back, grasp the end of the flap with the capsulorhexis forceps and pull the flap towards the centre. The rhexis will continue inwards

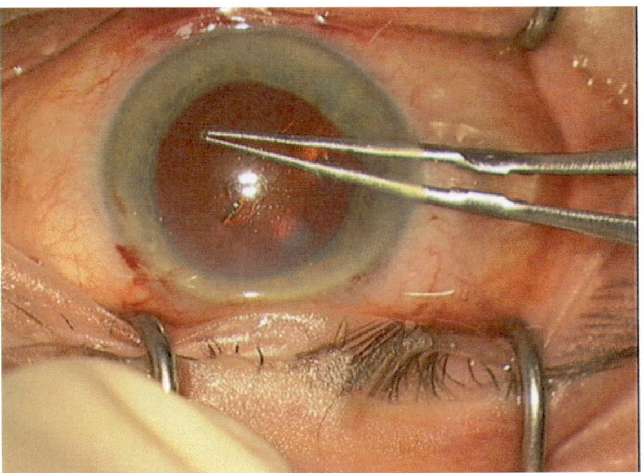

Fig. 5.27 Fold the flap back and continue with the rhexis

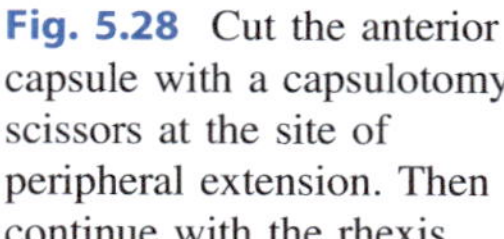

Fig. 5.28 Cut the anterior capsule with a capsulotomy scissors at the site of peripheral extension. Then continue with the rhexis

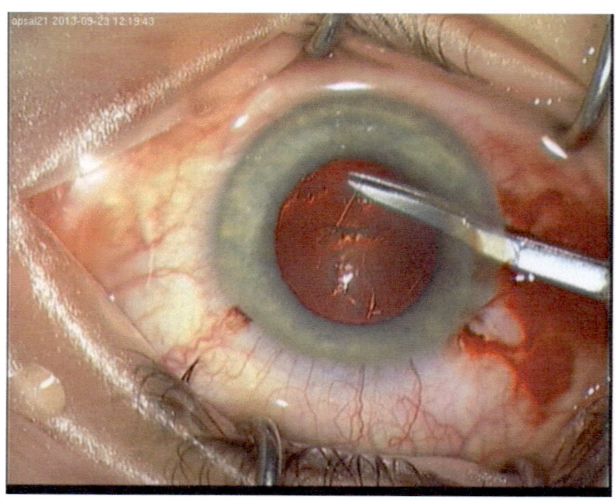

Pits and Pearls no. 8

Poor visualization of rhexis edge: If you lose the rhexis edge during capsulorhexis, you need to visualize the rhexis edge. Remove viscoelastics with I/A. Then inject trypan blue and after waiting a few seconds remove it with BSS. Inflate again the anterior chamber with viscoelastics. Now the rhexis is clearly visible. Finalize the rhexis.

(3) **Outside notch in the rhexis**

Instrumentation:

Capsulorhexis forceps

An outside notch is dangerous because the rhexis can extend peripherally at the notch. As soon you detect this defect, inject viscoelastic into the anterior chamber, grasp one side of the notch with the capsulorhexis forceps and make the defect round (Fig. 4.76). Only a round rhexis is stable. If you detect the outside notch during I/A, you can also grab (aspirate) the defect bit of rhexis with the tip of the aspiration handpiece and remove it by making a round movement.

Pits and Pearls no. 9

Incomplete rhexis: Pay attention that the rhexis is 100% round. If the rhexis is only 99% round, then you may aspirate the rhexis flap with the phacoemulsification handpiece and cause an anterior and posterior rupture of the lens capsule (Fig. 5.29).

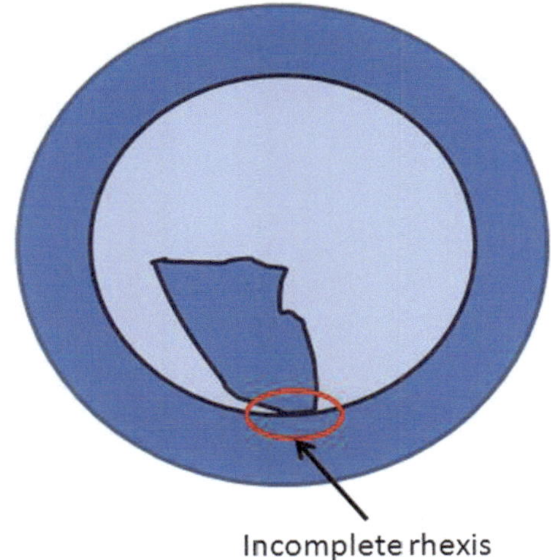

Fig. 5.29 Outside notch of capsulorhexis. Grasp the anterior capsule with the capsulorhexis forceps and pull the flap in the direction of the arrow. The aim is a round rhexi

Pits and Pearls no. 10

<u>Not round rhexis:</u> It does not matter whether the rhexis is circular or pear shaped, as long as it is round.

(4)   **White mature nucleus. Staining with VisionBlue®**

<u>Material:</u>

VisionBlue® (DORC)

<u>Procedure:</u> Begin with the injection of an air bubble into the anterior chamber (Fig. 5.30). The air bubble protects the endothelium from a possible toxic effect of vision blue (trypan blue). Inject next VisionBlue® (Fig. 5.30). Wait approximately 30 s and then irrigate the anterior chamber with BSS (Fig. 5.31). Inject at last viscoelastics and proceed with the rhexis (Figs. 5.32 and 5.33).

You will never regret to have used VisionBlue® (Fig. 5.33), but you often regret not to have used it. However, it is never too late to use VisionBlue®. If you notice during a rhexis that you need VisionBlue®, then remove the viscoelastic with I/A and inject VisionBlue®. Remove then the dye with BSS, inject viscoelastic and proceed with the rhexis.

Pits and Pearls no. 11

<u>Small pupil and white nucleus.</u> First insert iris retractors and then stain the nucleus. If you first stain the pupil, then you will only stain the central part of the nucleus.

You will never regret having used iris hooks but sometimes regret not to have used them. It is never too late to use iris retractors. If you cannot cope with a small pupil during phaco or I/A then don't hesitate to insert iris retractors. The same applies for VisionBlue.

Fig. 5.30 Inject first an air bubble in order to protect the endothelium and then the dye

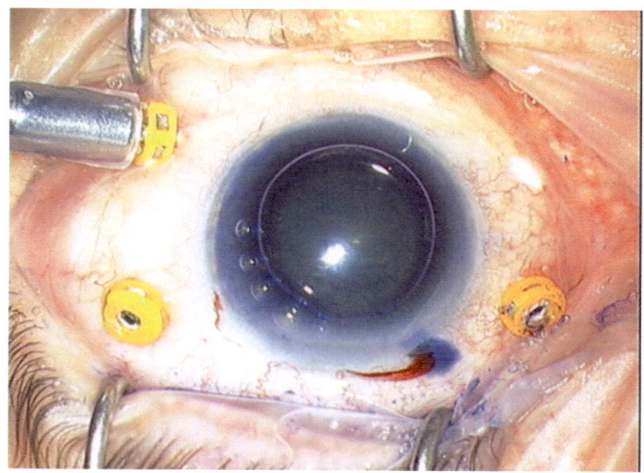

Fig. 5.31 Wait a few seconds and then remove the dye with BSS

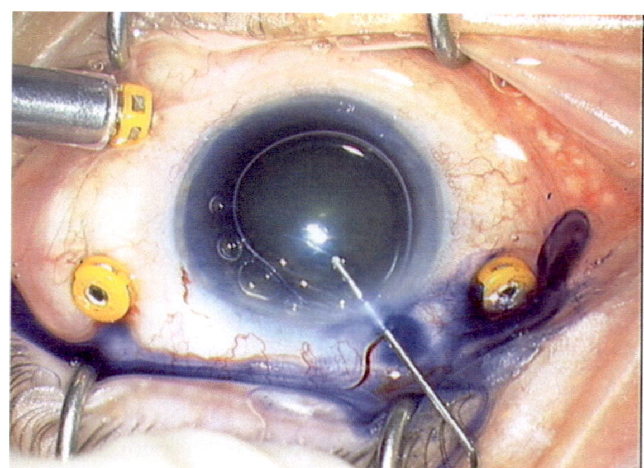

Fig. 5.32 Inject viscoelastics and remove the air bubble

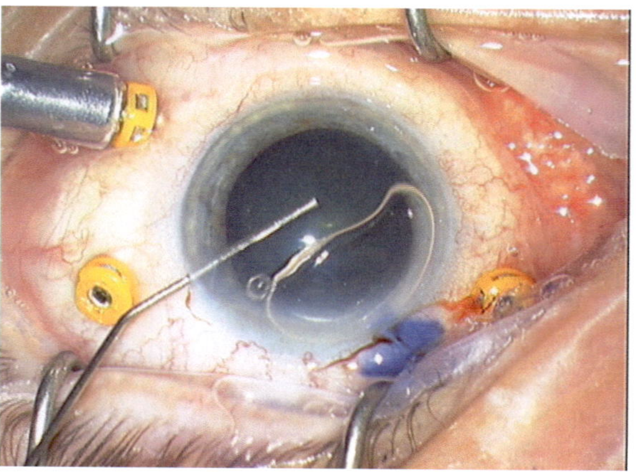

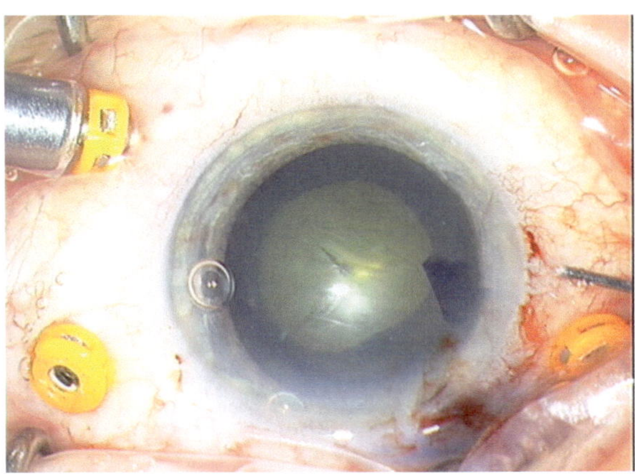

Fig. 5.33 You never regret using vision blue

5.8 Problems During Hydrodissection

(1) <u>Iris prolapse.</u>

An iris prolapse is caused by an increased intraocular pressure. A short tunnel incision, a flat anterior chamber and a tense patient aggravate the prolapse risk. If you then overinflate the anterior chamber with BSS, the iris presses towards the incisions (Fig. 5.34). What to do? Wait 5 min! Check with the finger if the eye gets soft. Then press carefully on the paracentesis incisions to release intracameral fluid. Then push the iris *gently* back (Fig. 5.33).

If the iris prolapse recurs, I recommend a new tunnel incision. The procedure is as follows: Reposition the iris prolapse, close the tunnel incision with an Ethilon 10–0 interrupted stitch and make a new and longer tunnel incision. If you continue

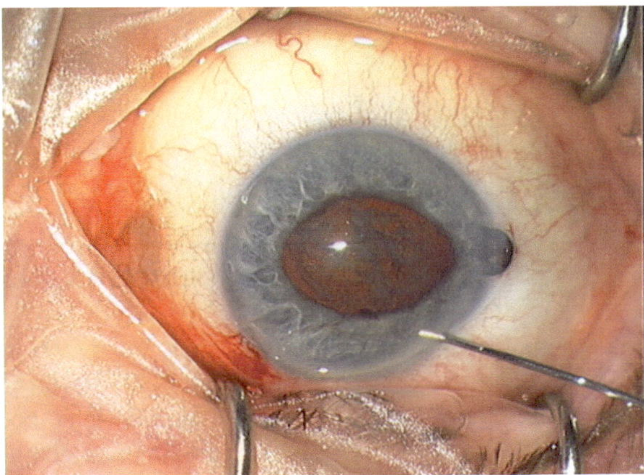

Fig. 5.34 Iris prolapse during hydrodissection

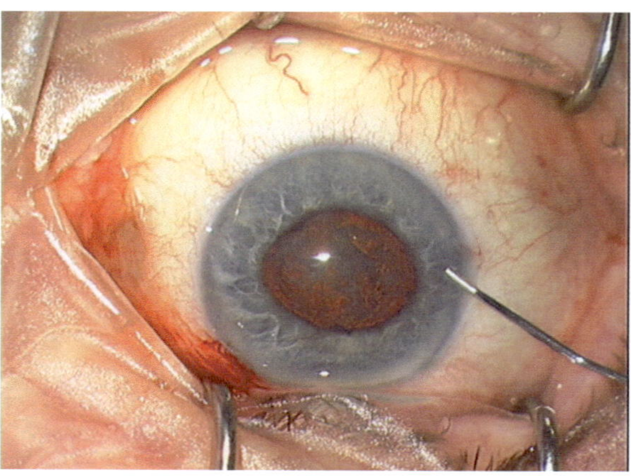

Fig. 5.35 Iris prolapse. Release fluid from the anterior chamber via the paracentesis. Check with the finger if the pressure is reduced. If not, release more fluid from the anterior chamber

with the same main incision you will cause a significant iris trauma and have continuous problems under phacoemulsification.

Remember: An iris prolapse is caused by increased intraocular pressure. It is therefore useless to push the iris prolapse back if the pressure is still high. You will not succeed! Reduce the intraocular pressure and the iris prolapse will disappear by its own (Fig. 5.35).

(2) Excessive pressure from behind during surgery.

In these cases, the anterior chamber is completely flat and I/A with maximal bottle height is not possible. There are two possible solutions: (1) Simply wait. Wait 10 min. The pressure from behind will disappear and you can continue with surgery. (2) Anterior/core vitrectomy. Insert a trocar 3.5 mm behind the limbus. Perform a short anterior vitrectomy from pars plana without infusion. Remove so much central vitreous until the globe is soft. Feel with your index finger. Then continue with phacoemulsification. For more details, see chapter "Anterior vitrectomy with trocars".

Pits and Pearls no. 12

Pressure from behind. If you work in topical anaesthesia, and the patient is tense, you should perform peribulbar anaesthesia to relax the eye and the patient.

5.9 Problems During Phacoemulsification

If you operate a myopic patient, then the anterior chamber may become very deep. Reduce irrigation to approximately 40–50 mmHg. In contrast, if you operate a hyperopic patient, the anterior chamber may become very shallow. Increase irrigation to 100–110 mmHg until the anterior chamber is sufficiently deep.

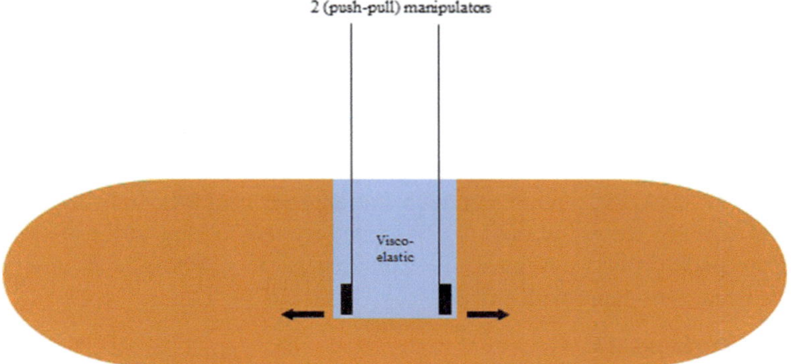

Fig. 5.36 Difficult cracking. In the case of a very dense nucleus, you may not succeed with the cracking manoeuvre although the groove is deep enough. Inject viscoelastics inside the groove. Place two manipulators at the bottom of the groove and proceed with the cracking movement

Fig. 5.37 Difficult cracking. It is essential to crack the groove. Do not proceed with a not or only partially cracked groove. You can only remove fragments, which are completely cracked!

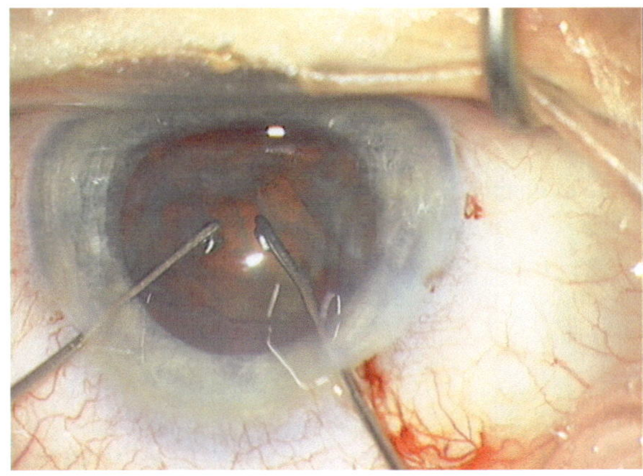

If you are right hand dominant and operate the left eye of a patient with a big nose, then a main incision at 9 o'clock may not be possible because you cannot insert the phaco handpiece. Try if a main incision at 10:30 allows sufficient manoeuvrability of the handpiece. If not, sit temporal and place the main incision at 12 or 3 o'clock.

Unsuccessful cracking. The reasons may be a dense nucleus or a groove, which is not deep enough. Inject viscoelastic into the groove. Take 2 manipulators (e.g. push–pull), one in each hand, place them at the bottom edges of the groove and crack the nucleus (Figs. 5.36 and 5.37). (Video available).

If you experience an iris prolapse, then tap aqueous from the side incision and reposition the iris prolapse in the main incision.

If the nucleus does not rotate during phaco, then remove the phaco handpiece and redo hydrodissection. The nucleus will rotate now.

Malignant glaucoma: A flat anterior chamber with iris prolapse through all incisions is a dangerous complication. It may be caused by a subchoroidal bleeding. You will see that the red reflex disappears. Terminate surgery and try to close the incisions with Ethilon 10–0. The most likely reason is a so called positive vitreous pressure. The reason is a short eye with flat anterior chamber and often an obese patient. There are two solutions: (1) Stop surgery. Redo surgery in peribulbar or general anaesthesia one day later. (2) Continue surgery: Perform an anterior vitrectomy from pars plana with trocar.

Pits and Pearls no. 13

<u>Soft nucleus:</u> Dislocate the nucleus through hydrodissection from the lens capsule into the anterior chamber. Remove it here with epinucleus mode.

<u>Pseudoexfoliation:</u> Eyes with pseudoexfoliation have weak zonules. Reduce the surgical stress as much as possible. Minimize mechanical stress during phacoemulsification, prevent a deep anterior chamber and use a capsular tension ring if necessary.

5.9.1 Posterior Capsule Rupture and Dropping Nucleus

If the nucleus begins dropping place a 27G needle cannula on a viscoelastic syringe, pierce the conjunctiva and sclera (like an intravitreal injection) 4 mm behind the limbus, place the cannula behind the nucleus and inject viscoelastics. Then elevate the nucleus into the anterior chamber. For details, see chapter "Posterior capsular rupture".

5.10 Problems During I/A—Implantation of Capsular Tension Ring

(1) <u>Reflux (backflush) function</u>

If you accidentally aspirate the lens capsule with the aspiration handpiece, then you need to release it. If you activate the backflush function, then the irrigation handpiece flushes out the aspirated material. It is essential to know this function because you will now and then aspirate the posterior capsule and unless you activate the backflush function the capsule will tear. Check, therefore, before you start with surgery how to activate the backflush function on the foot pedal. It is usually located on the lower right.

(2)   <u>I/A with small pupil</u>

An I/A is difficult if the pupil is small (Figs. 5.38). Take advantage of the bimanual I/A handpieces and move the iris to the side with the irrigation handpiece and aspirate the residual cortex with the aspiration handpiece (Fig. 5.39). If you have an aspiration handpiece with rough tip, you can place the aspiration handpiece so far in the periphery of the capsular bag until the rough tip is covered by the pupillary edge (Fig. 5.40). And again: If you do not feel secure during I/A because of a small pupil, then insert iris retractors.

(3)   <u>Zonular lysis. Implantation of a capsular tension ring (Videos available)</u>

If you detect a small zonular lysis (1 quadrant), then complete I/A and implant then the capsular tension ring. See also chapter 6.

<u>Instrumentation:</u>

Capsular tension ring with injector (Fig. 5.41).

<u>Capsular tension ring</u>: Indication: zonular lysis.

<u>Procedure</u>: Inflate the capsular bag with viscoelastic (Figs. 5.42, 5.43 and 5.44). Inject the capsular tension ring with an injector. It is important that you place the tip and the end inside the capsular bag and not in the sulcus. If the end (tail) is located in the sulcus and not in the capsular bag, then try to luxate the end with a Sinskey hook into the capsular bag or retract the capsular tension ring with the injector and reinject the ring.

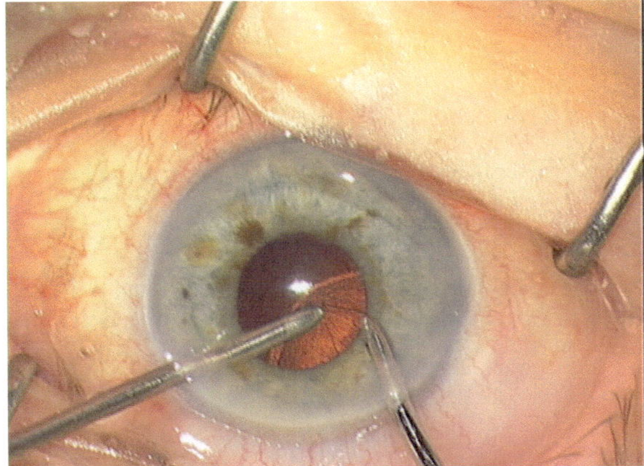

Fig. 5.38 Small pupil during I/A

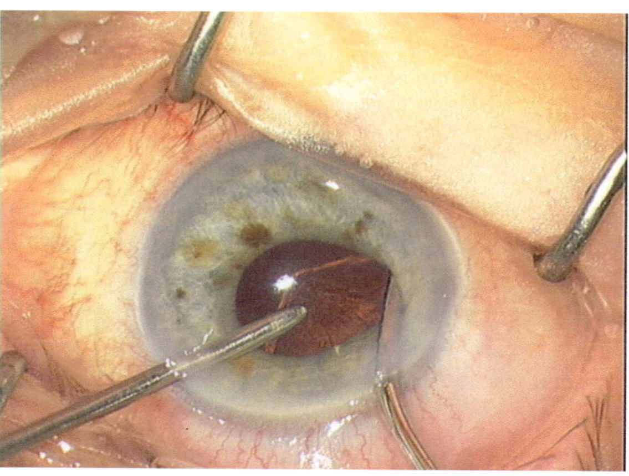

Fig. 5.39 Move the iris aside with the irrigation tip and remove the residual cortex

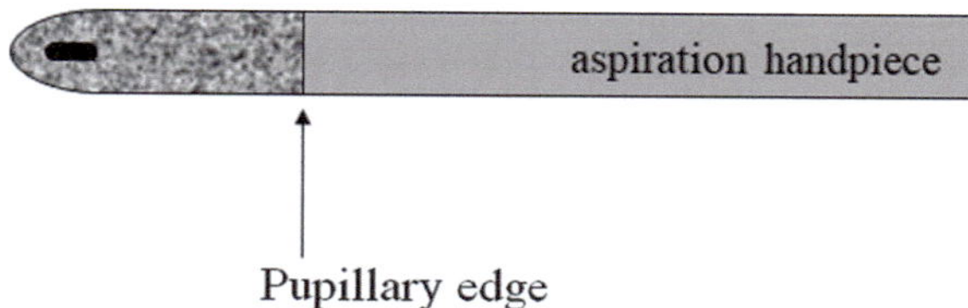

Fig. 5.40 Alternatively, you can move the aspiration tip so far behind the iris until the dusted part of the tip is completely behind the iris and then aspirate the residual cortex

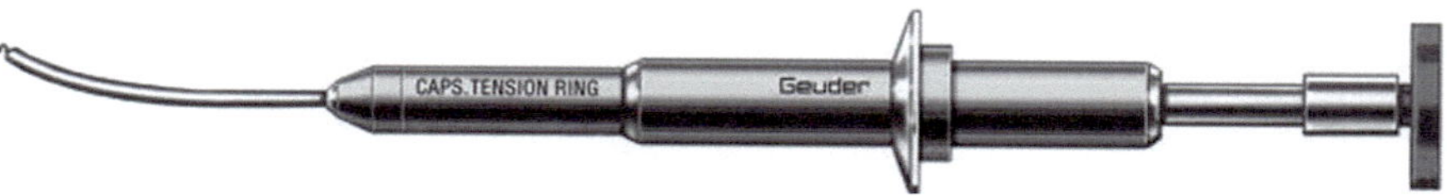

Fig. 5.41 Capsular tension ring. Indication: Zonular lysis. I recommend a preloaded capsular tension ring with injector. There are many providers, for example CROMA, AMO, Morcher, Arcadoptha, Geuder 32,955

Fig. 5.42 Tip of the capsular tension ring injector and the capsular tension ring

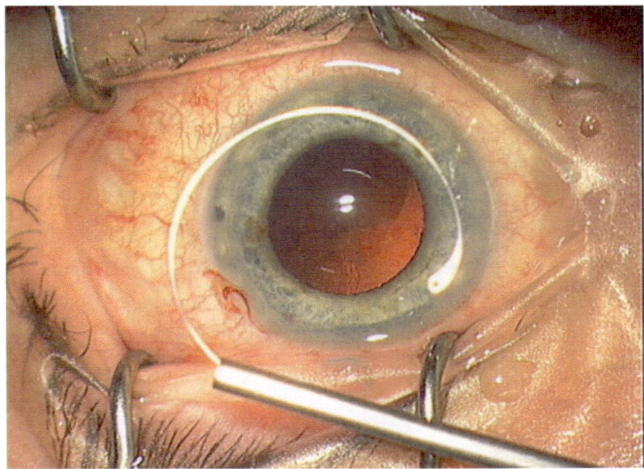

Fig. 5.43 It is important that the tip of the capsular tension ring is placed in the capsular bag and not in the sulcus

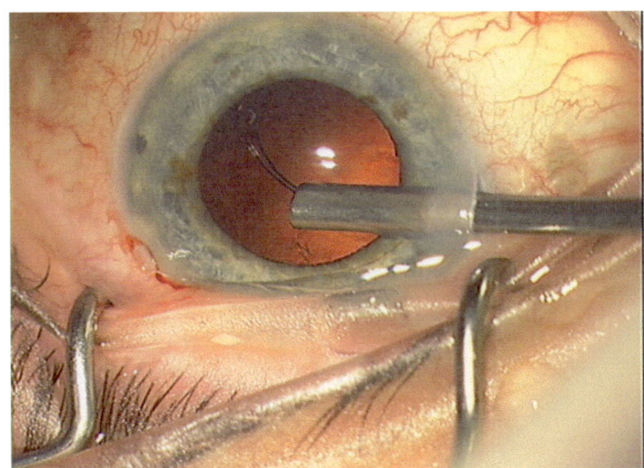

Fig. 5.44 Be also aware that the end of the capsular tension ring is located in the bag. If not, you can luxate it with a Sinskey hook into the bag

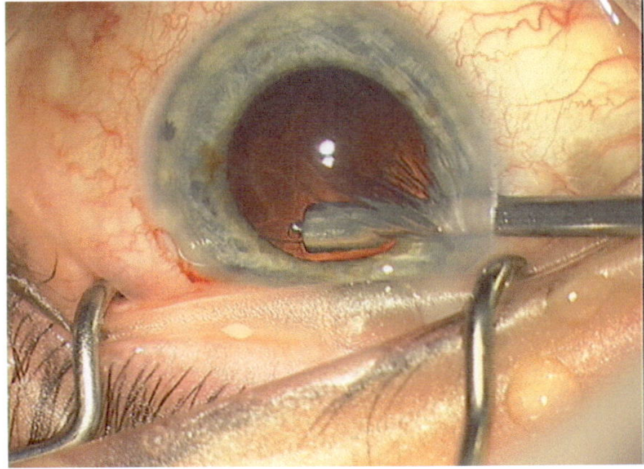

5.11   Problems During Removal of Cortex

<u>Residual cortex:</u> If a small cortical strand remains, leave it. Safety comes first. Do not insist on removing it and risking a posterior capsular defect.

But there are a few tricks to solve this problem. (1) The simplest solution is a paracentesis at the opposite side of the vitreous strand. Access the anterior chamber from the new paracentesis and remove the residual cortex (Figs. 5.45 and 5.46). (2) Implant the IOL in the capsular bag and rotate the IOL 360°. The haptics loosen the residual cortex. Remove finally the viscoelastic and the residual cortex with I/A. If you hold the aspiration tip above (not behind) the IOL, you do not risk injuring the posterior capsule.

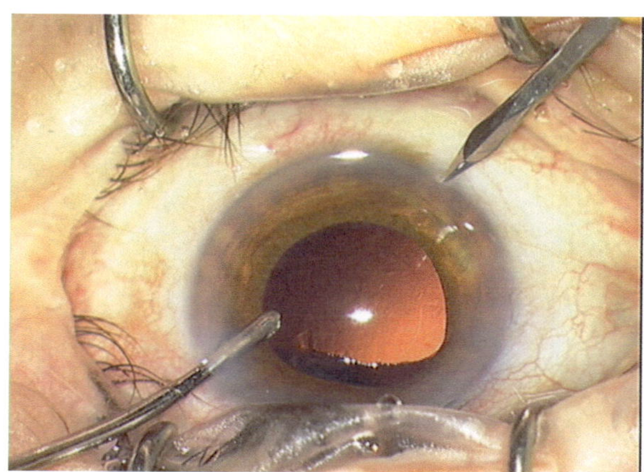

Fig. 5.45 Residual cortex at 12 o'clock. Perform a paracentesis at 6 o'clock

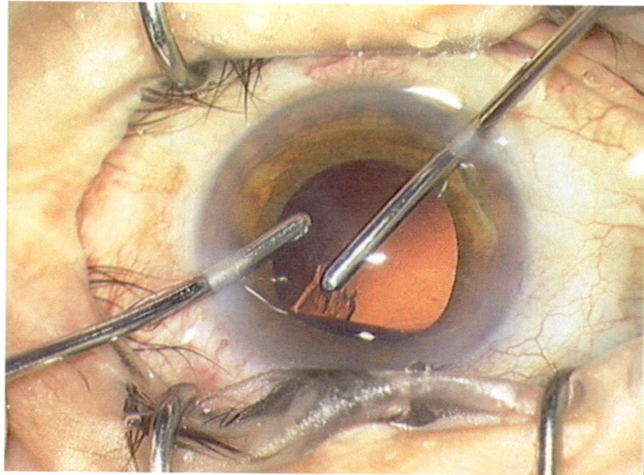

Fig. 5.46 Residual cortex at 12 o'clock. Insert the aspiration handpiece at 6 o'clock and remove the residual cortex

5.12 Problems During IOL Implantation

Today cataract surgery and IOL implantation are performed through very small incisions. If the cartridge is too big to introduce it into the main incision, a so called wound-assisted implantation is performed. This is usually the case with incisions smaller then 2.2 mm. After the eye is filled with OVD, the tip of the cartridge is connected to the main incision. It is very important to keep direct connection of the cartridge to the wound during the implantation. Most surgeons use a second instrument to stabilize and counterpressure the eye. Then the implantation is performed quickly. Sudden motion of the eye or patient, loss of counterpressure, soft eye and others can cause disconnection during the implantation. If this happens, the IOL unfolds within the main incision (butterfly phenomenon). Videos are available.

Instruments

1. **Anterior chamber maintainer or pars plana infusion**
2. **Tying forceps.**

Individual steps

1. **Insertion of permanent infusion or injection of more OVD**
2. **Decision making: continue implantation or explantation of IOL**
3. **If IOL was removed, refill with OVD and repeat IOL implantation**
4. **Remove OVD**
5. **Hydrate incision and if leaking suture main incision.**

If IOL is unfolding within the main incision, decision has to be made whether implantation is continued or aborted and IOL is removed from the main incision.

If less than one half is within the main incision, it is not possible to continue the implantation (Fig. 5.47). Removal is recommended. Even this could be very difficult. There could be a very high pressure within the main incision. This is the case if a hydrophobic IOL was used, or the incision was extremely small. Try just to pull at the outer part of the IOL. Create a counterpressure with a second instrument under the IOL or use side port incision (e.g. with the irrigation handpiece) (Fig. 5.48). If this is too traumatic, try to externalize the IOL haptic, which might be still within the folded optic. This will release some of the pressure and usually allow withdrawal of the IOL. Use a tying forceps or a toothed forceps (e.g. colibri forceps).

If more than one half is already through the main incision, it is better to complete the implantation (Fig. 5.49). Stabilize the anterior chamber with OVD or continuous irrigation. Then start to push the IOL with an atraumatic instrument (e.g. tying forceps). If this is not possible, the pressure within the main incision could be too high (Fig. 5.50). IOL haptic should be externalized from the main incision to reduce pressure within the main incision (Fig. 5.51). This should be performed very carefully. Inject some OVD into the folded IOL to reduce friction. Pull gently at the

Fig. 5.47 IOL is unfolding within the main incision, forceps is pulling, second instrument is creating a counterpressure and stabilizing the eye

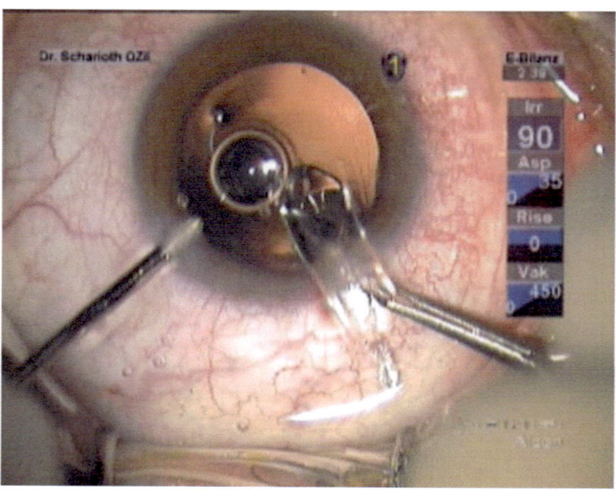

Fig. 5.48 IOL is explanted after haptic was removed from main incision

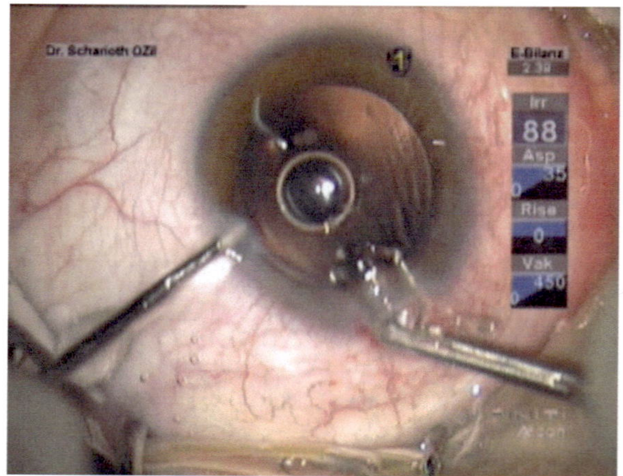

Fig. 5.49 IOL is unfolding within the main incision, more than 50% are already through

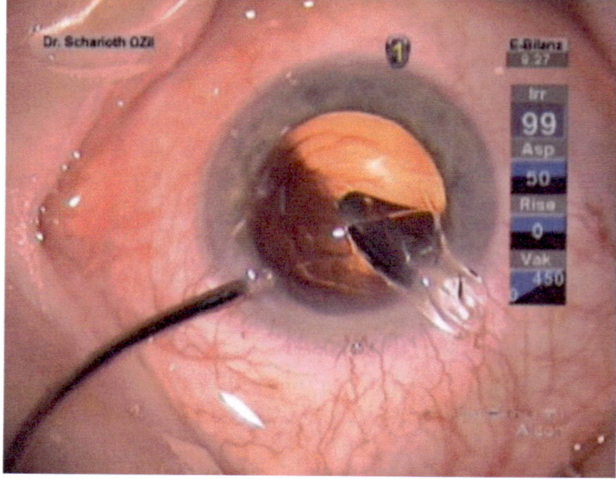

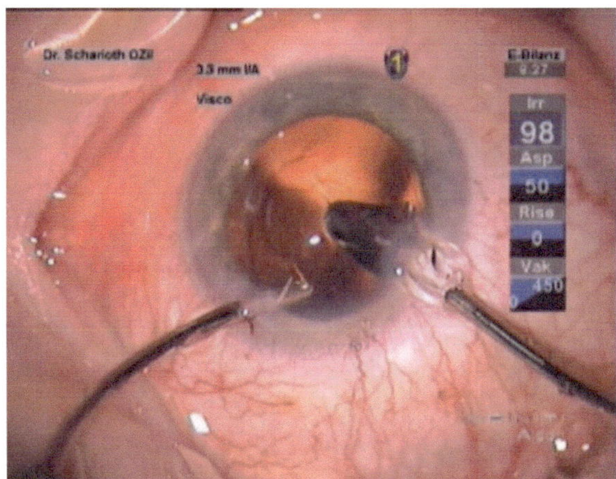

Fig. 5.50 Attempt is made to push the IOL through the main incision, but resistance is too high

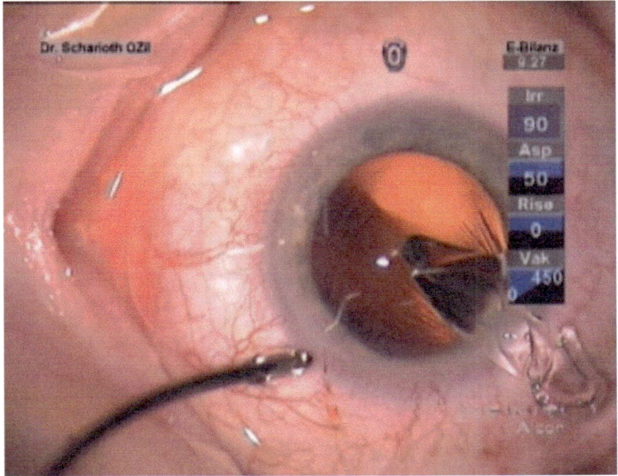

Fig. 5.51 IOL haptic is externalized, this releases some pressure from within the main incision

IOL haptic. Once it is externalized, start again to push the IOL through the main incision (Fig. 5.52). Now IOL is checked for damages. If IOL is undamaged, it is placed in the capsular bag (Figs. 5.53 and 5.54). If damages are affecting central visual axis or correct centration of the IOL, it should be exchanged.

Worst case is a so-called butterfly where the middle of the IOL optic is unfolding within the main incision. There sometimes it is not possible to move the IOL. The pressure within the main incision is so high that neither explantation nor implantation works. The only solution in this case is to enlarge the incision. Start with a side port incision next to the main incision and cut towards the main incision. Connection of both incisions will release pressure within the main incision, and IOL could be explanted.

Fig. 5.52 With a tying forceps IOL is folded and slowly pushed through the main incision, counterpressure is created with second instrument

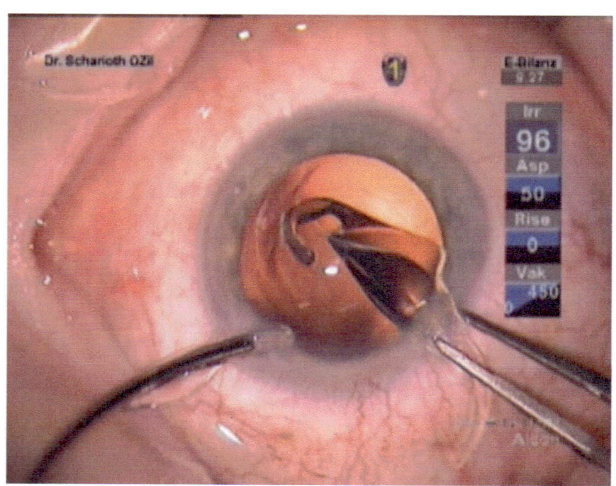

Fig. 5.53 Implantation is completed with bimanual irrigation and aspiration handpieces

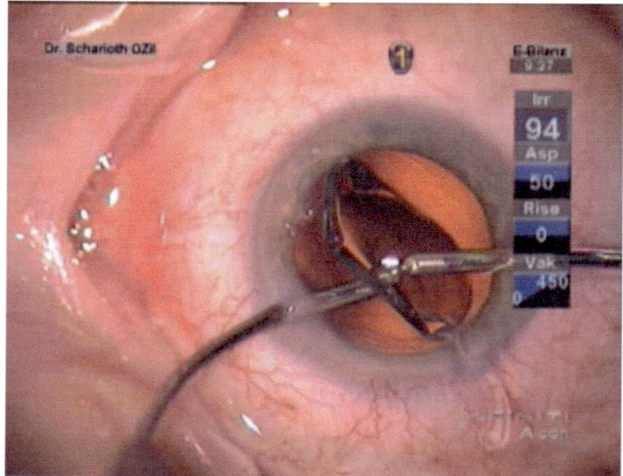

Fig. 5.54 IOL well centred within the capsular bag and IOL optic undamaged, after hydration incisions were self-sealing

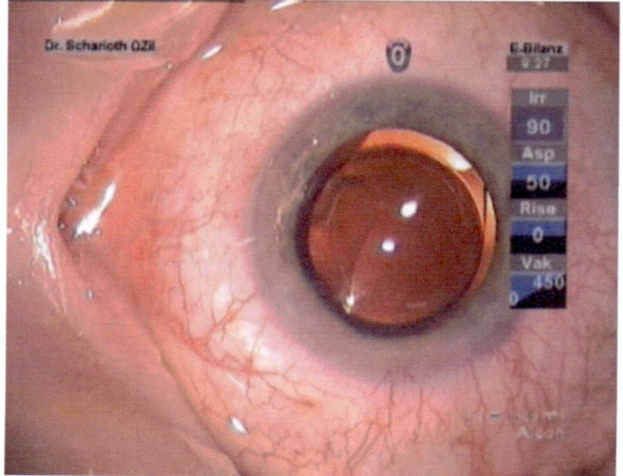

Finally check incisions for leakage. The main incision is often damaged and needs to be sutured with an Ethilon 10–0 interrupted stitch or a cross stitch.

Pits and Pearls no. 14

Wound-assisted IOL implantation can cause IOL unfolding within the main incision. Complete filling with OVD and continuous connection between IOL cartridge and main incision are mandatory. Create continuous pressure and counterpressure between the eye and the cartridge. Ensure patients cooperation.

If unfolding within the main incision occurred, explant the IOL if less than 50% are within the wound. Try to complete implantation if more than 50% are within the main incision.

Pits and Pearls no. 15

Double-check that both haptics are located inside the lens capsule. It may easily happen that one haptic is located in the lens capsule and the other haptic in the sulcus causing iris chafing. This is especially the case for a 1-piece IOL. These IOLs need have to be repositioned. Insert iris hooks when repositioning the IOL so that you can visualize the IOL and the rhexis edge.

5.13 Problems During Final Steps

If there is little leakage from main incision at the end of surgery, then inject an air bubble into the anterior chamber.

If there is significant leakage from the main incision, then it should be sutured. Suture the main incision with an interrupted stitch or even better with a cross stitch. The stitch can be removed one week postoperatively.

Suturing of tunnel incision.

Instrumentation:

(1)   Needle holder
(1)   Suturing forceps.
(2)   Tying forceps
(3)   Suture. Ethilon 10–0 (Ethicon).

Operation:

Grasp the upper lip of the main incision with the suturing forceps. Move the needle through the upper lip and then the lower lip of the main incision. Suture 3–2–1 knots with the needle holder and the tying forceps.

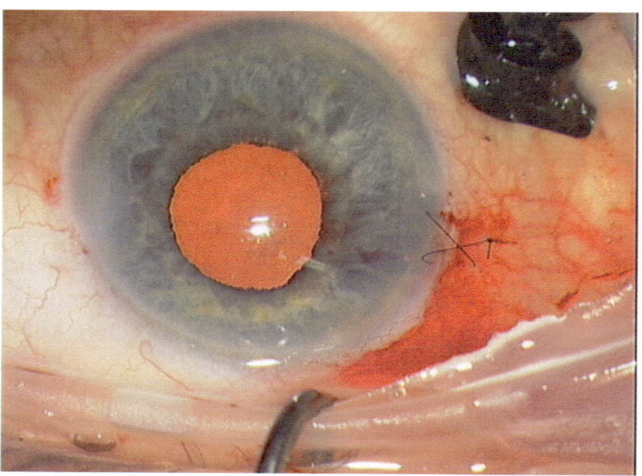

Fig. 5.55 Cross stitch on a main incision with Ethilon 10–0

More stable than an interrupted stitch is a cross stitch (Fig. 5.55). In general, a stitch on the main incision need not be too tight. The main incision should be form-stable in order to avoid leakage. Try to avoid corneal folds, otherwise you might induce astigmatism. You can remove the stitch after one week.

Part III

Complication Management with Trocar Cannulas

All videos of this part be found in a playlist of my YouTube channel:
https://www.youtube.com/playlist?list=PL0dKYclPD7yMJRuQAIt9Dr7pOtuI0
Seex

Anterior Vitrectomy and Other Surgeries with Trocars from Pars Plana

6

Contents

Abstract

This chapter explains in detail anterior vitrectomy for cataract surgeons. The anterior vitrectomy with trocars from pars plana is described in detail. All surgeries are performed with a phacoemulsification machine.

Keywords

Equipment · Trocar Surgery · Anterior segment · Trocar · Vitreous cutter

In the following part, we will describe a new technique for cataract surgeons, which increases your surgical spectrum immensely. Cases, which you sent to a retinal specialist, can be solved by yourself.

Insert a trocar into the sclera. That's all. Now you can perform an anterior vitrectomy from pars plana, which enables you to remove the anterior vitreous completely and reduces the risk of damaging the lens capsule. Secondly, you can recover a subluxated IOL by elevating the IOL from pars plana. Thirdly, you can

U. Spandau and G. B. Scharioth, *Complications During and After Cataract Surgery*,
https://doi.org/10.1007/978-3-030-93531-3_6

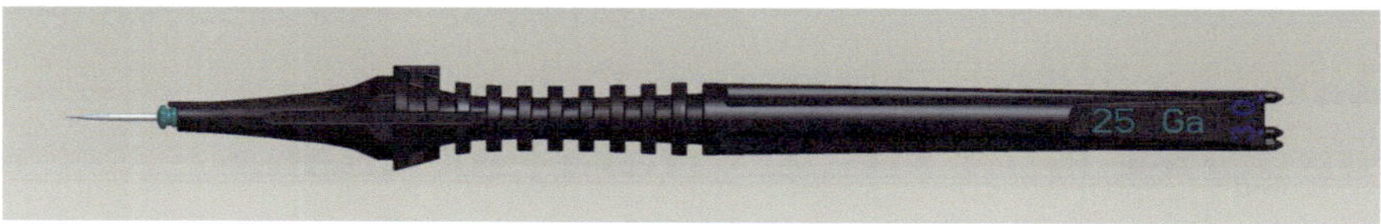

Fig. 6.1 Trocar with inserter (Alcon). The trocar is at the left side, the handpiece/inserter has a knife for the sclerotomy at the left side and a marker for the sclerotomy on the right side

rescue a dropping nucleus by recovering it from pars plana. Fourthly, you can remove a posterior capsular opacification (PCO) from pars plana with the vitreous cutter, if it cannot be removed with laser.

All videos of this part be found in a playlist of my YouTube channel:

https://www.youtube.com/playlist?list=PL0dKYclPD7yMJRuQAIt9Dr7pOtuI0Seex

An anterior vitrectomy is usually performed with an anterior vitreous cutter from the limbus (Figs. 6.1, 6.2 and 6.3). The disadvantage of this technique is that it is impossible to remove the anterior vitreous completely because the iris and the lens capsule are in the way resulting sometimes in a postoperative vitreous prolapse.

What is the advantage of an anterior vitrectomy from pars plana compared to a limbal approach? The advantage is that the anterior vitreous is much easier to remove from pars plana, because the iris and the lens capsule are not in the way (Figs. 6.2 and 6.3). In addition, the anterior vitreous can be completely removed from pars plana, but only partially from the limbus.

Fig. 6.2 Nuclear elevation from pars plana. In case of a posterior capsular defect and luxation of the nucleus, insert a trocar and inject viscoelastics posterior to the nucleus. Elevate then the nucleus with the viscoelastic cannula into the anterior chamber

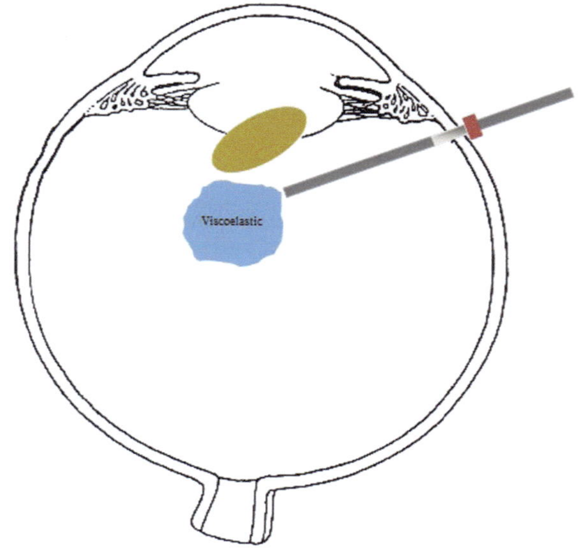

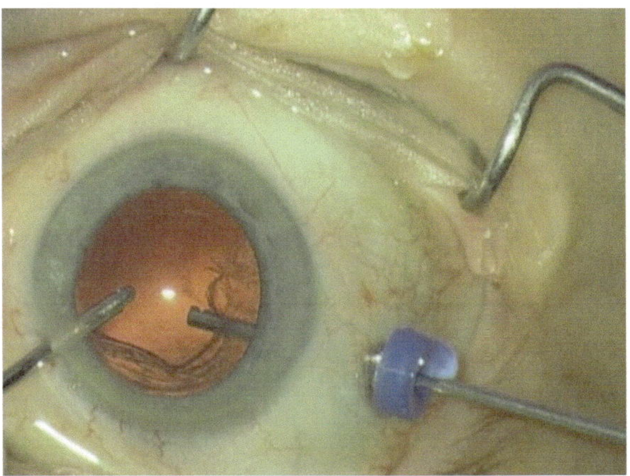

Fig. 6.3 An anterior vitrectomy from pars plana. Insert a trocar 3.5 mm behind the limbus. Then vitrectomize the anterior vitreous

The new technique enables an anterior vitrectomy from pars plana with a trocar, an anterior vitreous cutter, using a conventional phacoemulsification machine (Infinity, Alcon).

6.1 Equipment for Surgery of Anterior Segment with Trocars

The required equipment for trocar surgery of anterior segment is as follows (Video available):

(1) Phacoemulsification machine, (Fig. 6.4)
(2) Anterior vitreous cutter (23G), (Figs. 6.5 and 6.6)
(3) Trocars (23G), (Figs. 6.7 and 6.8)
(4) Infusion line (23G), (Fig. 6.9).

Phacoemulsification machines

You can use any modern phacoemulsification machine, Infinity (Alcon), Centurion (Alcon), Stellaris (B&L), all of them have powerful anterior vitreous cutters (Fig. 6.4). The cutting frequency of an anterior vitreous cutter for *Alcon Infinity* is 2500 cpm (cuts per minute), for *Alcon Centurion* 4000 cpm and for *Bausch & Lomb Stellaris* 5000 cpm. For the *Oertli Catarex 3* the cutting rate is 1200 cuts/min but the cutter cuts both ways, while going forward and backward, resulting in 2400 cpm. The Gauge of the anterior vitreous cutter is 23G (Fig. 6.5). There is no anterior vitreous cutter for 25G or 27G available. You can also use other phacoemulsification machines. The essential point is that the anterior vitreous cutter should be 23 Gauge and not 20 Gauge because there are no trocars available for 20 Gauge. There are only trocars available for 23 Gauge. In short, if your

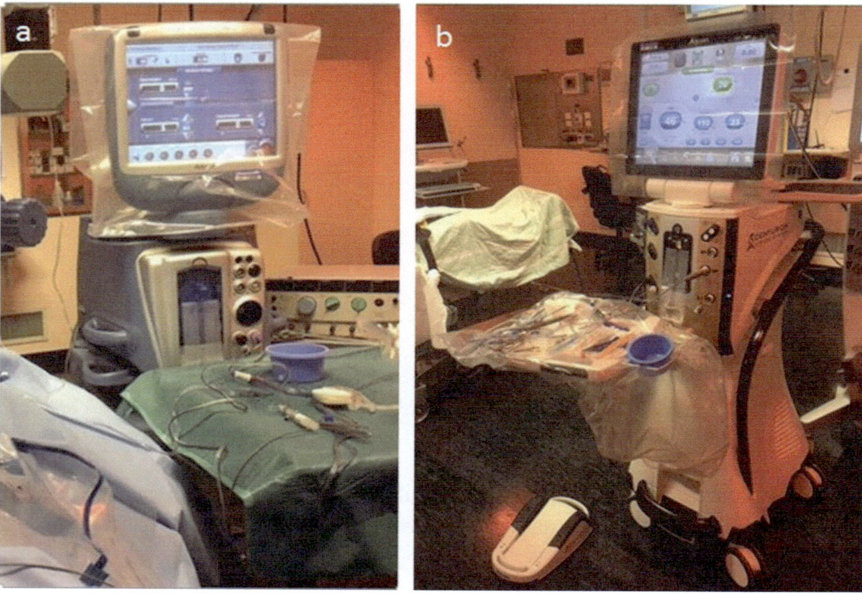

Fig. 6.4 Infinity machine (**a**) and Centurion machine (**b**). All modern phacoemulsification machines have a 23G anterior vitreous cutter

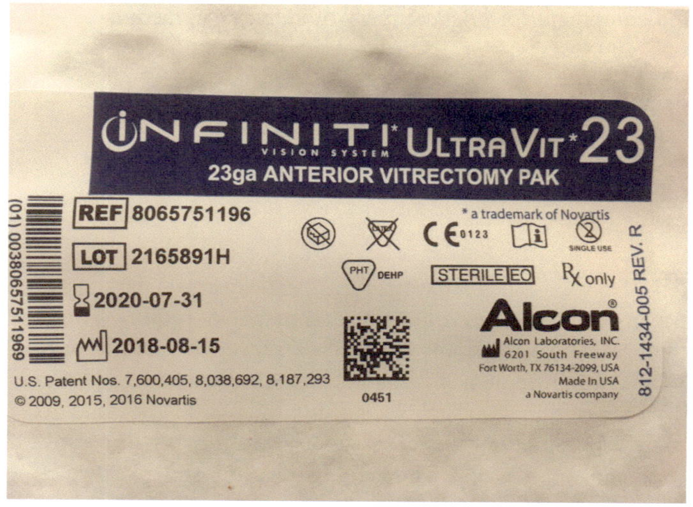

Fig. 6.5 Anterior vitreous cutter (23G) from Alcon. Anterior vitreous cutters come in two sizes, 20 Gauge and 23 Gauge. All modern anterior vitreous cutters are 23G

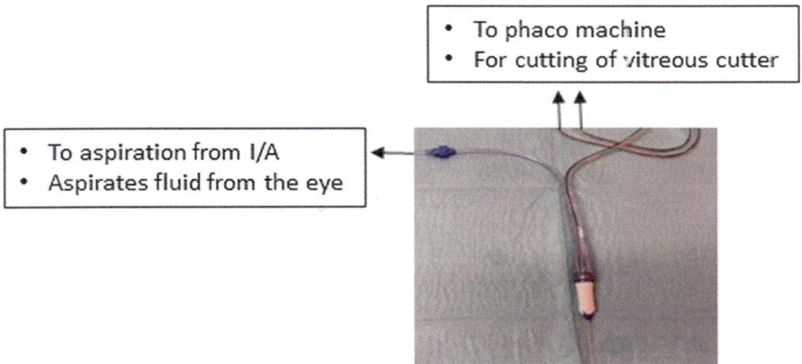

Fig 6.6 Three tubings are connected to the vitreous cutter. Two tubings are connected to the phacoemulsification machine. They steer the cutting function of the vitreous cutter. The third (blue) tubing is attached to the aspiration tube of I/A. This tubing aspirates the fluid from the vitreous cutter and transports it to the cassette. Remark: There is no irrigation inside the vitreous cutter. Irrigation is maintained by an irrigation handpiece or an infusion line

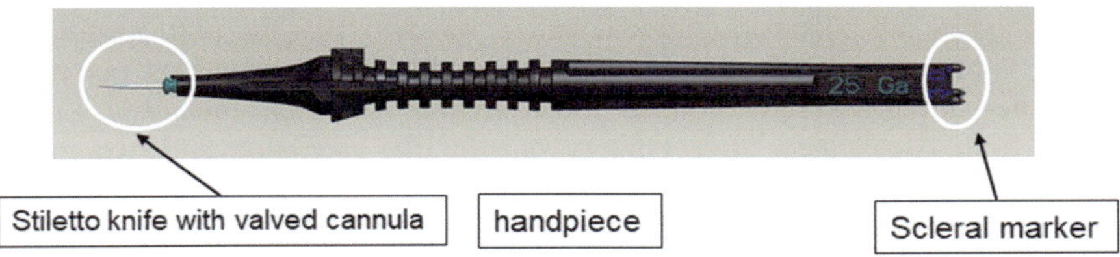

Fig. 6.7 A trocar. On the left side is the stiletto knife with valve. In the middle is the handpiece. On the right side is the scleral marker which marks the distance from the limbus

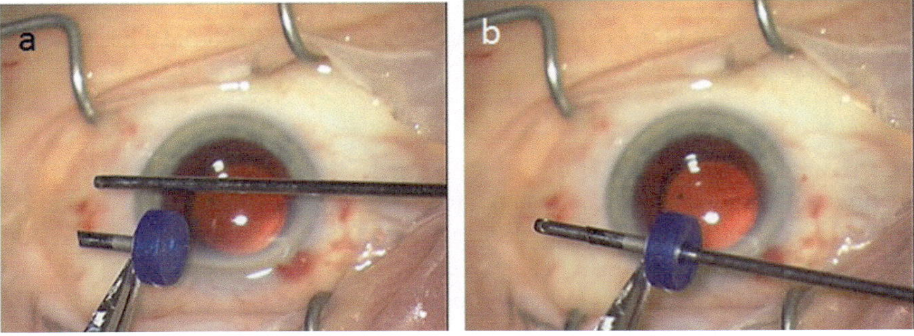

Fig. 6.8 a A trocar with blue valve (DORC) and a vitreous cutter. **b** The blue valve prevents outflow of intraocular fluid

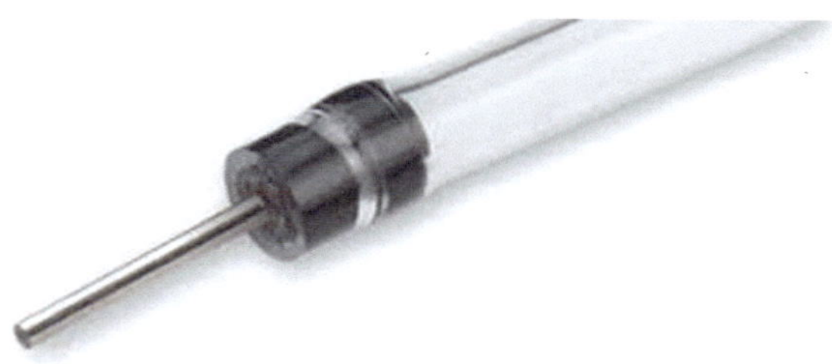

Fig 6.9 Infusion (=irrigation) line (23G, DORC)

phacoemulsification machine has a 23 Gauge anterior vitreous cutter, then you can perform all surgeries mentioned in this book.

Anterior vitreous cutter (Video available)

The *old* vitreous cutters were coaxial, i.e. the cutter was combined with irrigation. The *modern* cutters are not coaxial and have, therefore, *no* irrigation. Anterior vitreous cutter are pneumatic vitreous cutters meaning that the port opening and closing is controlled by air. Pneumatic spring cutters have two tubings, one tubing steers the cutting and the second is for aspiration. The dual pneumatic vitreous cutters from Alcon have three tubings, one for the aspiration and two for the dual-pneumatic drive (Figs. 6.5 and 6.6). The two tubings for the pneumatic drive are connected to the phacoemulsification machine. These tubes steer the opening and closing of the port of the vitreous cutter. The third tubing is connected to the aspiration port of the phacoemulsification machine and aspirates the fluid from the eye. There is *no* irrigation inside the cutter. The vitreous cutter aspirates fluid from the eye but does *not* irrigate the eye. Therefore, a separate irrigation handpiece is required to replace the aspirated fluid and maintain the IOP in the eye.

Caution: A vitrectomy without irrigation results in an under pressure of the globe. The choroidal vessels are injured and a dangerous subchoroidal haemorrhage with malignant glaucoma develops.

Trocars

Trocars are simple to use. A trocar has a trocar handpiece which consists of a stiletto knife and a valved cannula. Behind the handpiece is a scleral marker All modern 23G trocars include a handpiece, a knife with trocar and a marker (Fig. 6.7). Trocars are available from many companies. Trocar cannulas facilitate the insertion of instruments and protect the surrounding tissue. The valves prevent the outflow from intraocular fluid keeping the globe normotone (Fig. 6.8).

Anterior vitreous cutters of 23 G need to be used as it is compatible with 23 G trocars. You can purchase 23G trocars of any company, they can all be used with a 23G vitreous cutter (Fig. 6.8).

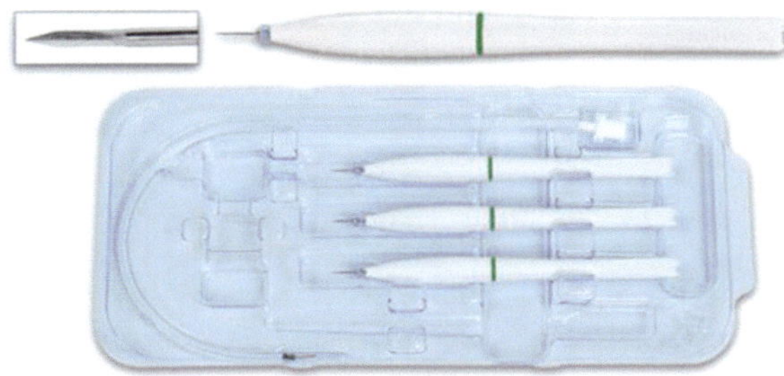

Fig 6.10   23G trocar from DORC No: 1272.ED206. This package includes three trocars and one infusion line (DORC, NL). Remark: DORC manufactures one step disposable valved 23 G trocars

For trocar surgery, you need at least one 23G trocar. This trocar is used for the vitreous cutter. It is, however, better and easier to work with two trocars. The second trocar can be used for the infusion line (Fig. 6.9). The infusion line replaces the irrigation handpiece. For the most surgeries, 1-2trocars are sufficient.

The trocars and infusion line are available as a kit from the following companies (Figs. 6.10, 6.11, 6.12 and 6.13).

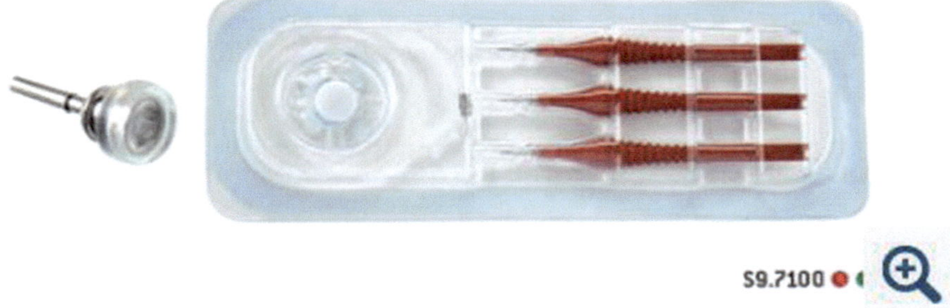

Fig. 6.11   This package includes three 23G trocars and one infusion (irrigation) line. (FCI, France No S9.7100.23)

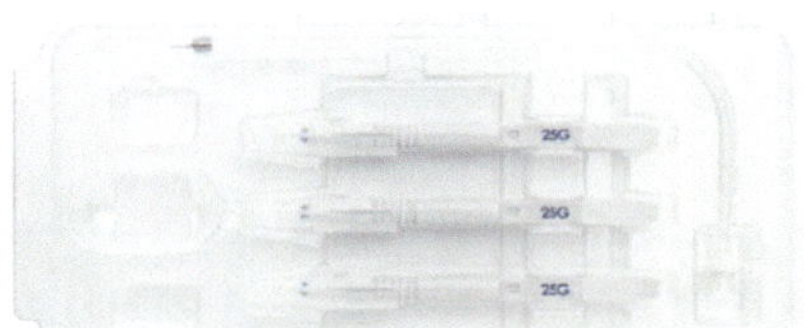

Product Name	Packaging	Order #
Trocar Kit 25G S	3 Kits / Box	MTK25S
Trocar Kit 23G S	3 Kits / Box	MTK23S

• Sterile 1 kit consists of 3 pcs. trocar with the valved cannula and 1 pc. infusion cannula.

Fig. 6.12   This package includes three 23G trocars and one infusion (irrigation) line. (Mani, Japan MTK23S)

Fig. 6.13 This package includes three 23G trocars and one infusion (irrigation) line. (Aurolab, India)

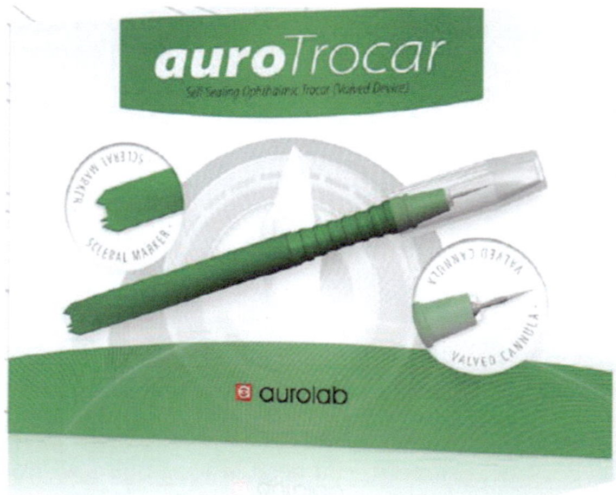

6.1.1   Setup of Anterior Vitreous Cutter

In the conventional setup, the anterior vitreous cutter is used with an irrigation hand-piece (Fig. 6.14a). Remember that the new vitreous cutters are non-coaxial. In trocar surgery, the irrigation handpiece is replaced by an infusion line (Fig. 6.14b). This infusion is included in the aforementioned packages (Figs. 6.10, 6.11, 6.12 and 6.13).

6.2   Surgical Setup for Trocar Surgery

The setup of the anterior vitreous cutter is very simple. Attach the two main tubings in the phaco machine and the short tubing to the aspiration tube from I/A (Fig. 6.15). If you want to perform an anterior vitrectomy with one trocar then

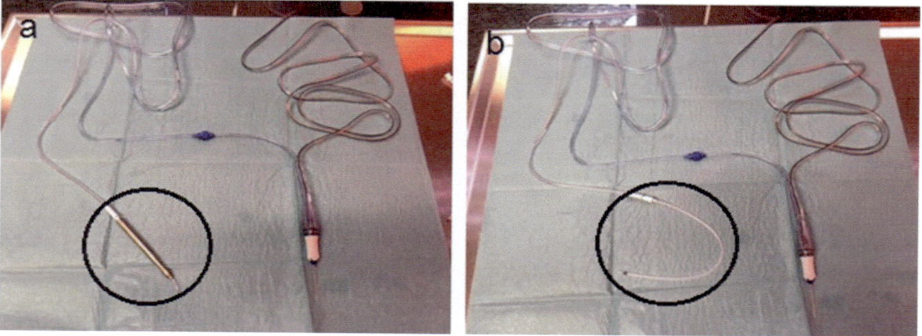

Fig. 6.14 a Conventional setup of anterior vitreous cutter with irrigation handpiece (circle). **b** Novel setup of vitreous cutter with infusion line for trocar surgery (circle)

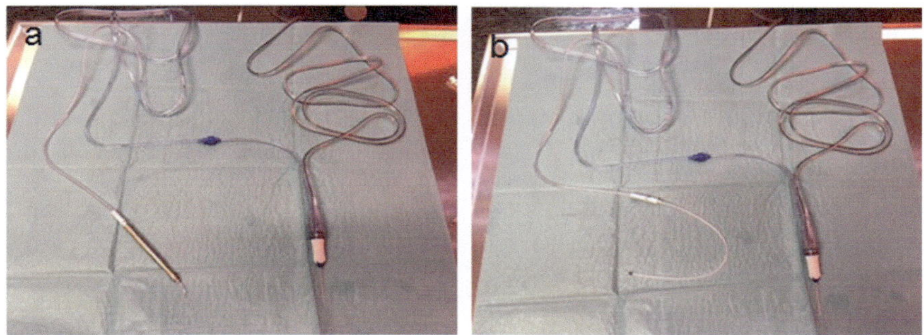

Fig. 6.15 **a** Conventional setup of anterior vitreous cutter. This is also the setup for trocar surgery with one trocar. **b** Novel setup of vitreous cutter with infusion (irrigation) line for trocar surgery with two trocars

attach an irrigation cannula or irrigation handpiece (Fig. 6.15). If you want to perform an anterior vitrectomy with two trocars, then attach an infusion line to the irrigation tube (Fig. 6.15).

Remark: Avoid the old coaxial vitreous cutters. Coaxial means irrigation and vitrectomy in one handpiece. A coaxial vitreous cutter hydrates the vitreous and causes further prolapse.

There are three possible setups for the irrigation:

(1)   Irrigation handpiece in anterior chamber (Fig. 6.16a)

The *advantage* is that it is easy to use, and the *disadvantage* is that you have no free hand.

(2)   Anterior chamber maintainer in anterior chamber (Fig. 6.16b)

The *advantage* is that you have a free hand, and the *disadvantage* is that the infusion is unstable and dislocates easily.

(3)   Trocar cannula in pars plana (Fig. 6.16c)

The *advantage* is that you have a free hand and the infusion is stable and does not dislocate. Also, you are exposing the cornea endothelium less to direct irrigation from fluids as your infusion is away from the cornea. There is no *disadvantage*.

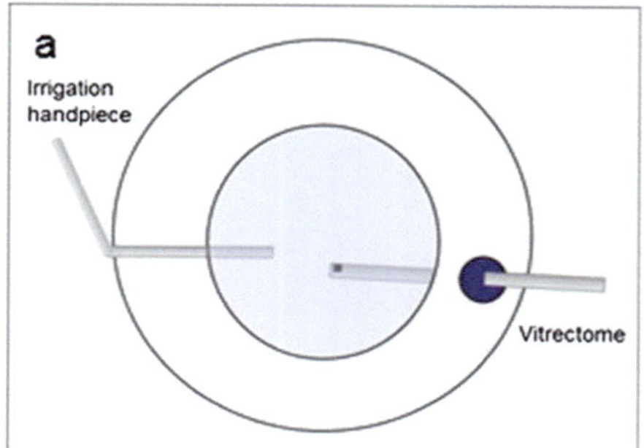

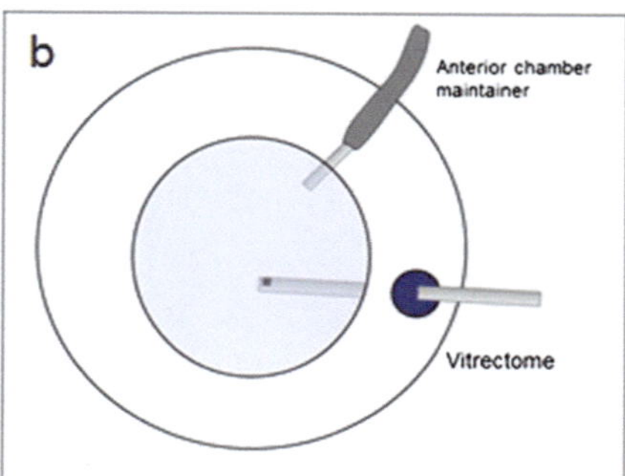

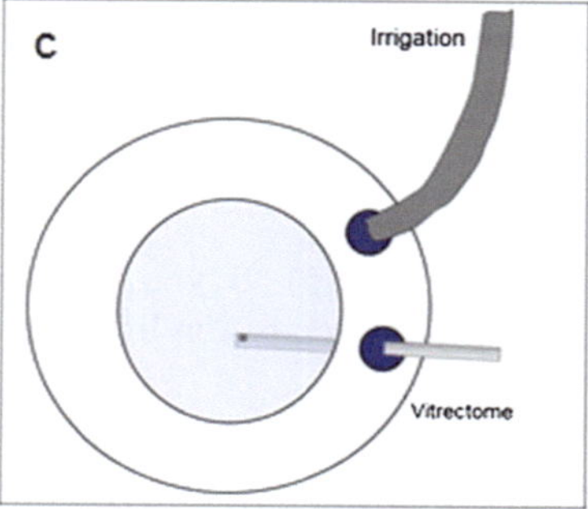

Fig. 6.16 a Conventional technique for anterior vitreous cutter with an irrigation handpiece in anterior chamber. **b** An alternative is the insertion of an anterior chamber maintainer. **c** The best technique is an infusion from pars plana. A second trocar cannula is inserted in the pars plana. The infusion line is inserted into the trocar cannula providing a stable infusion

6.3 Settings for Anterior Vitrectomy with Phacoemulsification Machine

Before operating on a complication on your own, you should have seen this complication managed by an experienced surgeon or in a surgical video. In addition, you have to know exactly the instrumentation and the machine settings for a vitrectomy on a phaco machine. I will therefore add some technical details:

  # Modern vitreous cutters are *not* coaxial. You need a separate infusion.

  # The Infinity and Centurion machines (Alcon) offer the following choices for anterior vitrectomy:

(1) Cutting-I/A;
(2) I/A-cutting;

Fig. 6.17 Settings for vitrectomy with an Infinity phacoemulsification machine. Note continuous irrigation, I/A-cut and cutting speed of 2500 cuts/min. The infusion pressure is reduced to 45–50 cmH$_2$O

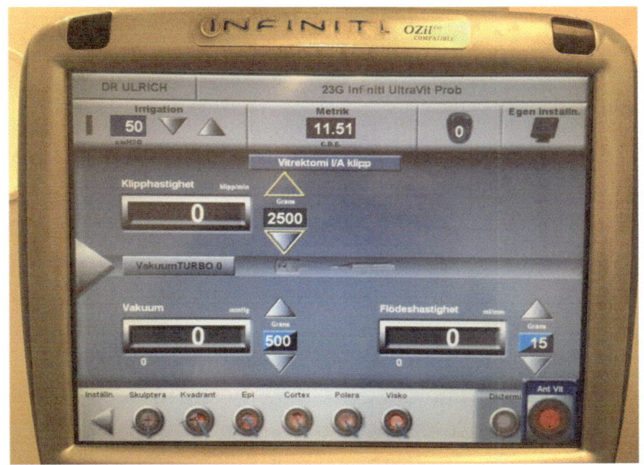

I recommend the I/A -cutting mode. When you step on the foot pedal slightly, you are in the aspiration mode, when you step firmly on the pedal, you are in the cutting mode. You can cause serious damage during cutting, which is not the case for the I/A mode. It is therefore prudent that a slight stepping on the foot pedal activates I/A (which causes little damage) and a firm stepping on the foot pedal activates vitrectomy (which can cause serious damage).

Settings for anterior vitrectomy

If you use two trocars with an infusion line we recommend using continuous irrigation. The globe has a stable IOP and you don't need to worry about irrigation (Fig. 6.17). The irrigation pressure is preset to 65 mmHg for Infinity machine.

6.4   Surgical Basics of Anterior Vitrectomy with Trocars

Intraocular pressure - clinical assessment and surgical action

The tonus of the globe is an essential element of anterior and especially of posterior segment surgery. As a surgeon, you must be able to assess the tonus of the globe and take adequate actions.

Assessment: The intraocular pressure can be assessed in the easiest way with the index finger. During posterior segment surgery, you check the globe pressure regularly with your index finger. There are also clinical signs for high and low IOP. If the IOP is too high, then the cornea becomes oedematous because the endothelium cannot pump out the excess intracorneal fluid. Further signs are an iris prolapse through the corneal incision and a flat anterior chamber. A low IOP presents with a globe losing its shape, scleral folds occur. In addition, a choroidal detachment develops. In the anterior segment, there are hardly signs for a low IOP except for folds in the cornea or a gaping scleral tunnel.

Another important factor is the presence of aphakia or not. If aphakia is present, then intraocular fluid can flow freely from posterior to anterior segment and vice versa. *Remark*: A PCR is more or less comparable to aphakia. In contrast, if a natural lens or in-the-bag IOL is present, then aqueous flows only slowly from posterior to anterior segment and vice versa. For example: In case of aphakia or PCR, an anterior chamber maintainer has the same effect as a pars plana trocar infusion because no barrier between anterior and posterior segment is present. If, however, a natural lens or an in-the-bag IOL is present, then an anterior chamber maintainer cannot maintain the IOP in the posterior segment. In case of pseudophakia (or natural lens), you cannot perform an anterior vitrectomy with an anterior chamber maintainer because the fluid flows too slowly from the anterior to the posterior chamber. If you perform in this situation a vitrectomy then an underpressure in the posterior segment will develop. This underpressure may result in a subchoroidal haemorrhage.

Surgical procedure: What to do if the IOP is too high? The simplest surgical procedure is a paracentesis. If a paracentesis is not possible because of a flat anterior chamber, then you can relieve pressure from the posterior segment (via pars plana). This can be achieved with a needle cannula or a vitreous cutter. If the IOP is too low, you can increase the IOP by injecting fluid into the anterior chamber or into the posterior chamber (like an intravitreal injection). Assess the effect of your action with the index finger. *Remark*: A normal eye tolerates an intravitreal injection of approximately 0,1 ml fluid without a paracentesis. If you inject 0,2 ml fluid into the vitreous, then a paracentesis is required. This is of course not valid for abnormally small eyes.

Location of vitreous prolapse

Vitreous prolapse can be from posterior segment to anterior segment or it can be localized in posterior segment (Fig. 6.19). In either case, it is best removed from pars plana with or without anterior approach. An only anterior approach will remove vitreous inadequately. If the vitreous prolapse is localized anterior to the iris (Fig. 6.18), then it can only be removed with a vitreous cutter placed anterior to the iris, i.e. from the anterior chamber. If the vitreous prolapse is localized posterior to the iris, then the vitreous can be only removed completely from pars plana (Fig. 6.19b). If a vitreous prolapse is present in the anterior chamber, then start with vitrectomy from pars plana (Fig. 6.19a) in order to remove the base of the vitreous prolapse. Then remove the vitreous prolapse from the anterior segment (Fig. 6.19b).

Conventional anterior vitrectomy limbus versus anterior vitrectomy from pars plana

A conventional anterior vitrectomy is performed from the limbus (Fig. 6.20). The disadvantage of this technique is that it is impossible to perform a complete anterior vitrectomy because the iris and the lens capsule are in the way. A conventional anterior vitrectomy results often in a postoperative vitreous prolapse because anterior vitreous is only partially removed.

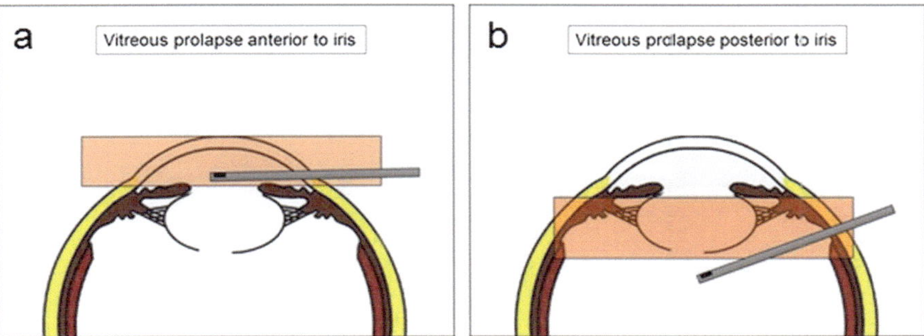

Fig 6.18 Vitreous prolapse anterior *or* posterior to iris. **a** The vitreous prolapse is localized anterior to the iris and is best removed from the anterior segment. **b** The vitreous prolapse is localized posterior to the iris and is best removed from pars plana

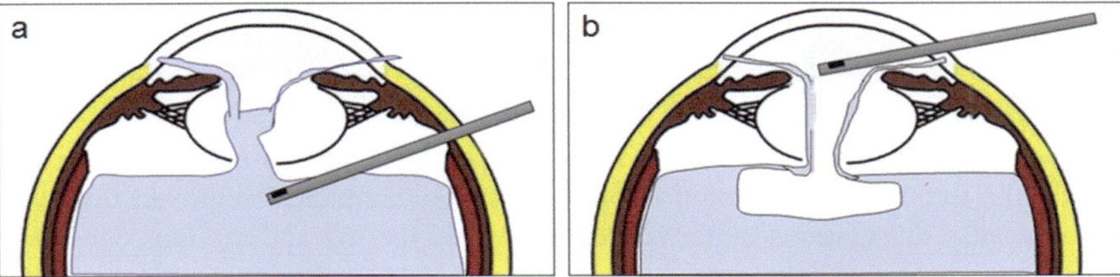

Fig 6.19 Vitreous prolapse anterior *and* posterior to iris. **a** Remove first the anterior vitreous from pars plana. **b** Then remove the vitreous strands from the cornea

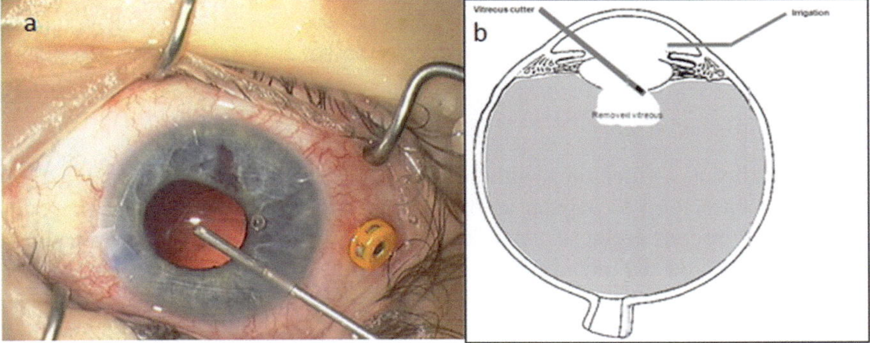

Fig 6.20   a An anterior vitrectomy from the limbus. Insert the anterior vitreous cutter through a paracentesis and remove the vitreous prolapse. Caution: Do not forget the infusion (not depicted). **b** Drawing of an anterior vitrectomy from the limbus. The disadvantage of this technique is that the anterior vitreous is only inadequately removed. In addition, the lens capsule can be easily damaged

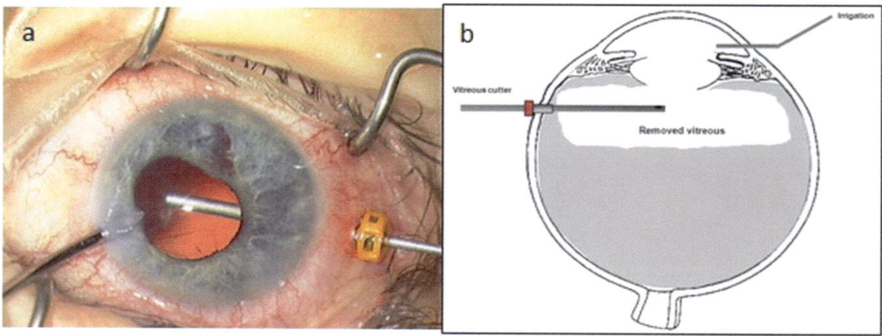

Fig. 6.21   **a** An anterior vitrectomy from pars plana. Place the infusion via a paracentesis in the anterior chamber. Then vitrectomize the anterior vitreous from pars plana. **b** Drawing of an anterior pars plana vitrectomy from pars plana. Insert a 23G trocar 3.5 - 4 mm behind the limbus. The advantage of this method is that the anterior vitreous can be completely removed, that the vitrectomy is easier to perform, and a damage of the lens capsule is unlikely.

What is the advantage of an anterior vitrectomy from pars plana compared to a limbal approach? The advantage is that the anterior vitreous is much easier to remove from pars plana, because the iris and the lens capsule are not in the way (Fig. 6.21). In addition, the anterior vitreous can be completely removed from pars plana because the vitreous cutter is located behind the iris and the lens capsule.

An anterior segment surgeon has not much experience with a vitreous cutter. A vitreous cutter is much less powerful than a phacoemulsification handpiece and can, therefore, cause less damage. Which damage can a vitreous cutter cause? If you touch the retina with the vitreous cutter you can damage the retina but that's unlikely. Which is the most common damage with the vitreous cutter? The anterior capsule. Try absolutely to avoid damaging the anterior capsule during anterior vitrectomy. Hold therefore the port of the vitreous cutter away from the lens capsule and point it towards the optic disc. You need an intact anterior capsule to implant a sulcus fixated IOL.

Dry versus Wet vitrectomy

Dry vitrectomy is a vitrectomy without irrigation, and wet vitrectomy is with irrigation. Dry vitrectomy is popular among elder cataract surgeons because irrigation increases the vitreous prolapse. I want to give here a very strong recommendation to my readers. If you are not an experienced VR surgeon, then use *never* a dry vitrectomy. I have seen many, many terrible complications from dry vitrectomy. What happens, if you do dry vitrectomy? You create an under pressure in the eye, the choroidal vessels rupture and subchoroidal haemorrhage develops with terrible consequences. There is one exception to my recommendation. In positive vitreous pressure, you need to do a dry vitrectomy. *Remark*: When you perform a vitrectomy, check the IOP with your index finger. If the globe is soft, then stop immediately with vitrectomy.

6.5   Trocar Surgery with One Trocar

Trocar surgery with one trocar is very simple. The setup of the vitreous cutter is identical as if you work without trocar; the infusion line is attached to the irrigation handpiece (Fig. 6.22). One trocar is inserted into the sclera on the temporal side (Fig. 6.23a). The vitreous cutter is inserted through this trocar, and the irrigation handpiece is placed in the anterior chamber (Fig. 6.23b). Now an anterior vitrectomy from pars plana is possible. The complete removal of the anterior vitreous is possible.

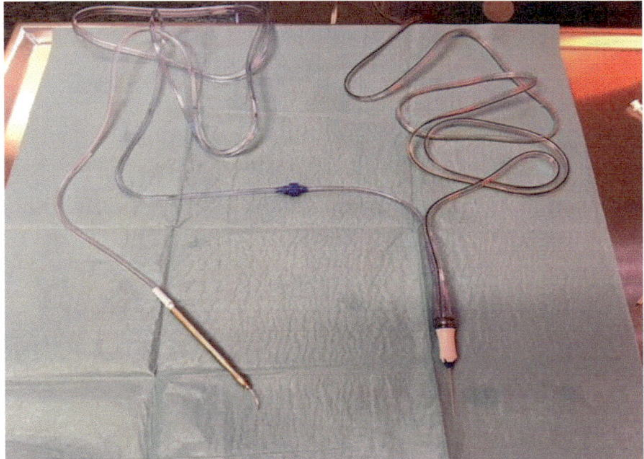

Fig. 6.22 Conventional setup for anterior vitrectomy with an Alcon machine. On the right side, you see the anterior vitreous cutter and on the left side the irrigation handpiece

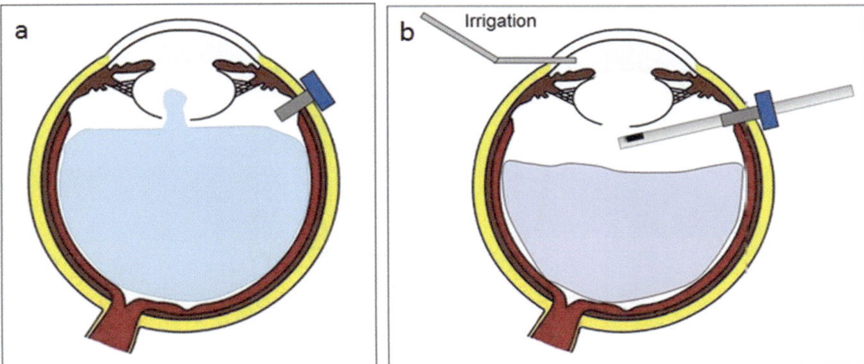

Fig. 6.23 **a** One trocar is inserted on the temporal side. The vitreous cutter is inserted through the trocar and removes the anterior vitreous. **b** An irrigation handpiece is held in the anterior chamber

6.6 Trocar Surgery with Two Trocars

The advantage of two trocars is that the second hand is free. The irrigation hand-piece is replaced by an infusion line (Fig. 6.24). The infusion line is inserted into one trocar and establishes a stable pressure inside the eye globe (Figs. 6.25 and 6.26). Two trocars are inserted on the temporal side; at 2 and 4 o'clock for the left eye and at 8 and 10 o'clock for the right eye. One trocar is used for the infusion line, and the second trocar is used for the vitreous cutter (Fig. 6.23). Alternatively, you can use an anterior chamber maintainer. The disadvantage of an anterior chamber maintainer is that it dislocates easily if you rotate the eye. In contract, a pars plana infusion is stable and does not dislocate. Start trocar surgery with one trocar but move soon over to two trocars. The best trocar surgery technique is with two trocars. The infusion line is placed in the second trocar (Fig. 6.24).

Summary:

Start this technique with one trocar cannula. Get acquainted with anterior vitrectomy with one trocar and an irrigation handpiece. Then insert two cannulas and insert an infusion line in the second trocar. Finally get acquainted to perform an anterior vitrectomy with an infusion line (See Fig. 6.27).

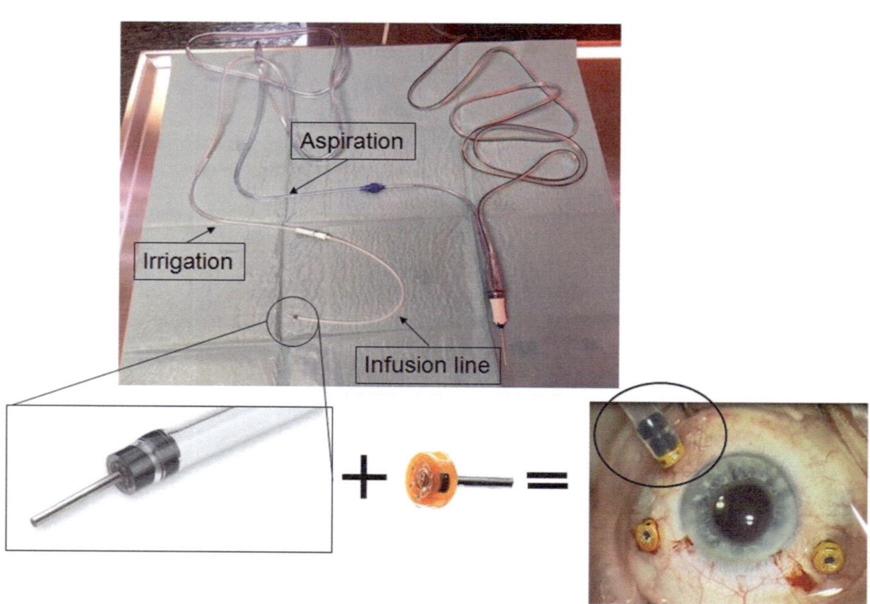

Fig. 6.24 In this setup, the irrigation handpiece is replaced by an infusion line. The infusion line is inserted in a trocar. This setup is for *two* or three trocars

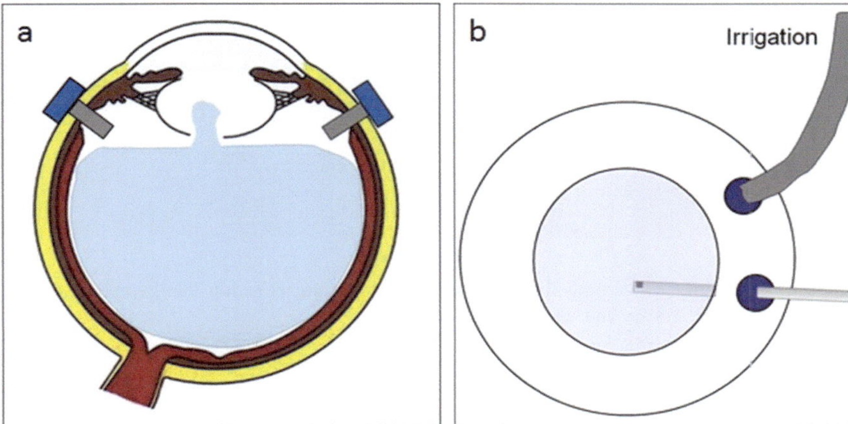

Fig. 6.25 (**a**, **b**) Trocar surgery with two trocars. One trocar is used for the vitreous cutter, and the second trocar is used for the infusion line

Fig. 6.26 An anterior chamber maintainer is a good alternative to the irrigation handpiece

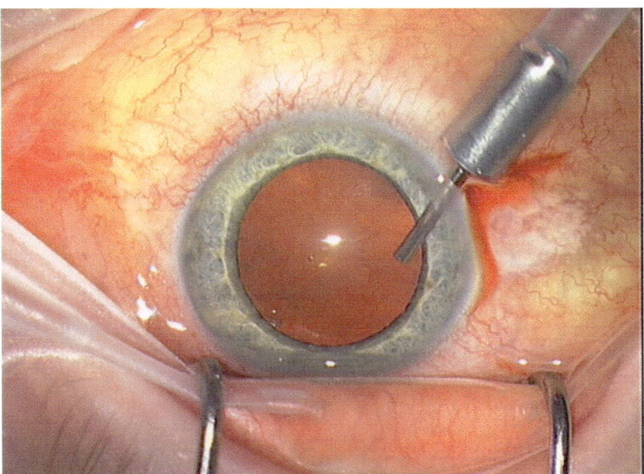

6.7 Anaesthesia

For cataract surgery, we use topical and intracameral anaesthesia, and for trocar surgery, we use retrobulbar/peribulbar anaesthesia. For the latter, we use 50% Carbocaine (mepivacain 20 mg/ml) and 50% Marcaine (bupivacaine 5 mg/ml). Inject 5 cc (ml) inferotemporal through the inferior eyelid.

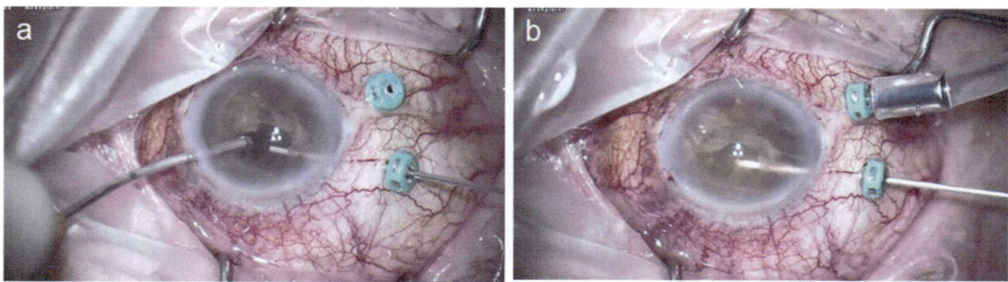

Fig. 6.27 **a** Anterior vitrectomy through one trocar with an irrigation handpiece. **b** Anterior vitrectomy with two trocars and an infusion line

Fig. 6.28 Inject 3 ml (cc) Carbocaine through the caruncle

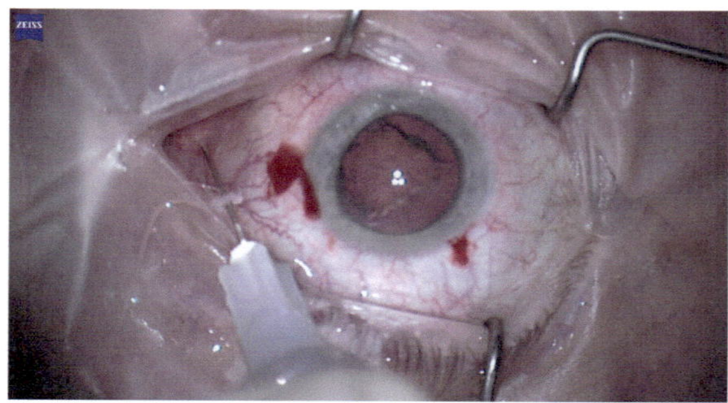

Tipps & tricks:

If you want to add anaesthetics during an ongoing surgery, then inject 3 ml Carbocaine through the caruncle (Fig. 6.28). The caruncle is further away from the sclera which makes it a safe place to inject. In addition, the anaesthetic reaches the retrobulbar space. Wait one minute before you continue.

6.8   The Surgical Technique of Insertion of Trocar Cannulas

The insertion of trocar cannulas is technically easy and fast to learn. It is similar to an intravitreal injection. See one, do one.

6.8.1   Anatomy of Pars Plana

The trocar cannulas are placed in the pars plana. Pars plana is a landmark in the ocular wall, but the surgery is done in the vitreous. The pars plana is located between the ciliary body and the retina and devoid of retina (Fig. 6.29). This feature

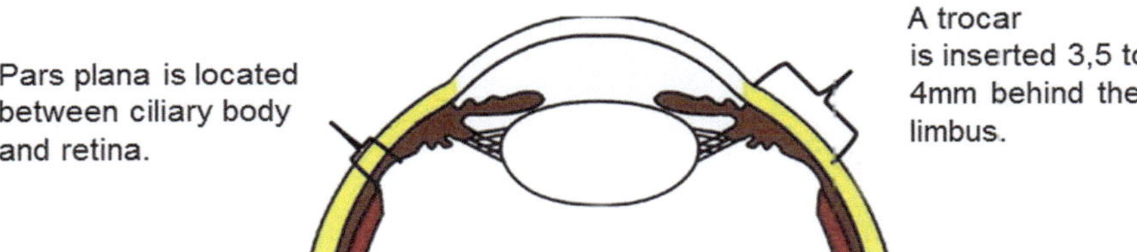

Fig. 6.29 Pars plana is located between ciliary body and retina. The retina is absent at the pars plana region. This feature makes the pars plana the perfect anatomic place for insertion of instruments into the posterior segment of the eye

makes the pars plana an excellent place for insertion of trocars or instruments into the posterior cavity.

Two types of sclerotomy

There are two types of sclerotomy (Fig. 6.30). The first (traditional) sclerotomy is performed perpendicular. Open the conjunctiva and perform a perpendicular sclerotomy (ideally with a V-lance from Alcon). This sclerotomy is 20G big and is used for fragmatome. No trocar cannula is inserted in this sclerotomy. This sclerotomy is not watertight and requires a suture, ideally a X-stitch. The second (new) sclerotomy is lamellar. A trocar is inserted in a 15 deg angle through conjunctiva and sclera. A trocar cannula is left in this 23G sclerotomy. This lamellar sclerotomy is watertight after removal of the trocar cannula. A suture is usually not required.

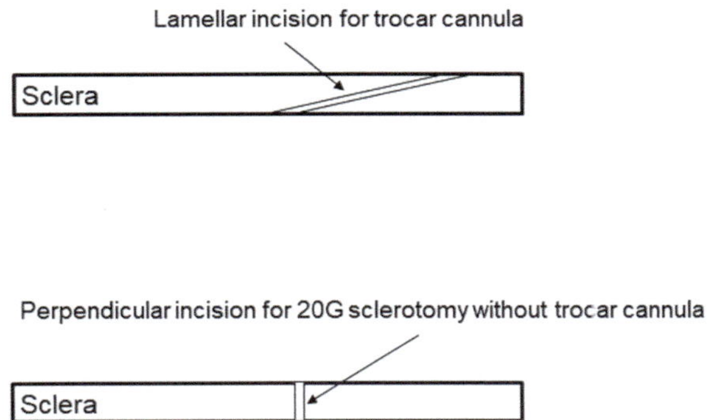

Fig. 6.30 There are two types of sclerotomy. In case of a trocar cannula, the sclerotomy is lamellar resulting in a watertight closure of the sclerotomy. In case of a 20G sclerotomy without trocar cannula, a perpendicular incision is made. This sclerotomy is not watertight and has to be consequently sutured

6.8.2 Insertion of Trocar Cannulas

Instruments:

Trocars (Mani, FCI, DORC, Aurolab).

1. **Mark the sclerotomy**
2. **Insertion of the trocar**

Insert a trocar at 3 or 9 o' clock. Measure and mark the sclerotomy with a scleral marker (Fig. 6.31a), a calliper or with the trocar 3.5–4 mm posterior to the limbus. It is advisable to fixate the eyeball simultaneously with forceps or a cotton wool swab. Insert the knife in an angle of 15° to the limbus and stab the knife through the conjunctiva and the sclera (Fig. 6.31a). If you are half way through (Fig. 6.31c), raise the inserter and stab the knife for the second half in direction of the middle of the eye (perpendicular) (Fig. 6.31d, e). Then fixate the trocar with a cannula holding forceps or an anatomic forceps or cotton swab and pull out the trocar handpiece (Fig. 6.31e).

1. **Removal of trocar**

Remove the trocar cannula with a trocar forceps (DORC) or an anatomical forceps. Then press the tip of the forceps against the sclera so that the wedges of the sclerotomy get attached to each other. A suture is usually not required. In case of a suture, close the sclerotomy with a Vicryl 8-0 suture.

Tips & tricks

Insertion of trocars: The insertion of a trocar is almost identical to an intravitreal injection. The only difference is that an injection is performed completely perpendicular (to the middle of the eye), whereas the trocar is inserted for the first half lamellar and the second half perpendicular.

Summary

The insertion of a trocar cannula at pars plana increases the surgical spectrum of a cataract surgeon immensely: Anterior vitrectomy from pars plana, the recovery of a dropping nucleus, the elevation of a dislocated IOL in anterior vitreous and removal of a PCO. All these procedures can be performed with a regular phacoemulsification machine.

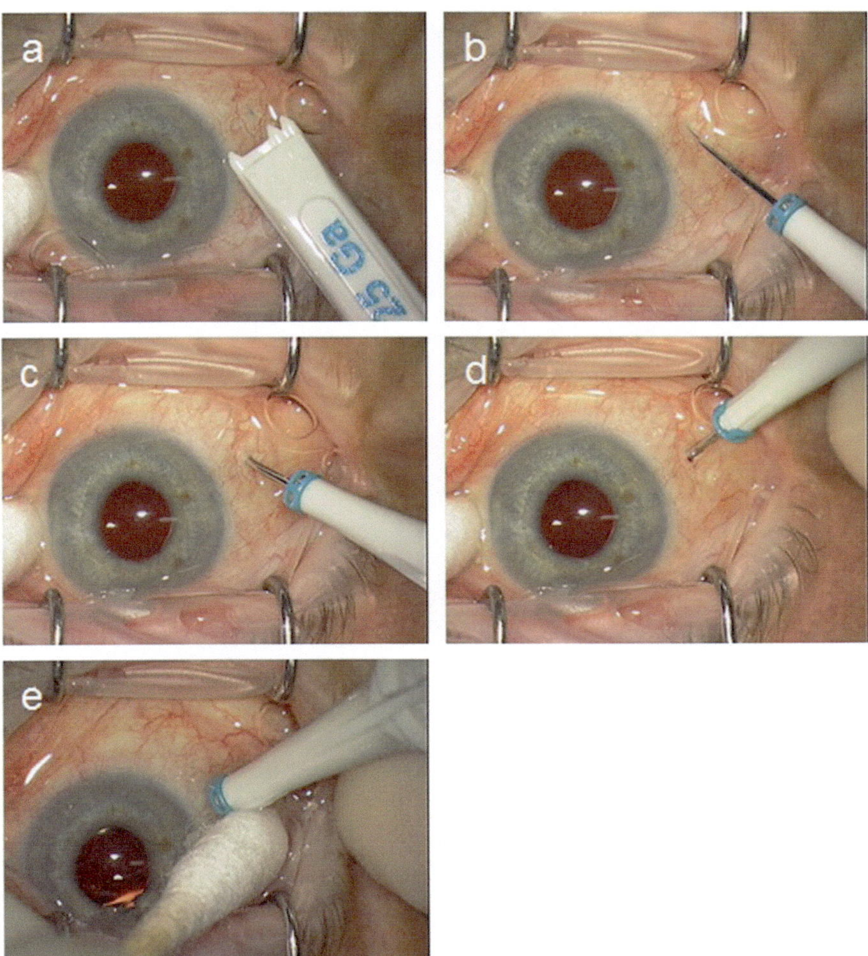

Fig. 6.31   Insertion of a trocar: **a** Fixate the globe with a cotton swab. Mark the sclerotomy with the trocar marker (3.5–4 mm). **b** Insert the trocar in an angle of 15-20° through the conjunctiva and sclera. **c, d** Then insert the second half in direction of the middle of the eye. **e** Fixate the cannula with a forceps and remove the handpiece. The trocar cannula remains in the sclera

How to Approach a Surgical Complication

7

Abstract

This chapter gives a short introduction how to approach a surgical complication during phacoemulsification surgery.

Keywords

Phacoemulsification · Complication

If a complication such as posterior capsular defect occurs (Fig. 7.1), the following procedure is recommended:

Remove the instruments.
Inject viscoelastics.
Think.

Then ask yourself the following questions:

What is the problem?
Can I solve the problem myself?
Do I have the required equipment?
Do I have enough time to solve the complication now?

If you are uncertain whether you can solve the problem yourself, then you should remove the viscoelastic from the anterior chamber and send the patient to an experienced clinic. It is psychologically difficult to stop the surgery, but it is a laudable decision. It is much easier to continue with surgery than to stop. But if you do not master the complication, you are doing no service to the patient; on the

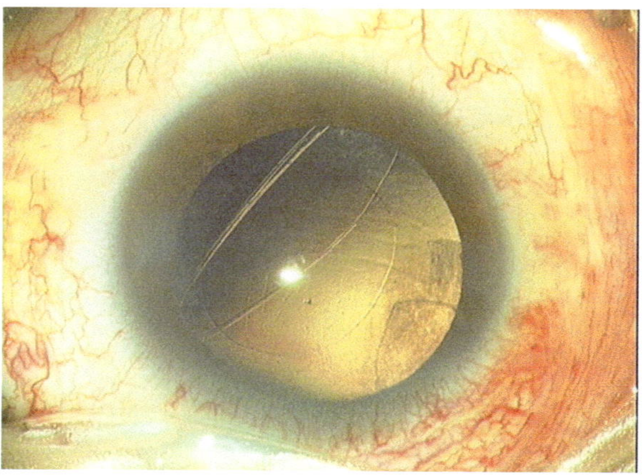

Fig. 7.1 An eye with a posterior capsular defect. The anterior capsule is intact, and no zonular lysis is present

contrary, you can make the situation worse. In addition, you might increase the surgical trauma, which makes the second operation more difficult.

Another consideration for you to master the complication surgically is the availability of time, equipment and anaesthesia required. Time because additional 10–20 patients have to be operated, equipment, and anaesthesia, because a vitrectomy cannot be carried out in topical anaesthesia. If a vitrectomy is necessary, I recommend stopping the ongoing surgery and scheduling the vitrectomy one week later with retrobulbar anaesthesia.

For the preoperative assessment of a complicated cataract surgery such as a dropped nucleus, reflect about the following three main issues:

(1)   Status of lens capsule.
(2)   How hard is the nucleus?
(3)   Status of the cornea; how soon can the eye be operated?

Status of the lens capsule:

If the nucleus together with the lens capsule is luxated (e.g. zonular lysis), you cannot implant the IOL into the sulcus but must perform a scleral fixated or iris fixated implantation. If the nucleus is luxated without the lens capsule and this is usually the case, then you have to examine the anterior capsule. Here are two important points: (1) Is the rhexis intact? (2) Are the zonules intact?

How do you examine an anterior capsule? Examine the anterior capsule with a maximally dilated pupil at the slit lamp. Sometimes, in a small pupil, this is not possible. In this case, you have to examine the anterior capsule during surgery and be prepared for a sulcus implantation as well as an iris or scleral fixated implantation. Inject viscoelastics intraoperatively into the anterior chamber and examine the anterior capsule with one or even better with two push–pull instruments, by moving the iris with the instruments to the periphery (Fig. 7.2). Alternatively, you can use iris retractors.

If the rhexis is intact and the zonules are intact, you can implant the IOL into the sulcus.

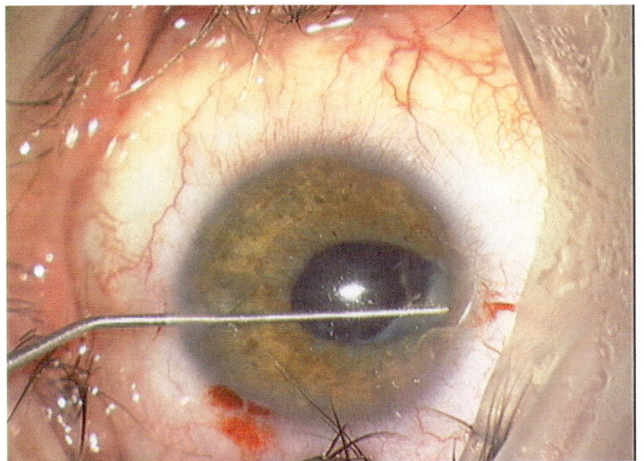

Fig. 7.2 Examine the rhexis and the anterior capsule with a manipulator

It is essential that the haptics are located in an area without capsular rift, ideally at 12 and 6 o'clock. If an anterior capsular rift is present inferiorly between 5 and 7 o'clock, then a sulcus implantation is not possible because the inferior haptic is not stable. An anterior rift at 3 or 9 o'clock is however acceptable. For details, see Fig. 7.3.

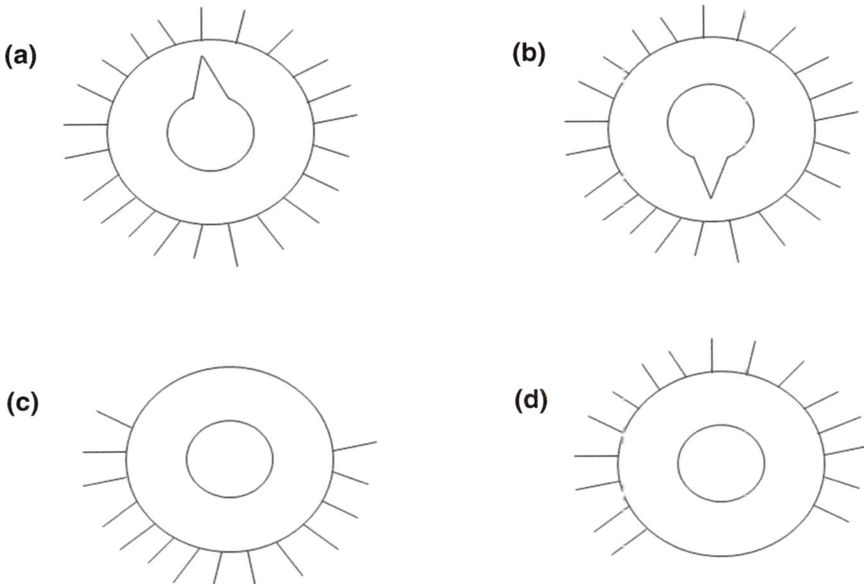

Fig. 7.3 Posterior capsule is defective in all cases (**a–d**). **a** Superior rift in the anterior capsule with intact zonules. A sulcus implantation is possible. **b** An inferior rift in the anterior capsule with intact zonules. A sulcus implantation is risky but may function. **c** Intact rhexis with a superior zonular defect. A sulcus implantation is possible. **d** Intact rhexis with an inferior zonular defect. A sulcus implantation is not possible

<u>Status of the cornea:</u>

If a pronounced corneal oedema is present, you cannot operate. Treat the patient first conservatively. The surgical planning depends on the size of the dropped nucleus. If 50–100% of the nucleus is luxated, we would operate within a few days. The nucleus can cause a substantial intraocular inflammation, and the nucleus may stick to the retina. If small nuclear fragments are luxated, we would operate within 2 weeks, if the intraocular inflammation can be controlled with cortisone drops.

Posterior Capsular Rupture

8

Contents

Abstract

This chapter explains step-by-step the surgical management of posterior capsule rupture. Alle instruments are presented and the surgical approach is explained in theory and practice.

Keywords

Posterior capsule rupture · Surgery · Complication

8.1 Management of Posterior Capsule Rupture

For the subsequent surgical procedure, it is important during which step of phacoemulsification the posterior capsule was ruptured. If the posterior capsule ruptured during phacoemulsification, then nuclear fragments remain and have to be removed first. See the treatment algorithm Fig. 8.1. If you continue with phacoemulsification, the nuclear fragments will drop into the vitreous cavity. You can prevent this to happen by first injecting viscoelastic behind the posterior capsule defect. Now you can proceed in two ways. You can place a lens glide or an IOL as scaffold behind the lens fragments and then continue cautiously with

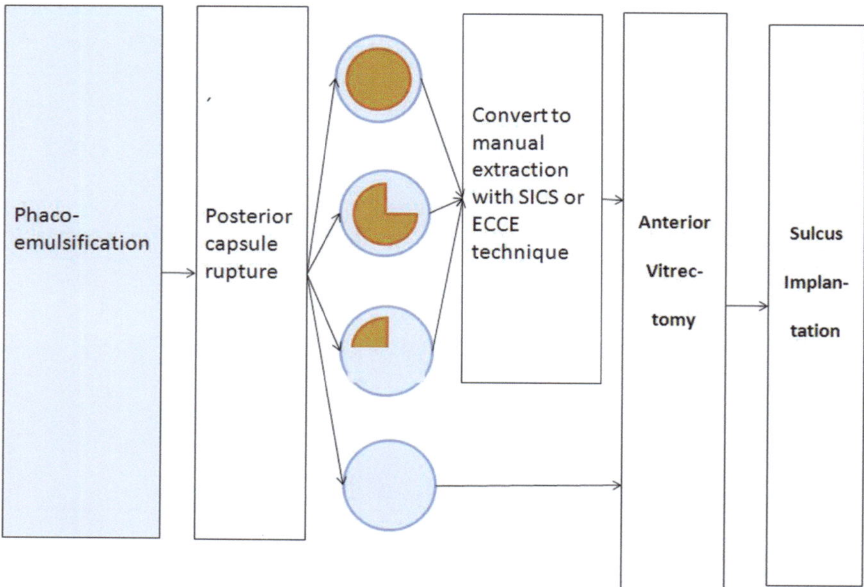

Fig. 8.1 Our treatment algorithm for a posterior capsular rupture. Depending on the timing of the capsular defect and the size of the nucleus, different techniques are recommended

phacoemulsification. Or you can remove the fragments manually without use of phacoemulsification (videos available).

The safest procedure is to remove the lens fragments manually. Luxate the fragments into the anterior chamber and place them on the iris. Then you have to widen the main incision according to the size of the nuclear fragment. See the treatment algorithm Fig. 8.2. The fragments can then be removed with the fragment forceps or viscoelastics. If the posterior capsule ruptured during I/A, then only the residual cortex has to be removed. This is best done with the vitreous cutter.

Instruments

1. Fragment forceps (Fig. 8.3)
2. Vitreous cutter for phaco machine
3. Trocar.

Dye

Triamcinolone (Fig. 8.4).

Individual steps

(1) Viscoelastics into the lens capsule
(2) Luxation of lens fragments into the anterior chamber

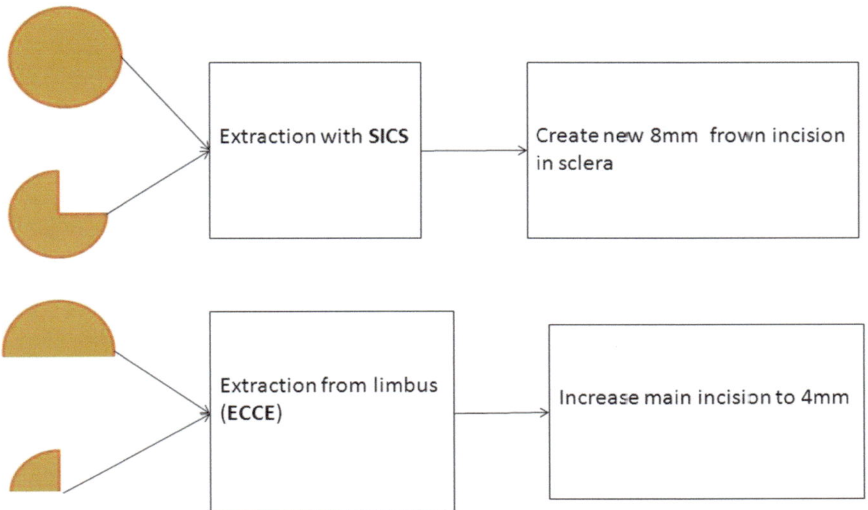

Fig. 8.2 Depending on the size of the nucleus the extraction is performed from the old main incision or a new scleral incision

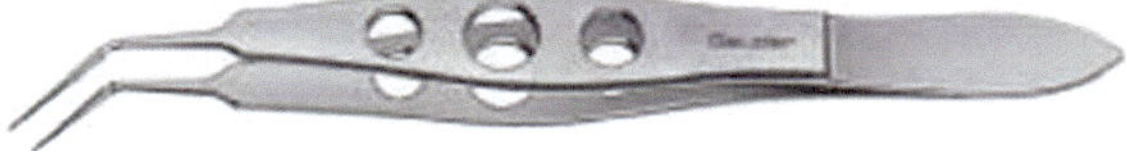

Fig. 8.3 Fragment removal forceps after Gaskin. Indication: removal of nuclear fragments during a complicated cataract surgery. Geuder, 31624

Fig. 8.4 Kenalog® (Triamcinolone) from Squibb stains the vitreous well

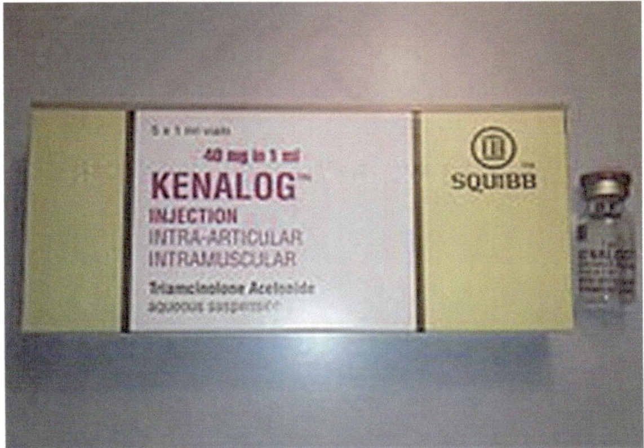

  (3)   Widen main incision
  (4)   Extraction of nuclear fragments
  (5)   Insertion of trocar cannulas
  (6)   Anterior vitrectomy and removal of cortex
  (7)   Triamcinolone into the anterior chamber
  (8)   Exclusion of a vitreous strand
  (9)   IOL implantation
(10)   Trocar removal
(11)   Lens capture.

The surgery step by step:

1. **Viscoelastics into the lens capsule**
2. **Luxation of lens fragments into the anterior chamber**

Inject viscoelastic into the capsular bag, so that the vitreous prolapse is pushed back (Fig. 8.5). The vitreous together with the viscoelastics will be a barrier for the nuclear fragments. If nucleus fragments are still present in the capsular bag, luxate the nuclear fragments with a nucleus manipulator from the lens capsule onto the iris (Figs. 8.6 and 8.7).

3. **Widen main incision**
4. **Extraction of nuclear fragments**

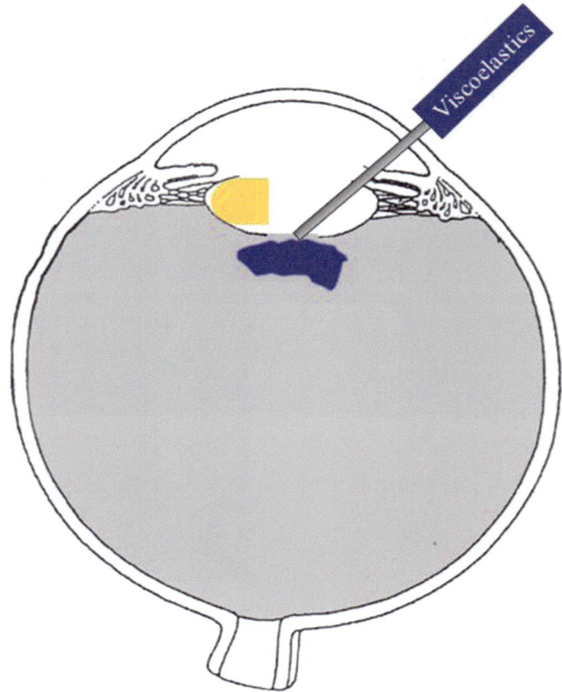

Fig. 8.5 If you detect a posterior capsular defect inject first viscoelastics to push, the vitreous prolapse back and to stabilize the lens capsule with the nucleus

Fig. 8.6 Then lift the nuclear fragments up with a nucleus manipulator and place them on the iris

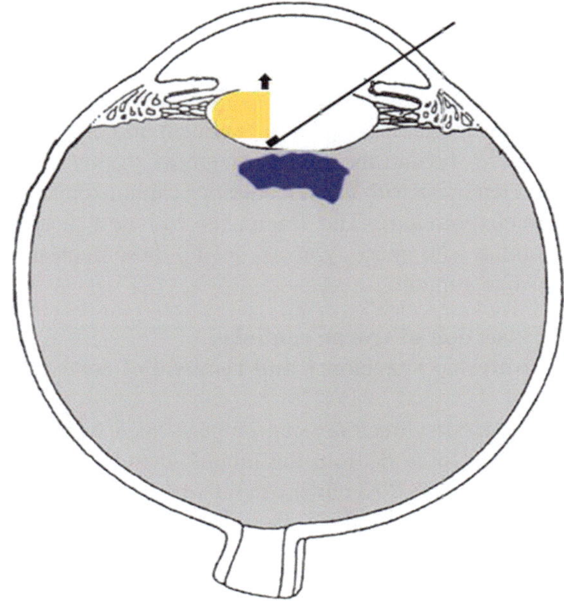

Fig. 8.7 Place the nuclear fragments safely on the iris. If you inserted iris hooks, then remove them now in order to constrict the pupil

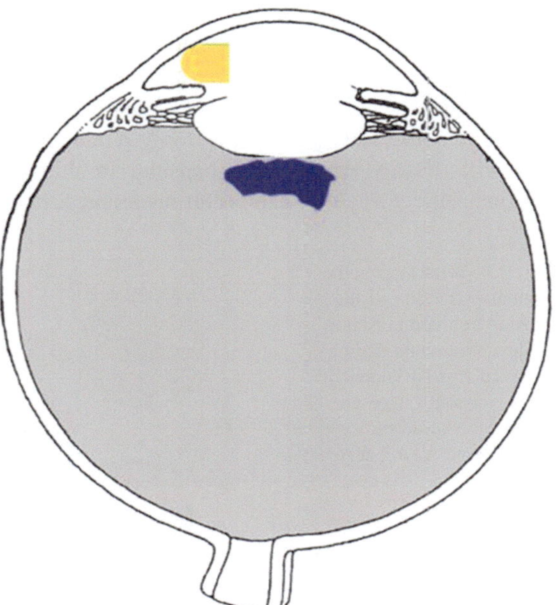

Continue with widening of the main incision according to the size of the nuclear fragment. See treatment algorithm Fig. 8.8. If 75–100% of the nucleus has to be extracted, then perform a scleral 8 mm frown incision. If 25–50% of the nucleus has to be removed, then widen the corneal main incision to 4 mm. Extract the nucleus fragments with the fragment forceps. Alternatively, you can inject viscoelastics behind the nuclear fragment so that it moves towards the main incision and then press with the viscoelastics cannula on to the lower lip of the main incision (viscoexpression). The fragments will now leave the anterior chamber. If you continue with phaco, you risk losing these nuclear fragments through the posterior capsular rupture.

5. **Insertion of trocar cannulas**
6. **Anterior vitrectomy and removal of cortex**

The anterior vitrectomy can be performed from the limbus or from pars plana. If you want to work from the limbus, then insert the 23G vitreous cutter through a paracentesis. A 20G cutter can only be inserted through a main incision. If you want to work from pars plana, then insert first a trocar (Figs. 8.9, 8.10 and 8.11).

Then start with the anterior vitrectomy (Figs. 8.12, 8.13, 8.14 and 8.15). Regarding vitrectomy, the machine settings are important. Remove first the vitreous behind the capsular rupture (use I/A Cut mode). Rotate the vitreous cutter port slowly in a circular fashion in order to remove as much vitreous body as possible. As a beginner, you tend to remove too little anterior vitreous; you need approximately 5 min for complete removal of the anterior vitreous. The visualization of the vitreous with triamcinolone is a good help. Then carefully remove the remaining cortex with the vitrector (aspiration mode) or I/A handpieces. Be careful that you do not accidentally activate the vitrectomy mode during removal of the cortex because you will destroy the anterior capsule. In this manoeuvre, you have to switch between vitrectomy and aspiration back and forth.

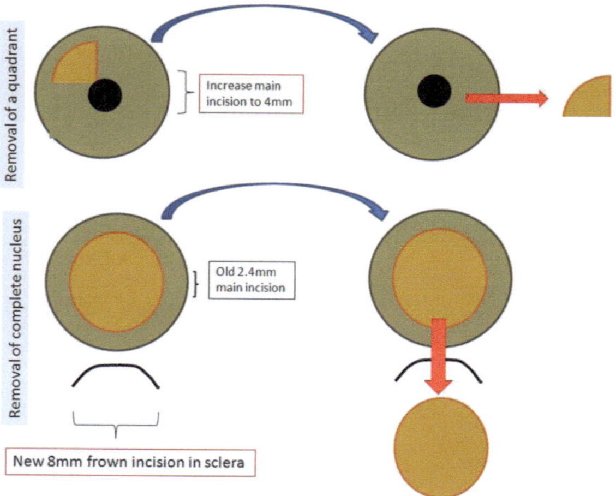

Fig. 8.8 Next step is the manual extraction of the nuclear fragments. Small nuclear fragments can be removed from a widened main incision. Large nuclear fragments should be removed from a large scleral frown incision

Fig. 8.9 Mark the sclerotomy 3.5–4 mm behind the limbus

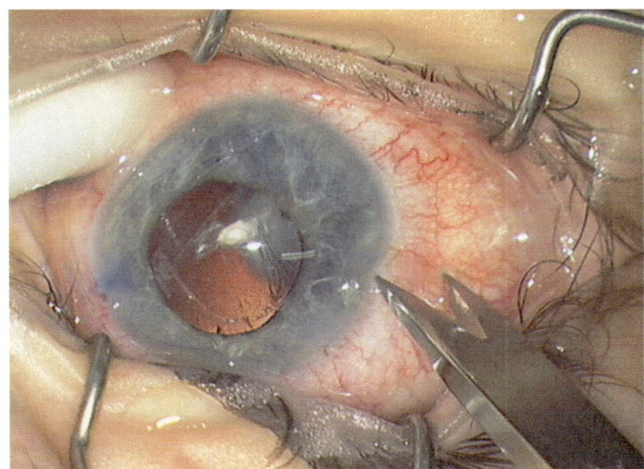

Fig. 8.10 Insert the trocar (lamellar sclerotomy)

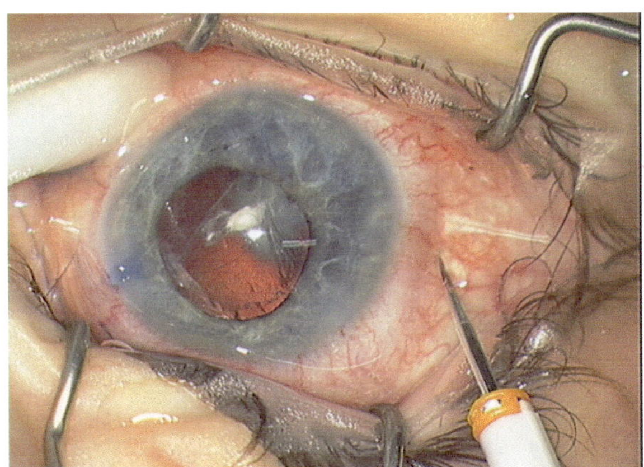

Fig. 8.11 Fixate the trocar with a cotton swab and remove the inserter

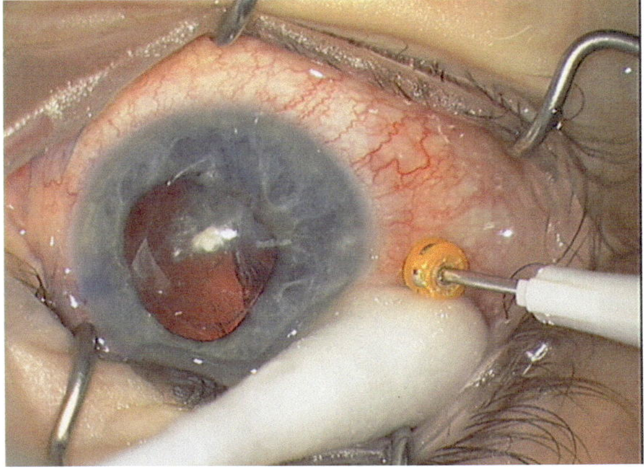

Fig. 8.12 Place the infusion handpiece in the anterior chamber and begin with the anterior vitrectomy from pars plana. If epinucleus is present inside the lens capsule, then try to remove it first; it might drop otherwise into the vitreous cavity

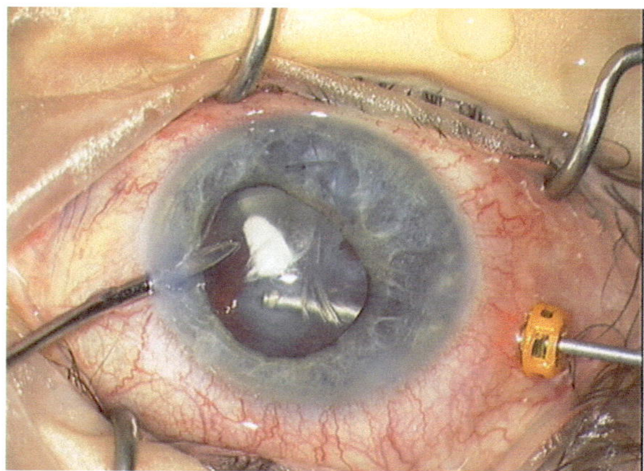

Fig. 8.13 Then continue with removal of cortical cortex. You can use I/A for cortex removal but switch back to the vitreous cutter if you aspirate vitreous

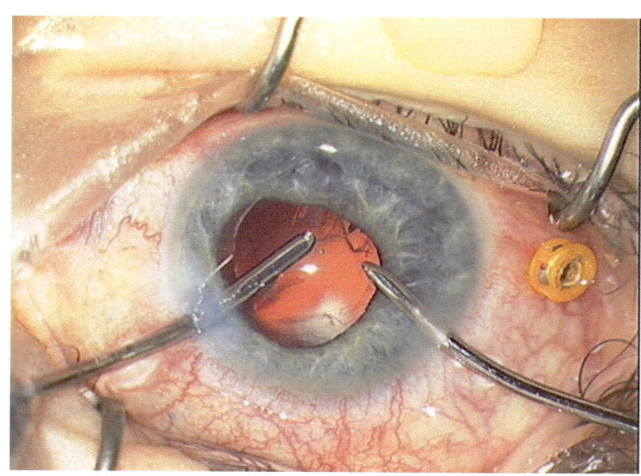

Fig. 8.14 A 23G vitreous cutter must be used with caution when removing cortex. If you remove vitreous then work in the cutting mode. But if you remove cortex then work in the aspiration mode. You will otherwise destroy the anterior capsule. You need the anterior lens capsule for the sulcus implantation

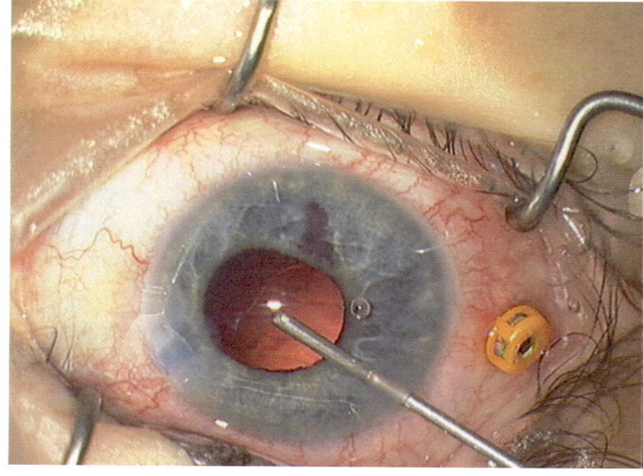

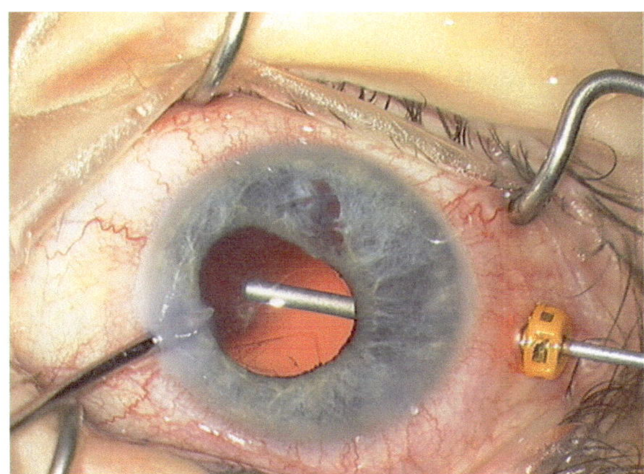

Fig. 8.15 Tip of the vitreous cutter should always be visible when it moves behind the pupil. Cut the vitreous for approximately 5 min. The beginner tends to remove too little vitreous

7. **Triamcinolone into the anterior chamber**
8. **Exclusion of a vitreous strand**

Check with a push–pull instrument or an iris spatula, if the vitreous is completely removed. Inject approximately 0.1 ml of triamcinolone (30% triamcinolone and 70% BSS) into the anterior chamber. The triamcinolone crystals visualize the vitreous very well (Figs. 8.16 and 8.17). The vitreous strands are incarcerated into the corneal wounds (paracentesis or main incision) and can be identified by a distorted pupil. If necessary, inject again triamcinolone. Insert a spatula instrument through a paracentesis and rotate it in a circular fashion in the complete anterior chamber and check, especially the incision sites. Perform the same manoeuvre from the second paracentesis but not from the main incision. If you detect vitreous strands, then remove them with the vitreous cutter.

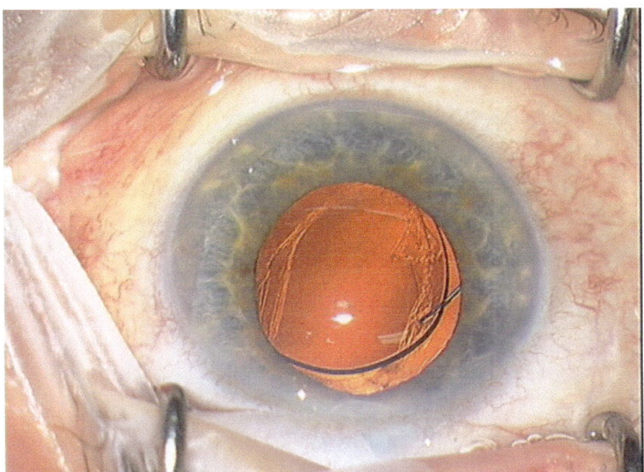

Fig. 8.16 Is the vitreous completely removed?

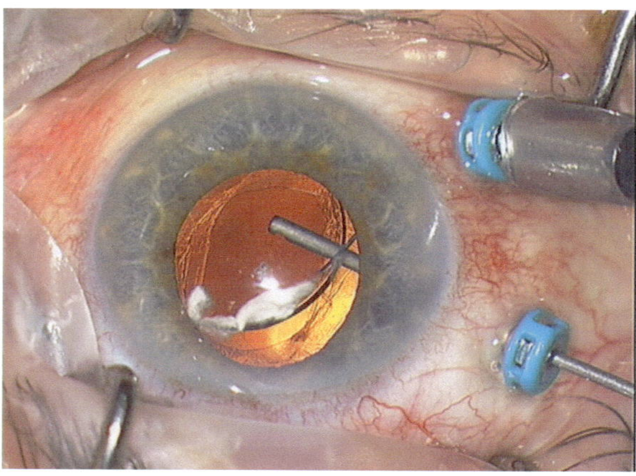

Fig. 8.17 Stain with triamcinolone and you will be surprised. There is vitreous!

9. **Implantation of the IOL**

Inject viscoelastics into the anterior chamber and into the sulcus. It is important to visualize the anterior capsule during this step. If the pupil is not sufficiently dilated, then implant iris hooks. Implant a 3-piece IOL and try to place the leading haptic onto the iris. Then rotate the trailing haptic into the sulcus and continue with the second haptic. Remarks: If you place the leading haptic first into the sulcus instead on the iris, then the haptic tends to dislocate into the posterior capsular rupture.

10. **Removal of trocar cannulas**

If the main incision was extended for the extraction of nuclear fragments, you should suture it with an Ethilon 10–0 cross-stitch. Hydrate the side incisions and remove finally the trocar cannula (Figs. 8.18 and 8.19).

11. **IOL capture**

In case of a posterior capsule tear, the best position for an IOL is "optic in, haptic out" (lens capture). The haptics are in the sulcus and the optic behind the rhexis of the anterior capsule (Figs. 8.20 and 8.21). The IOL is well centred, the iris–lens diaphragm is stabilized and the IOL is less myopic than in the sulcus. Another advantage relates to retinal surgery: a tamponade in the vitreous cavity cannot enter the anterior chamber.

Instrumentation:

(1)   2x manipulators (e.g. push–pull, Kuglen hook)

Procedure: Two paracentesis at an angle of about 90 degrees to the haptics. If the haptics are located at 12 and 6 o'clock, then place the paracentesis at 3 and 9 o'clock. Take two push–pulls, one push–pull presses one side of the IOL behind the

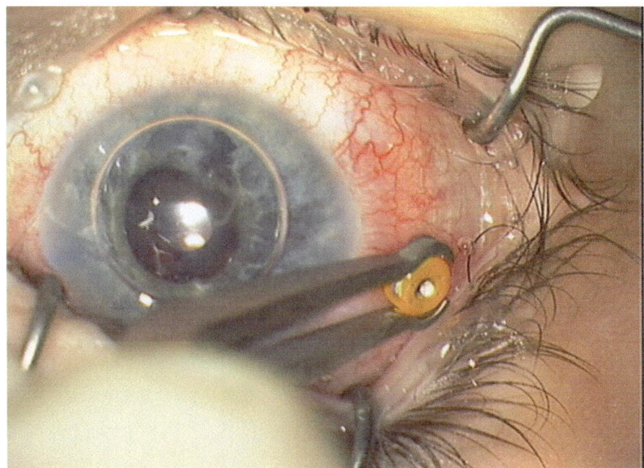

Fig. 8.18 Inject an air bubble to stabilize the anterior chamber if necessary and remove finally the trocar with an anatomic forceps or a trocar forceps

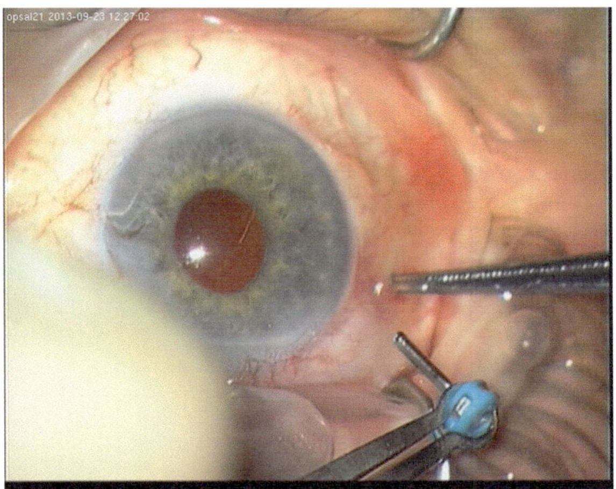

Fig. 8.19 Compress the wedges of the sclerotomy with the forceps for a few seconds

anterior capsule, while the other push–pull stabilizes the IOL (Fig. 8.21). Then, the same manoeuvre on the other side. Then, examine with the push–pull instruments whether the rhexis margins are located before the IOL. When properly performed, the rhexis takes an oval shape.

Pits and Pearls no. 16

Postoperative distorted pupil with incarcerated vitreous strand. A vitreous strand should be removed because it causes a distorted pupil, a vitreous wick syndrome with an increased risk of infection and vitreous dragging with Irvine Gass syndrome or retinal tears. There are different methods:

Fig. 8.20 Drawing of a lens capture. The posterior capsule is defective. The IOL is first placed in the sulcus, and the optic is buttonholed behind the rhexis. The haptics remains in the sulcus. The round rhexis takes an almond shape

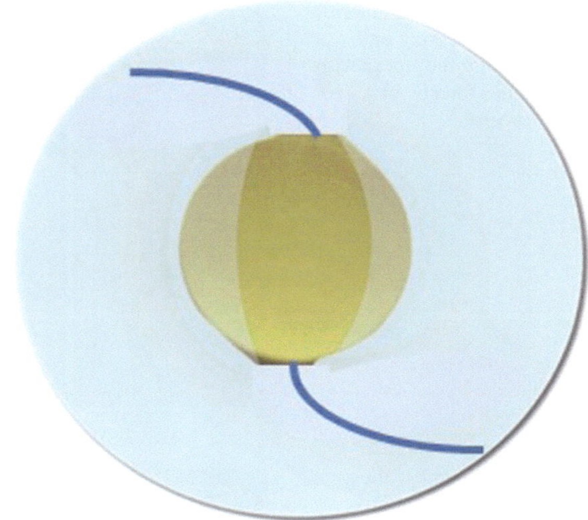

Fig. 8.21 Lens capture manoeuvre. Work bimanually with two push–pulls or iris spatulas and press the optic at one side behind the rhexis while stabilizing the optic at the other side and then the same manoeuvre at the other side

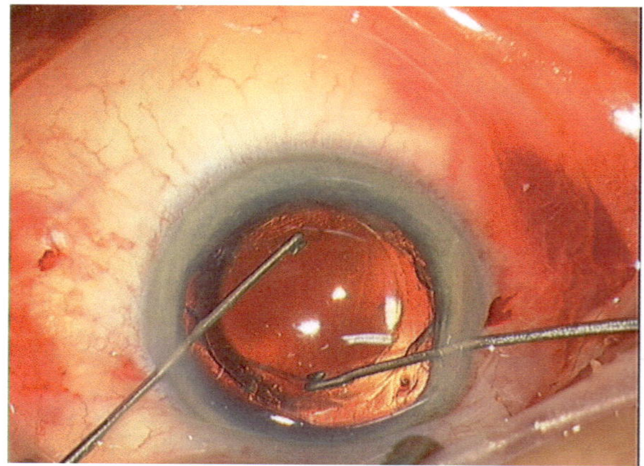

(1) You cannot relieve the vitreous strand from the same corneal incision. You have to remove it from a second incision. Insert a manipulator (e.g. iris spatula) into a second paracentesis and remove the vitreous strand with a circular movement. The strand remains in the anterior chamber but causes no traction. (2) YAG—laser treatment. Especially if the vitreous strand is pigmented, you may succeed with a laser treatment. (3) Anterior vitrectomy. Remove the vitreous strand with the vitreous cutter.

8.2   IOL Scaffolding for Residual Lens Pieces in Capsular Rupture (Agarwal Technique)

An alternative technique is the implantation of an IOL into the sulcus (IOL scaffolding. IOL scaffolding is a good technique to prevent loss of nuclear fragments through the pupil into vitreous cavity. (Video available).

Individual steps

1. Placing lens fragment onto the iris
2. Stabilizing lens fragment with OVD or second instrument
3. Implantation of IOL in the posterior chamber and behind the lens fragment
4. Refill anterior chamber with OVD
5. Phacoemulsification of remaining lens fragments in anterior chamber
6. Removal of OVD.

The operation step for step

1. **Placing lens fragment onto the iris**
2. **Stabilizing lens fragment with OVD or second instrument**

If a larger posterior capsule break occurs during phacoemulsification, remaining lens fragments could be lost into the vitreous cavity (Fig. 8.22). Surgeon should stop without retracting the phaco tip from anterior chamber and analyse the situation. It is important to move the remaining lens fragment to a safe area (e.g. anterior chamber angle) (Fig. 8.23). This could be done with a second instrument and/or OVD. The OVD is injected through the side port incision and should be placed also behind the capsular defect to create a barrier. This will not work in vitrectomized eyes. Here, a bimanual irrigation handpiece placed through the side port incision could be helpful (Fig. 8.24).

3. **Implantation of IOL in the posterior chamber and behind the lens fragment**

After the lens fragment is secured, the phaco tip could be withdrawn from anterior chamber. Now, preferably, a 3-piece IOL is placed into the ciliary sulcus and behind the remaining lens fragment to prevent posterior loss of the pieces (Figs. 8.25, 8.26 and 8.27). In case of an anterior capsule tear, the IOL haptic could be placed in the anterior chamber angle.

4. **Refill anterior chamber with OVD**
5. **Phacoemulsification of remaining lens fragments in anterior chamber**
6. **Removal of OVD**

Anterior chamber is refilled with OVD to prevent excessive endothelial cell loss. Phacoemulsification of the remaining lens pieces is performed in front of the IOL (Fig. 8.28). Anterior segment is checked for vitreous prolapse, and if necessary,

Fig. 8.22 Large posterior capsule defect with remaining retroiridal nuclear fragment is manipulated bimanually

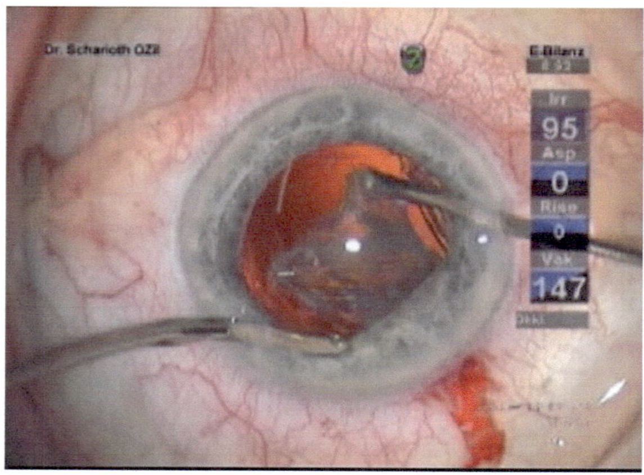

Fig. 8.23 Nuclear fragment is safely positioned in the anterior chamber angle, eye is already vitrectomized; therefore, manipulations are performed with bimanual I/A handpieces

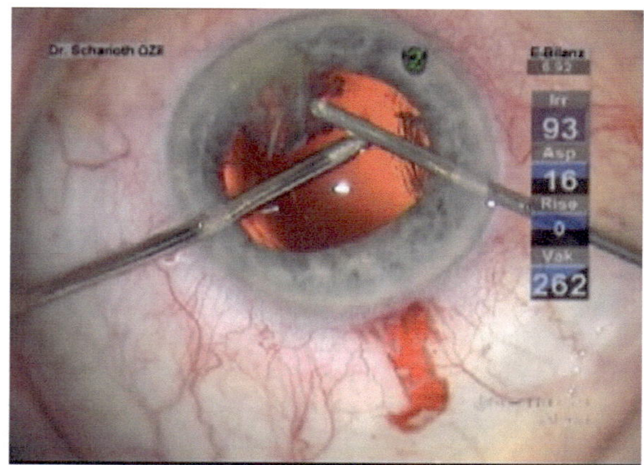

Fig. 8.24 Nuclear fragment is stabilized with the irrigation handpiece, while the aspiration is used to remove residual cortex

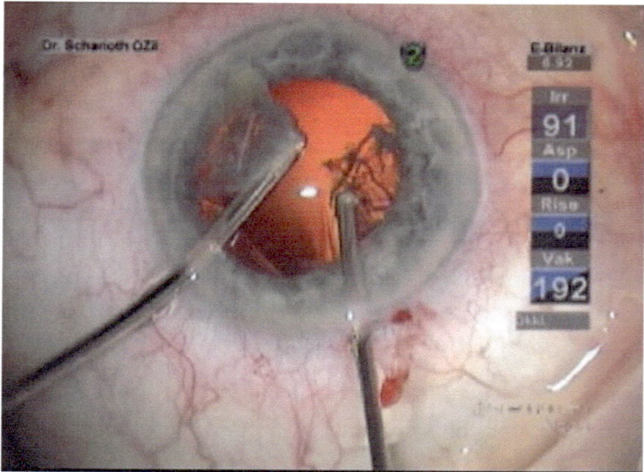

Fig. 8.25 Irrigation handpiece is "locking" the nuclear fragment in the anterior chamber angle, while a three-piece IOL is implanted in the ciliary sulcus

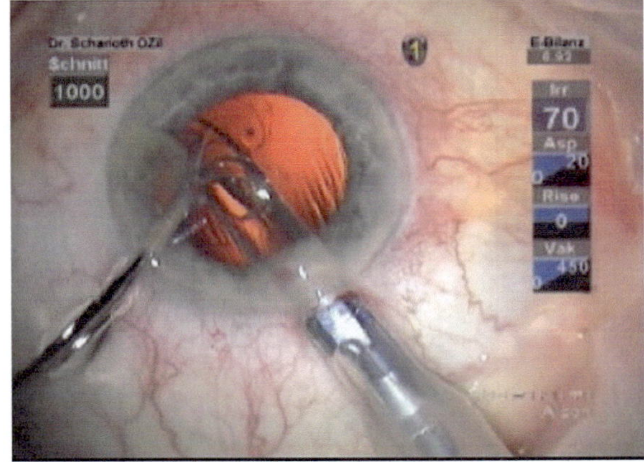

Fig. 8.26 Trailing haptic is implanted and lens fragment is in the anterior chamber and cannot luxate into the vitreous cavity

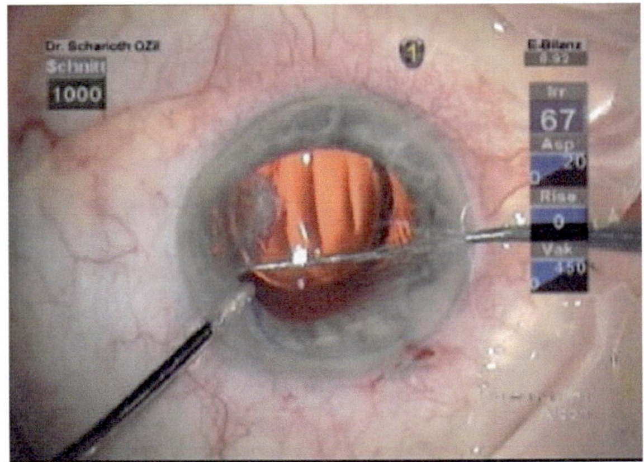

Fig. 8.27 IOL scaffolding (Agarwal technique), anterior chamber is filled with OVD, lens fragment is in front of the IOL

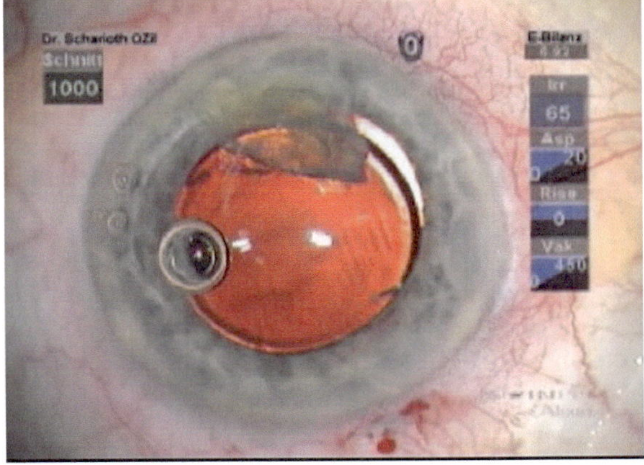

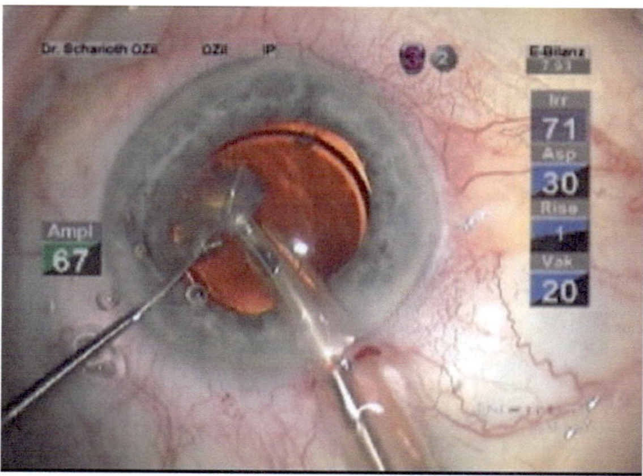

Fig. 8.28 Phacoemulsification is performed in the anterior chamber, and corneal endothelium is protected with OVD

Fig. 8.29 IOL is placed in the ciliary sulcus and well centred

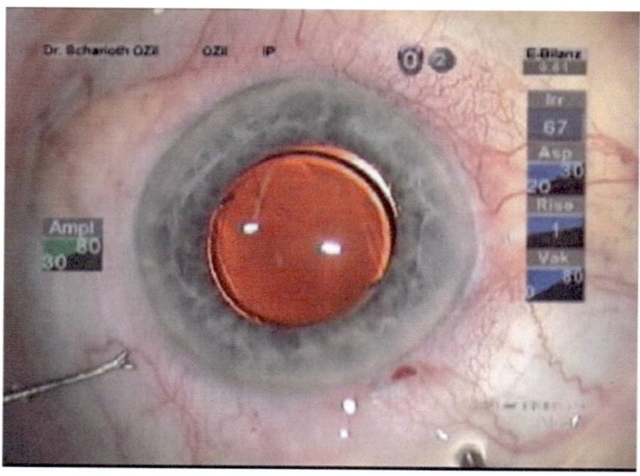

anterior vitrectomy is performed. If IOL was not perfectly positioned, it is placed now in the ciliary sulcus and centred (Fig. 8.29). If anterior capsulorhexis is intact, a posterior optic capture should be performed. OVD is removed. Finally, incisions are hydrated and checked for leakage.

Pits and Pearls no. 17

<u>IOL scaffolding</u> could be used for any size of remaining lens fragments in case of posterior capsule break. It reduces the risk for loss of lens fragments into the vitreous cavity. Before IOL implantation, the remaining lens fragment should be placed in anterior chamber angle.

Remark: An alternative to an IOL scaffold is a lens glide (Figs. 8.30 and 8.31).

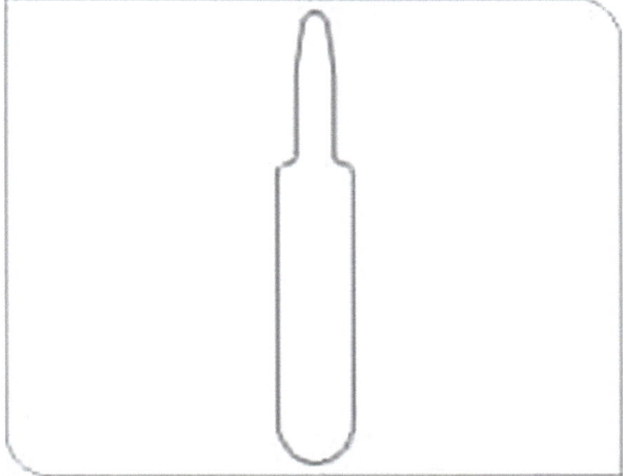

Fig. 8.30 Lens glide. Indication: Scaffold to prevent dislocation of nuclear fragments into the vitreous cavity. The lens glide is placed over the posterior capsular defect. BD Visitec 581,033

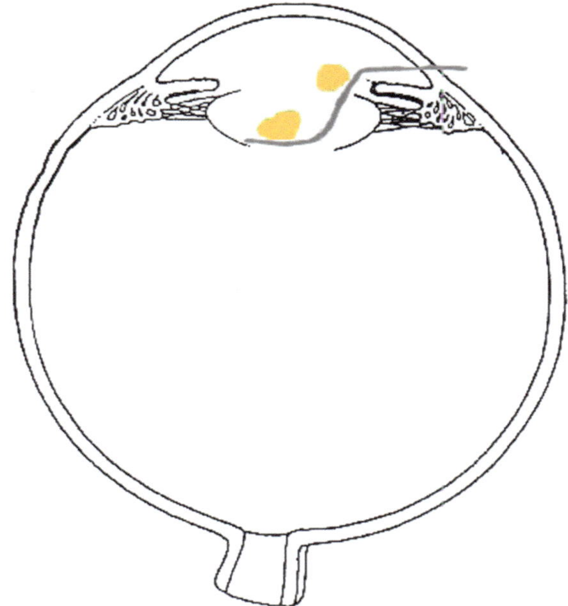

Fig. 8.31 Drawing for use of lens glide. The lens glide is placed as a scaffold inside the bag in order to prevent the dislocation of nuclear fragments into the vitreous cavity

Summary: The management of a posterior capsular rupture depends on the timing of the rupture. If the rupture happens during phacoemulsification , then convert to manual extraction of nuclear fragments. An alternative method is the IOL scaffolding. If the rupture happens during I/A, then you can convert directly to anterior vitrectomy. Train yourself to perform an anterior vitrectomy from pars plana with a trocar.

Surgical Management of Subluxated IOL from Pars Plana

9

Abstract

This chapter explains in detail the surgical management of a subluxated IOL. The surgery is explained step-by-step and only a phacoemulsification machine is required.

Keywords

Trocar Surgery · Trocar · Pars plana · Subluxated IOL

A subluxated IOL cannot be elevated from the limbus, but an elevation is easy from pars plana.

Surgical technique of removal of PCO from pars plana:

Insert one or two trocars 3.5 mm behind the limbus on the temporal side. Insert the vitreous cutter and place the tip behind the IOL. Then, elevate the IOL into the anterior chamber (Fig. 9.1). An anterior vitrectomy may be necessary (Fig. 9.2).

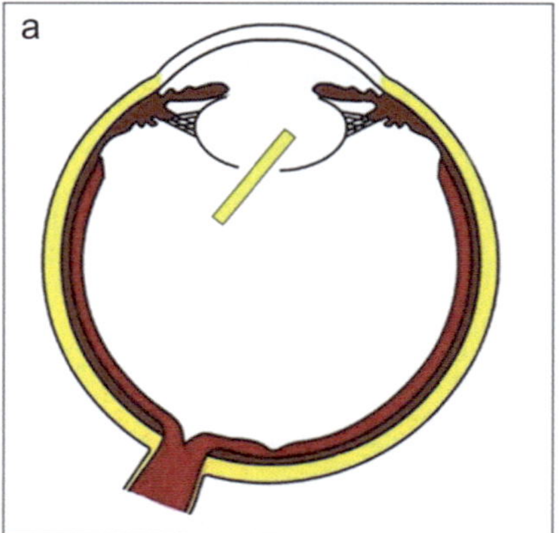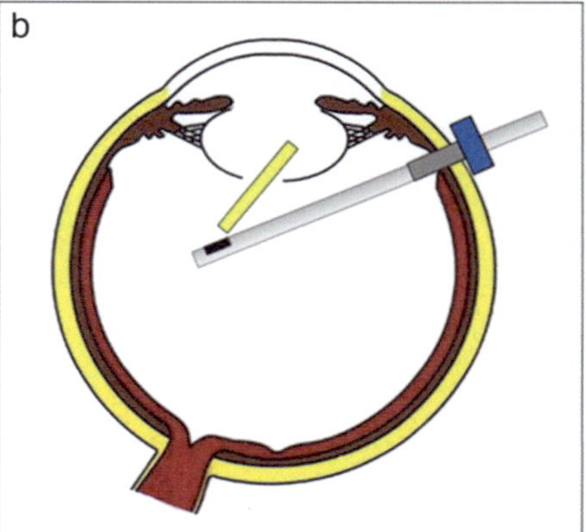

Fig. 9.1 *Subluxated IOL:* **a** The recovery of a subluxated IOL is difficult and in the most cases impossible from the limbus. **b** From pars plana, the recovery is easy. Insert an instrument at pars plana and lift the IOL into the anterior chamber

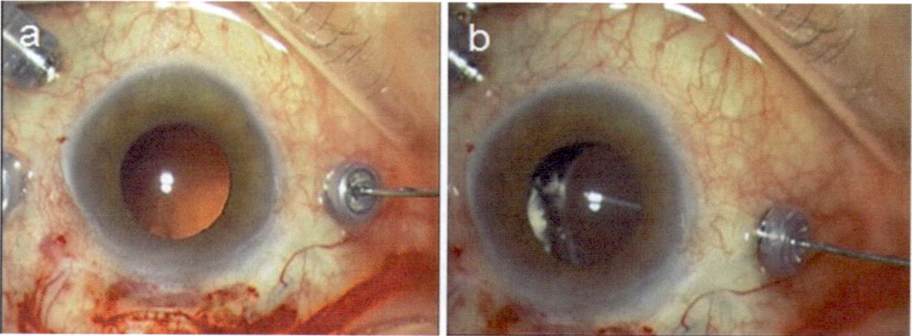

Fig. 9.2 **a** Dislocated IOL secondary to zonular lysis. The IOL cannot be elevated from the limbus into the anterior chamber. **b** After insertion of a trocar, the IOL can be easily elevated with the vitreous cutter. This maneuver is only possible from pars plana

Surgical Management of Dislocated Cortical Fragments

10

Abstract

Cortical fragments may dislocate into the Berger space in an uneventful cataract surgery or during a posterior capsular rupture. This chapter reports about the surgical management of dislocated cortical fragments from pars plana.

Keywords

Berger space · Trocar · Dislocated cortical fragments · Pars plana · PCR

Cortical or nuclear fragments may dislocate behind the lens capsule into the so-called Berger space (Fig. 10.1). The Berger space is the space between the patellar fossa of the vitreous and the lens. In case of a zonular defect, cortical fragments may dislocate through the zonular defect into the Berger space (Figs. 10.1 and 10.2). A removal from the anterior chamber is not possible. The only possibility to remove a cortical fragment at this location is from pars plana (video available).

Surgical technique

<u>Instruments:</u>

1. One or two 23G trocars
2. One anterior vitreous cutter

The surgery in detail:

Insert one or two trocars at the temporal side. Place the tip of the vitreous cutter behind the cortical fragment and cut cautiously in order not to injure the lens capsule (Fig. 10.2).

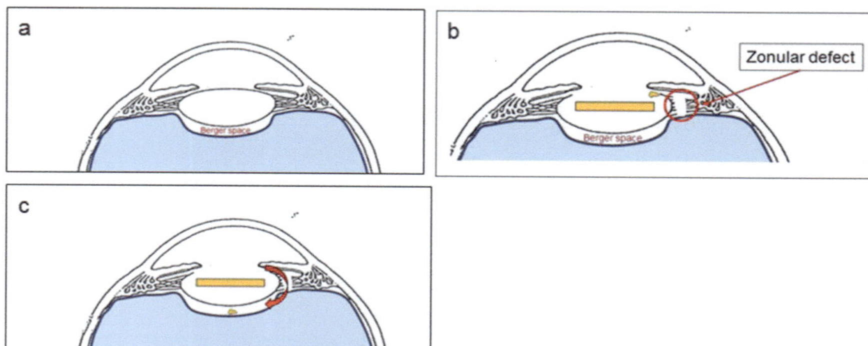

Fig. 10.1 **a** The Berger space is the space between the anterior hyaloid and the lens. **b** A cortical or nuclear fragment may dislocate through a zonular defect into the Berger space. **c** The lens capsule is intact. It is impossible to remove the fragment from the anterior chamber; it can only be removed from pars plana

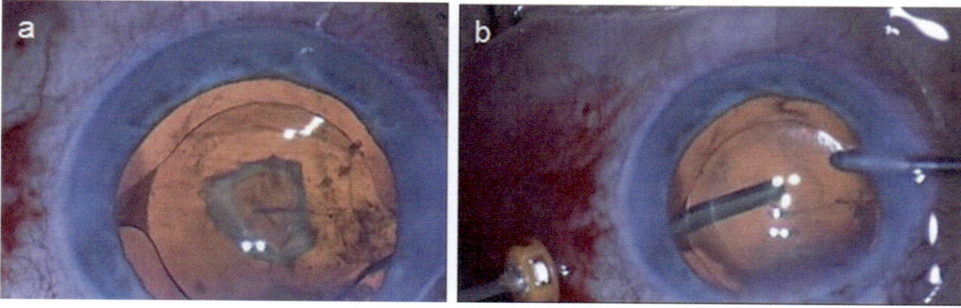

Fig. 10.2 **a** Cortical fragment is located behind the intact lens capsule. **b** A trocar cannula is inserted on the temporal side. The cortical fragment is removed with a 23G anterior vitreous cutter (Alcon)

It may happen that a posterior capsular rupture occurs when cortical material is still present in the eye. The surgeon implants the IOL in the sulcus. The cortical material is located behind the IOL. Then. he refers the patient for removal of cortical fragments. You can try to remove the cortical material with I/A from corneal incision, but the vitreous prolapse makes cortex removal difficult. The best technique is, therefore, the removal from pars plana (Fig. 10.3). Insert one or two trocars on the temporal side. Place the tip of the cutter behind the cortical fragments. It may happen that the cortical material drops through the capsular rupture. In this case, be prepared to continue vitrectomy with three trocars, viewing system and light fibre.

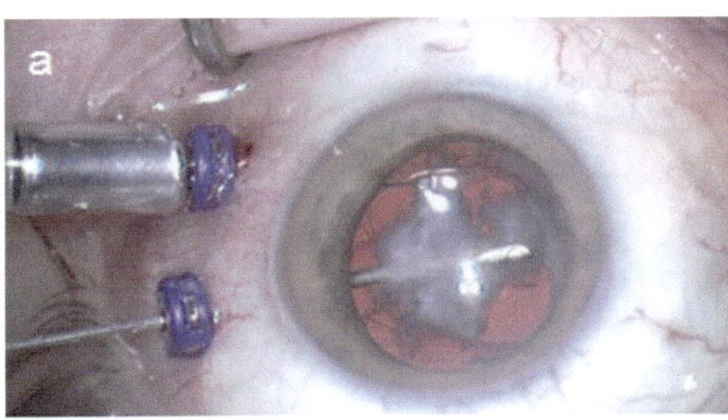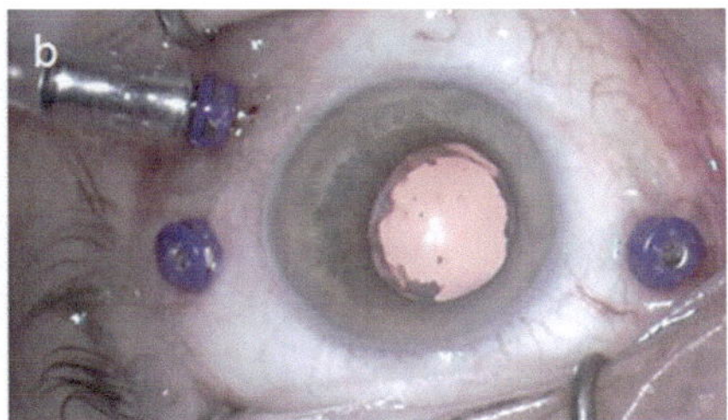

Fig. 10.3 **a** Cortical material is located behind the IOL. A posterior capsular rupture is present, and the IOL is located in the sulcus. **b** Insert one or two trocars and remove the cortical material from pars plana. If cortical material drops, then you insert three trocar cannulas in order to remove the dropped cortex from the posterior cavity

Remark: In case of a PCR when cortical or nuclear fragments are present, it is advisable to place the IOL behind the fragments to prevent a drop through the capsular rupture (IOL scaffold).

Surgical Management of Posterior Capsular Opacification from Pars Plana

11

Abstract

This chapter reports about the surgical management of posterior capsular opacification from pars plana. The surgery can be done with a phacoemulsification machine.

Keywords

Trocar surgery · Trocar · Pars plana · Posterior capsular opacification · PCO

In children or handicapped patients, a YAG capsulotomy cannot be performed. An alternative is a capsulectomy from pars plana (video available).

Vitrector settings

200 cuts per min, normal vacuum.

Surgical technique of removal of PCO from pars plana:

Insert one or two trocars 3.5 mm behind the limbus at 3 o'clock or 9 o'clock. Perform round circular movements with the vitreous cutter until a central and round opening is present (Fig. 11.1). An anterior vitrectomy is not necessary.

Postoperative treatment:

Combined Dexamethasone-Gentamicin drops 3 × daily for 3 weeks. Mydriatics are not necessary.

a

b

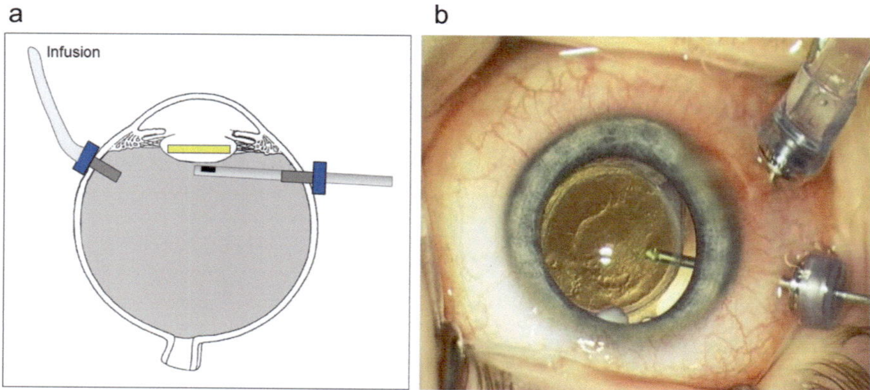

Fig. 11.1 **a** A thick PCO is present. **b** Removal of posterior capsular opacification from pars plana

Surgical Management of Positive Vitreous Pressure (PVP) During Cataract Surgery

Contents

Abstract

Positive vitreous pressure during cataract surgery is a dreaded complication. This chapter shows step-by-step the surgical management of positive vitreous pressure during cataract surgery.

Keywords

Trocar surgery · Trocar · Pars plana · Positive vitreous pressure · PVP

When the anterior chamber becomes shallow during phaccemulsification, the surgeon must promptly evaluate its potential cause. A decisive determinant in the differential diagnosis is the hardness of the globe, which the surgeon must palpate. Firmness signals positive vitreous pressure (PVP); softness indicates its absence. PVP is a phenomenon characterized by forward displacement of the lens-iris diaphragm during phacoemculsification that can lead to a cascade of intraoperative complications, potentially with devastating results. Cataract surgeons need to understand the causes of a shallow anterior chamber (Chronopoulos et al. (2017; Fishkind 2009). (Video available under https://www.youtube.com/playlist?list= PL0dKYclPD7yMJRuQAIt9Dr7pOtuI0Seex).

Pathomechanism of PVP is an aqueous misdirection; the misdirection of BSS behind the lens capsule or behind the nucleus. The latter case, misdirection of BSS behind the nucleus occurs commonly during hydrodissection. The typical cascade of surgical mistakes goes like this: an inexperienced surgeon performs a too small rhexis. Then he/she continues with hydrodissection. There is no effect because the

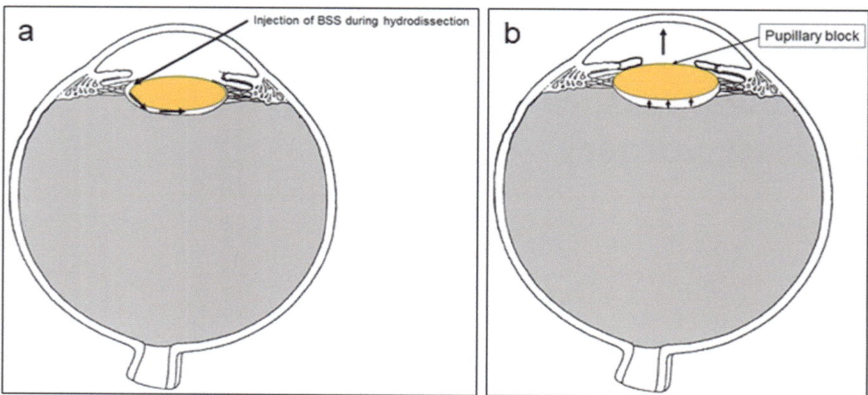

Fig. 12.1 **a** Beginner cataract surgeon performs a small capsular rhexis. During hydrodissection, he/she injects a high volume of BSS into the lens capsule. The BSS cannot escape due to the too small rhexis. **b** The lens capsule is inflated and creates a ciliary block and pupillary block. The iris–lens diaphragm is pushed forwards resulting in a shallow anterior chamber

nucleus cannot move due to the small rhexis. Now comes the mistake: the inexperienced surgeon injects additional BSS into the lens capsule. The BSS inflates the lens capsule (Fig. 12.1a) and pushes the nucleus towards the iris creating a pupillary block. This leads to an angle closure as the lens and iris shift forward, exacerbating the elevation of IOP (Fig. 12.1b).

In the past, surgeons used 3 ml or even 5 ml syringes for hydroprocedures leading to tremendous amount of vitreous hydration in case of a posterior capsular rupture. A particular mention is for small pupil cases where the surgeons blindly do a hydroprocedure and inadvertently inject fluid over the CCC behind the lens capsule. This fluid can go through the zonules into the vitreous cavity leading to a PVP due to vitreous hydration particularly if you inject copious amount. A PVP, however, may also occur during IOL implantation. There is no explanation available in the literature. The patient can strain and squeeze eyelids resulting in PVP, or if having cough, thereby increasing intrathoracic pressure and causing PVP.

Surgical treatment of PVP:

The anterior chamber is shallow, and the iris prolapses through the incisions. Remove slowly all instruments. Now you can do three things: (1) wait approximately 15–20 min. The intraocular fluid will slowly resorb, the IOP will decrease, and you can try to continue surgery. (2) Stop surgery. Give the patient two acetazolamide tablets and continue surgery a few hours later. (3) Perform a dry anterior vitrectomy (Fig. 12.2). Dry vitrectomy means a vitrectomy without irrigation. You perform a short core vitrectomy until the pressure of the globe has normalized. It is very important to perform only a short vitrectomy. <u>Remark</u>: If you remove too much vitreous resulting in an under pressure, then a suprachoroidal haemorrhage may develop.

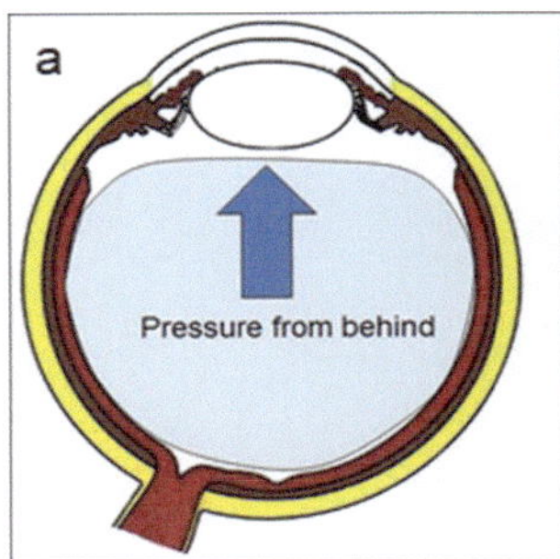

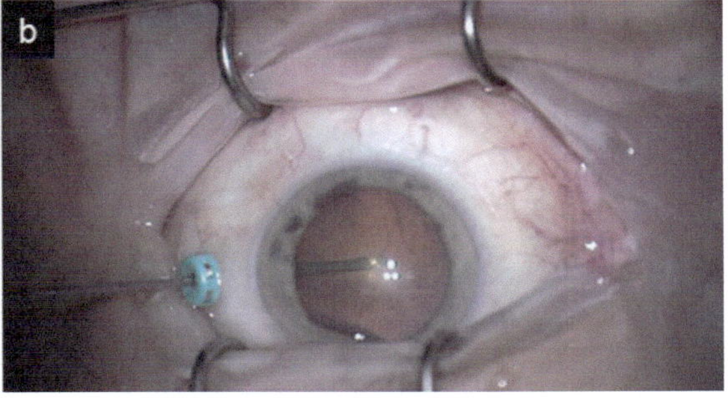

Fig. 12.2   **a** Positive vitreous pressure during cataract surgery. **b** Perform an anterior vitrectomy from pars plana to relieve pressure. Note that there is no infusion

Surgery of dry vitrectomy:

Insert one trocar on the temporal side. An irrigation is not required because it will increase the IOP even more. Then place the vitreous cutter behind the nucleus, hold it stable and perform vitrectomy. The opening of the vitreous cutter is pointed towards the optic disc. During vitrectomy, place your fingertip on the limbus to feel the pressure of the globe. In the beginning of the procedure, the globe is hard, but after a few seconds, the globe becomes soft. If the globe has approximately an IOP of 10 mmHg, stop with vitrectomy. Inflate the anterior chamber with BSS and continue surgery.

Tips and tricks (Fig. 12.3):

A vitreous decompression can also be performed with a needle cannula. Attach a 23G or 25G needle cannula to a 3 cc syringe. Insert the cannula 3.5 mm behind the limbus and push the cannula forward until the tip of the needle is located in the middle of the eye. Then, aspirate 0,2–0,3 ml of fluid. Inflate next the anterior chamber with BSS and continue with cataract surgery.

Remark: The technique may cause vitreous traction. It should therefore only be performed in old patients. In this age group, the PVD is usually complete and the vitreous is sufficiently liquefied. In contrast, this technique may fail in young eyes because the vitreous is intact and no fluid can be extracted.

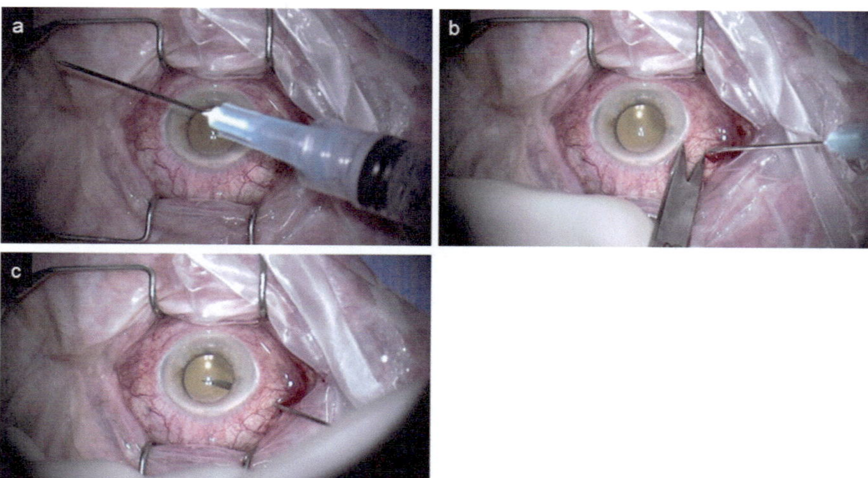

Fig. 12.3 **a** Attach a 23G or 25G needle cannula to a 3 cc syringe. **b** Insert the needle 3,5 mm behind the limbus. **c** extract fluid from vitreous cavity

References

Chronopoulos A, Thumann G, Schutz J. Positive vitreous pressure: pathophysiology, complications, prevention, and management. Surv Ophthalmol. 2017;62:127–133
Fishkind WJ. Positive pressure. J Cataract Refract Surg. 2009

All videos of this part be found in a playlist of my YouTube channel:
https://www.youtube.com/playlist?list=PL0dKYclPD7yMJRuQAIt9Dr7pOtuI0
Seex

Part IV: SICS technique
Part IV: Zonular lysis and phacoemulsification
Part IV: Traumatic cataract with inferior zonular lysis
Part IV: ICCE and iris claw IOL
Part IV: SICS and inferior zonular lysis
Part IV: Small pupil and phacodonesis

Small Incision Cataract Surgery (SICS = Modified ECCE)

13

Contents

Abstract

This chapter explains step-by-step the surgery of a SICS. SICS is a modified ECCE and the standard cataract surgery in Africa and Asia. The main indications for this technique in developed countries is a rockhard nucleus and phacodonesis.

Keywords

SICS · ECCE · Cataract surgery · Rockhard nucleus · Phacodonesis

The knowledge and mastering of the SICS technique open new surgical possibilities for cataract surgeons. SICS is a modification of the old ECCE technique. The main difference is that no corneal incision is created but a scleral incision. The complete nucleus can be removed from the scleral incision. The SICS technique can also be used as alternative to the ICCE technique. The ICCE technique is required in eyes with zonular lysis.

In addition, we will show a technique to save a dropping nucleus. The technique is simple but effective.

Learn the three techniques, phacoemulsification, SICS (modified ECCE) and the saving of a dropping nucleus from pars plana and you do not need help from a posterior segment surgeon. You will be a cataract surgeon master. All videos of this part be found in a playlist of my YouTube channel:

© The Author(s), under exclusive license to Springer Nature Switzerland AG 2022
U. Spandau and G. B. Scharioth, *Complications During and After Cataract Surgery*,
https://doi.org/10.1007/978-3-030-93531-3_13

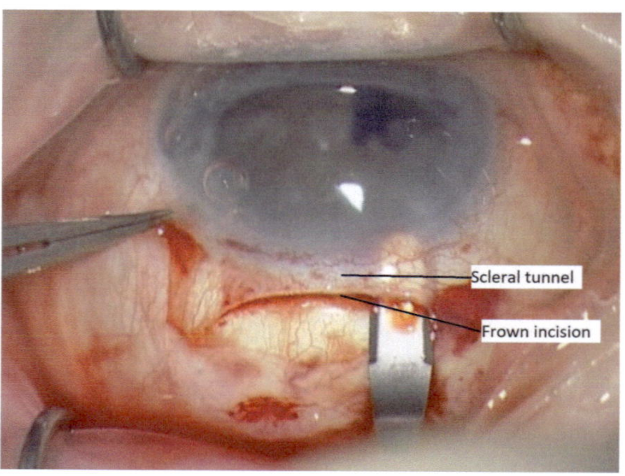

Fig. 13.1 SICS surgery. 8 mm wide frown incision

https://www.youtube.com/playlist?list=PL0dKYclPD7yMJRuQAIt9Dr7pOtuI0 Seex

If the nucleus is too dense for phacoemulsification and you risk a corneal decompensation, you can remove the nucleus faster and with fewer complications in toto. An excellent technique is SICS (modified ECCE). The main difference between SICS and ECCE is the main incision (Fig. 13.1). In ECCE, a limbal incision from 10 o'clock to 2 o'clock is performed; in SICS, a frown incision of the sclera is performed. A frown incision is tighter and more stable than a corneal incision. A suture is usually not necessary. We prefer to suture the frown incision with a Vicryl 8-0 cross-stitch. We recommend performing the surgery in peribulbar anaesthesia.

13.1 Standard Instruments for SICS

Phaco set

Phaco handpiece and IOL injector are not needed.

Frown incision

Westcott scissors (Fig. 13.2).

Calliper

Indication: Marking of main incision and sclerotomy. The main incision for the implantation of an iris-fixated PMMA IOL is 6 mm wide. Calliper by Castroviejo, Geuder 19135.

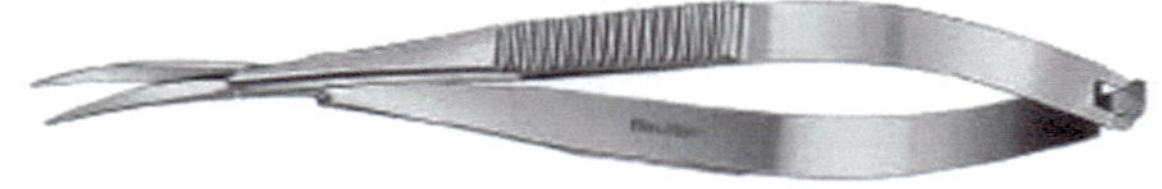

Fig. 13.2 Westcott scissors. Indication: Limbal peritomy. Geuder 19750

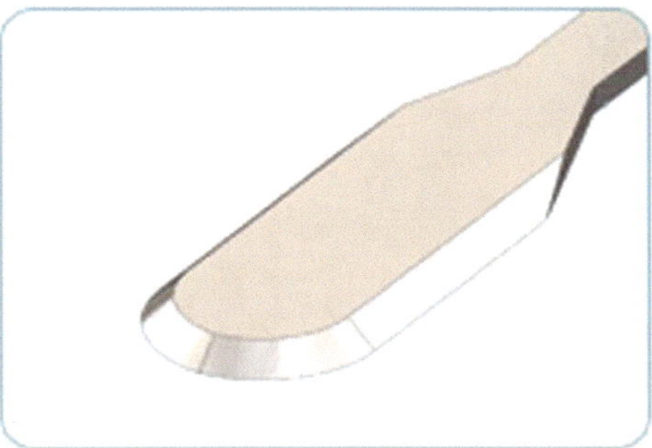

Fig. 13.3 Crescent angled bevel-up knife. Indication: Dissection of a scleral tunnel. (Alcon 8065990002, Beaver Visitec 373835, DORC 51.1118 or Aurosleek crescent bevel up (Aurolab))

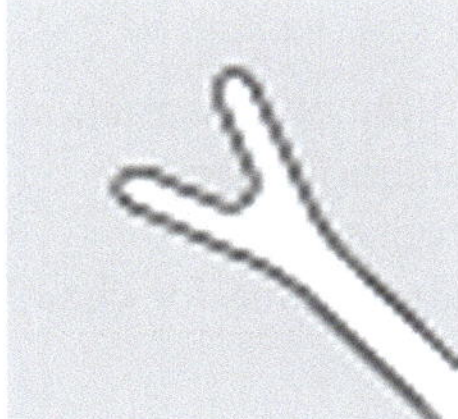

Fig. 13.4 Y-manipulator or nucleus rotator. Indication: Rotation of nucleus, very useful during SICS surgery for luxation of the nucleus into the anterior chamber. Nucleus rotator after Neuhann, Geuder 32160

Crescent angled bevel-up knife (Fig. 13.3).

Rotation of nucleus

Y-manipulator or nucleus rotator (Fig. 13.4).

Extraction of nucleus

Lens extraction hook (Fig. 13.5).

Alternative: (1) 27G grey cannula. Bend a 27G cannula to a fish hook. (2) Lens loop or Vectis (Serrated lens loop, Geuder 15620).

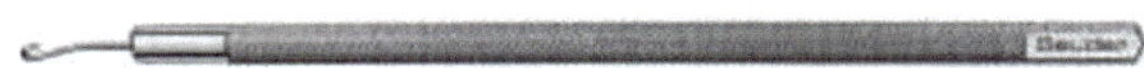

Fig. 13.5 Lens extraction hook. Indication: Extraction of nucleus. Lens extraction hook after Henning/Friedrich, Geuder 32034

13.2 SICS Surgery

<u>Instruments</u>

1. I/A
2. Lens nucleus rotator
3. 15° knife
4. Crescent bevel-up knife
5. 2.4 mm tunnel knife also known as keratome
6. Calliper
7. Lens extraction hook (Geuder, Germany) or serrated lens loop (Geuder, Germany)

Individual steps

 (1) Capsulorhexis
 (2) Limbal peritomy
 (3) Frown incision and scleral tunnel construction
 (4) Luxation of nucleus into anterior chamber
 (5) Inflate lens capsule with viscoelastics
 (6) Rotation of the nucleus into the anterior chamber
 (7) Extraction of the nucleus
 (8) I/A
 (9) Implantation of a 3-piece IOL
(10) Suturing of frown incision and conjunctiva

The surgery step by step

(1) Capsulorhexis

Begin with a paracentesis at 10 and 2 o'clock and inject viscoelastics (Viscoat®) into the anterior chamber. Perform then a large rhexis because the nucleus must be dislocated from the capsular bag (Fig. 13.6).

(2) Limbal peritomy

(3) Frown incision and scleral tunnel construction

Continue with a limbal peritomy from 11 o'clock to 1 o'clock with a Westcott scissors. Cauterize bleeding vessels and mark an 8 mm wide incision with a calliper (Fig. 13.7a). Perform an arc-shaped and 50% scleral thickness incision with the 15° knife (Fig. 13.7b). Dissect a scleral tunnel with the crescent angled bevel-up knife (Fig. 13.8). Do not dissect too deep (iris prolapse) but not too thin either (flap defect). If the blade is shining through the sclera, it is at the correct depth. Then, open the main incision with the 2.4 mm tunnel knife (Fig. 13.8). Move the knife 1–2 mm inside the clear cornea before entering the anterior chamber (Fig. 13.7c). Be aware that the scleral tunnel has a V-shape and not a U-shape like the normal tunnel

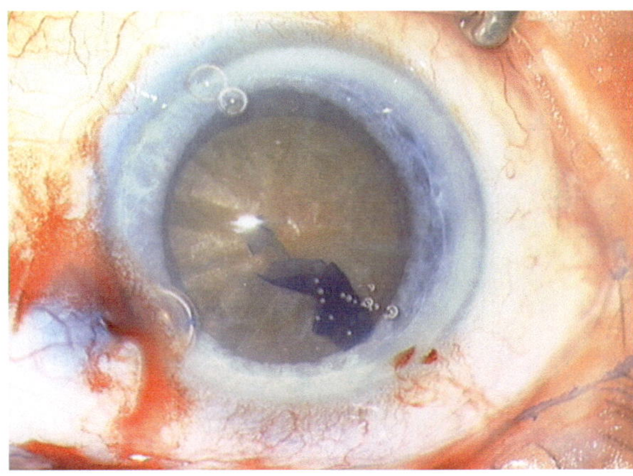

Fig. 13.6 Perform a large rhexis. A large rhexis is necessary to luxate the nucleus out of the lens capsule

incision (Fig. 13.7c); i.e., the scleral tunnel widens from the sclera to the anterior chamber.

Tips and tricks

Caution: The scleral tunnel in SICS surgery has a "V" shape. The scleral tunnel in iris-claw implantation surgery has the shape of a "U" (Fig. 13.7c).

(4) Luxation of nucleus into anterior chamber

(5) Inflate lens capsule with viscoelastics

(6) Rotation of the nucleus into the anterior chamber

Non-dominant hand: Y-manipulator

Dominant hand: Viscoelastics syringe

Continue with hydrodissection. If the rhexis is large enough, the nucleus prolapses out due to hydrodissection from the capsular bag. If the nucleus fails to prolapse from the capsular bag during hydrodissection, then you need to luxate the nucleus manually into the anterior chamber. Place the tip of the Y-manipulator at the superior edge of the nucleus and lift the nucleus up. Inject with the other hand viscoelastics (Viscoat®) behind the nucleus in order to inflate the lens capsule (Fig. 13.9). Then lift the nucleus completely into the anterior chamber. It is important to inject viscoelastics behind the nucleus in order to avoid a posterior capsular defect.

(7) Extraction of the nucleus

For nucleus extraction, use a lens extraction hook (Geuder, Germany). Use alternatively a lens loop. Before extracting the nucleus assure yourself that there is viscoelastics (Viscoat®) above and behind the nucleus in order to protect the lens capsule and the endothelium. Then insert the fish hook with the hook pointed to the

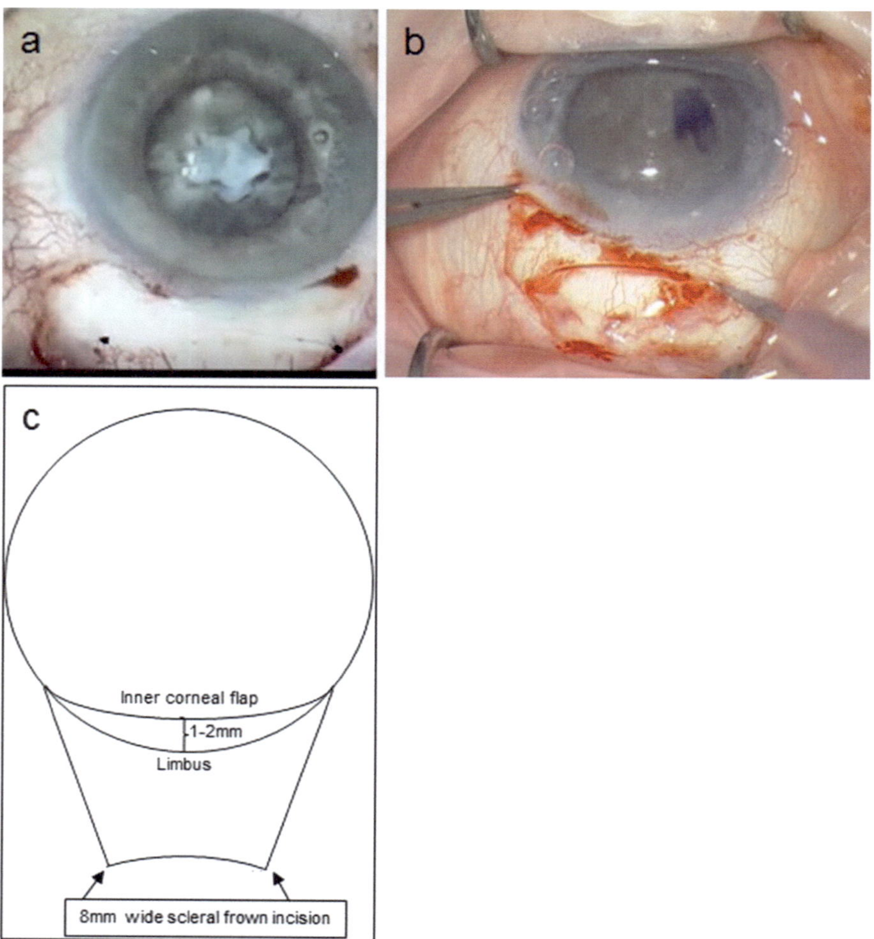

Fig. 13.7 **a** Mark an 8 **mm** long incision on the sclera. **b** Perform an 50% scleral thickness incision with the 15° knife. **c** Drawing of a frown incision. The incision is 8 mm broad and the tunnel has a "V" shape

side. Place the hook behind the middle of the nucleus, turn the hook into an upright position and draw the nucleus slowly out (Fig. 13.10). Check first that you did not catch the inferior iris with the fish hook. If the nucleus gets stuck in the frown incision, then do not insist; reinject viscoelastics and enlarge the frown incision with the 2.4 mm tunnel knife and repeat the extraction manoeuvre.

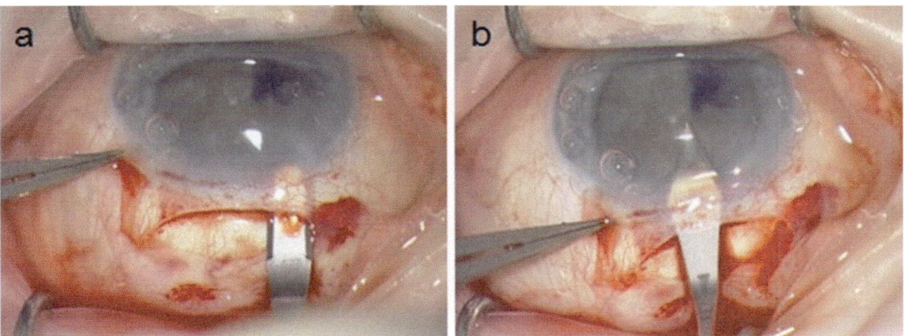

Fig. 13.8 **a** Dissect a scleral flap with a crescent bevel-up knife. If the blade of the knife is visible through the tissue you are on the right level. **b** Open the anterior chamber with a 2.4 mm blade. Do not enter the anterior chamber too close to the limbus; otherwise, the iris will prolapse

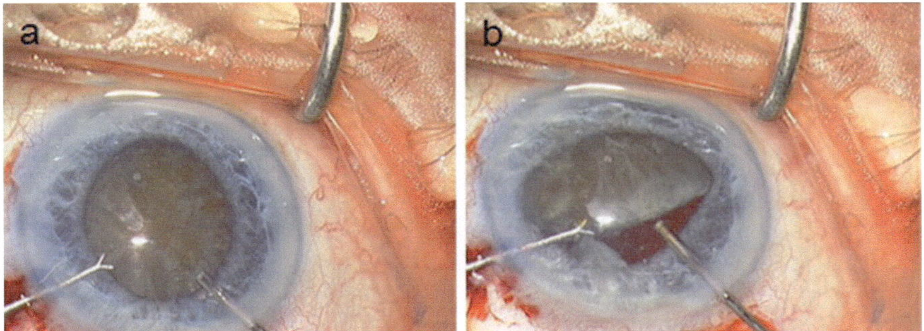

Fig. 13.9 **a** The left hand holds a Y-manipulator or Sinskey hook manipulator and the right hand viscoelastics. Place the Y-manipulator on the superior edge of the nucleus. **b** Then lift the nucleus up with the Y-manipulator and inject viscoelastics into the open space between nucleus and lens capsule in order to inflate the lens capsule

(8) I/A

(9) Implantation of a 3-piece IOL

(10) Suturing of the frown incision and conjunctiva

Continue with I/A. Then implant a 3-piece IOL because of the large rhexis (Fig. 13.11). The IOL requires no folding, because the main incision is sufficient large. Proceed to suture the main incision with a Vicryl 8-0 cross-stitch. If necessary, suture also the conjunctiva (Fig. 13.11). Remove the viscoelastics with I/A from the anterior chamber.

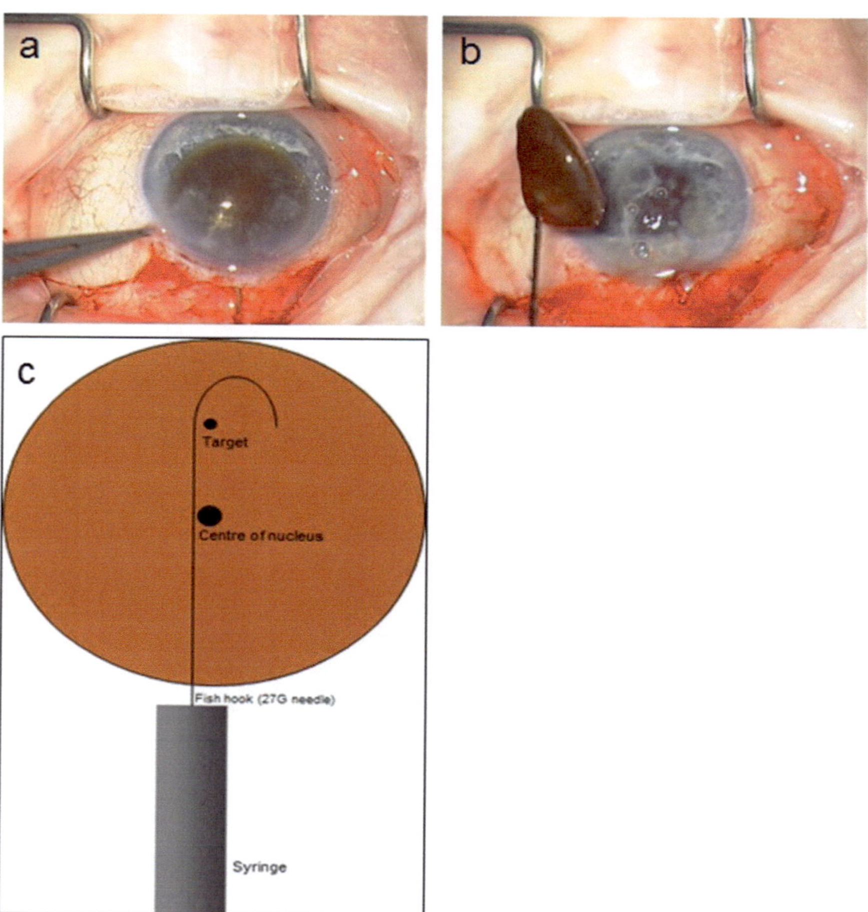

Fig. 13.10 **a** Inject viscoelastics between the nucleus and the lens capsule and between the nucleus and the endothelium. Insert the fish hook with the hook facing to the right. If you reach the extraction position (see Fig. 13.10c), then turn the cannula so that the hook faces the nucleus. **b** Remove the nucleus. **c** Drawing: Position the fish hook behind the nucleus as depicted

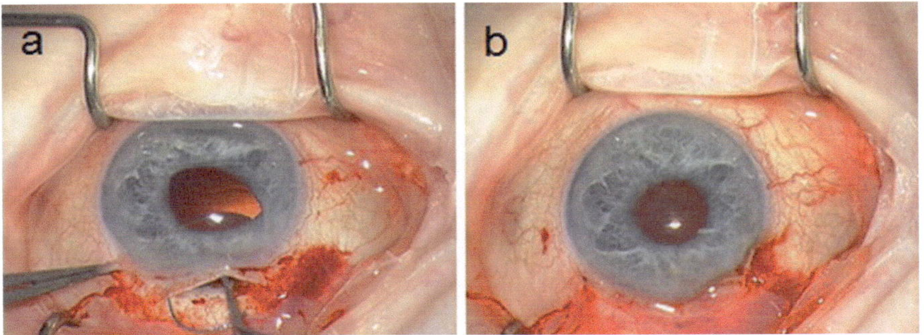

Fig. 13.11   **a** Implant a 3-piece IOL. An injector is not necessary. **b** Close the conjunctiva with a Vicryl 8-0 interrupted stitch

Caution: Keep an eye on the frown incision during surgery. Avoid that the incision is gaping because this may lead to a choroidal detachment. Close therefore the incision as soon as possible with a suture.

Complication: If the nucleus gets stuck during extraction, then do not insist. You will cause an iris damage. Reposition the nucleus and widen the scleral incision to 9 mm.

Summary

Train yourself with the three techniques, phacoemulsification, SICS (modified ECCE) and the saving of a dropping nucleus from pars plana, and you do not need help from a posterior segment surgeon. You are now a cataract surgeon master.

Surgical Management of Zonular Lysis

14

Contents

Abstract

This chapter reports about the surgical management of a small and big zonular lysis. A big zonular lysis (=phacodonesis) is the biggest challenge for a cataract surgeon. The surgery is desctibed step-by-step.

Keywords

Trocar surgery · Trocar · Pars plana · Zonular lysis · Vitreous prolapse · phacodonesis · ICCE

14.1 Cataract Surgery with Zonular Lysis

A cataract with zonular lysis is the most difficult cataract to operate (Fig. 14.1). Always check during the preoperative assessment, if a phacodonesis is present or not. If you are a beginner, you should rather send the patient to a hospital with retinal backup. The nucleus may drop and you should, therefore, be capable to convert to a SICS and to save a dropping nucleus from pars plana. See treatment

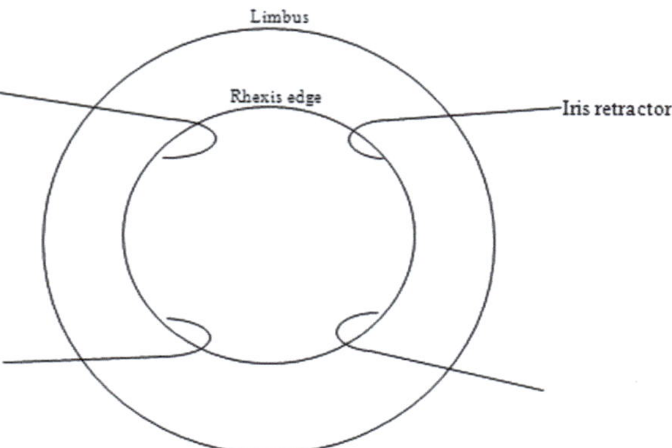

Fig. 14.1 In case of a zonular lysis, insert four iris hooks into the rhexis edge and try carefully to perform a phacoemulsification. If the zonular lysis is bigger than expected, then convert to a SICS surgery

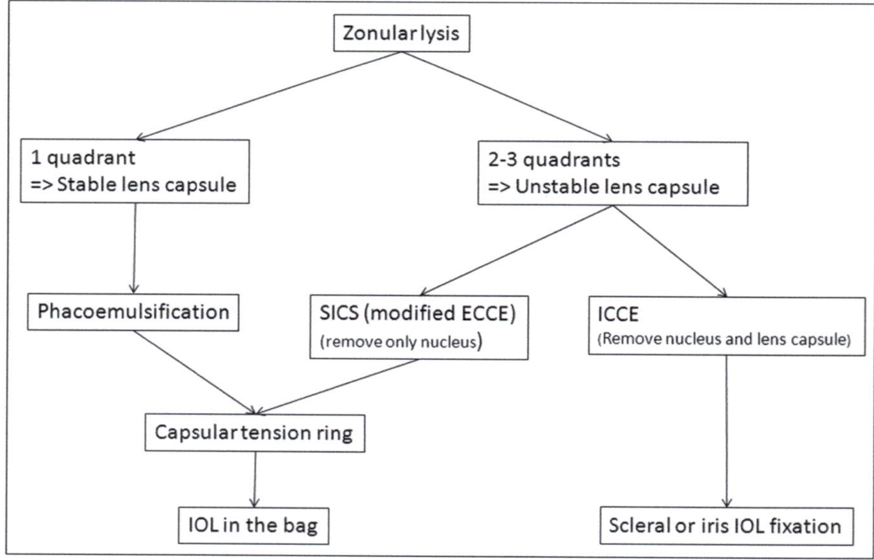

Fig. 14.2 Treatment algorithm for zonular lysis

algorithm Fig. 14.2. If you note a zonular lysis after starting your cataract case, then first assess the extent of the zonular lysis (Fig. 14.1). Insert iris hooks and inject triamcinolone to assess the size of the zonular lysis and the amount of vitreous prolapse.

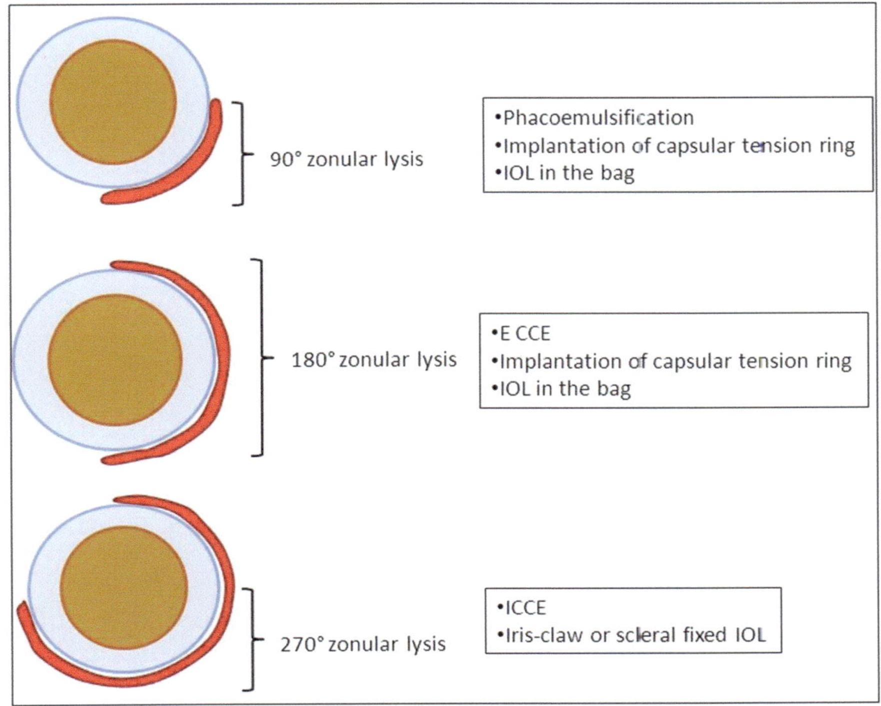

Fig. 14.3 Treatment algorithm for zonular lysis. Depending on the size of the zonular lysis different surgical techniques are recommended

A moderate zonular lysis of 1 quadrant is often discovered under I/A. Implant a capsular tension ring after I/A or insert the IOL with one haptic pressing against the loose quadrant.

If the zonular lysis is very advanced (2–3 quadrants), we prefer to perform a SICS (modified ECCE). A phacoemulsification on this situation is technically very difficult and risk full. All surgical possibilities are demonstrated in Fig. 14.4. (See treatment algorithm Fig. 14.3).

14.2 Zonular Lysis of 1 Quadrant

Instrumentation:

Maybe: Iris retractors (Fig. 14.4).
Capsular tension ring (Fig. 14.5).

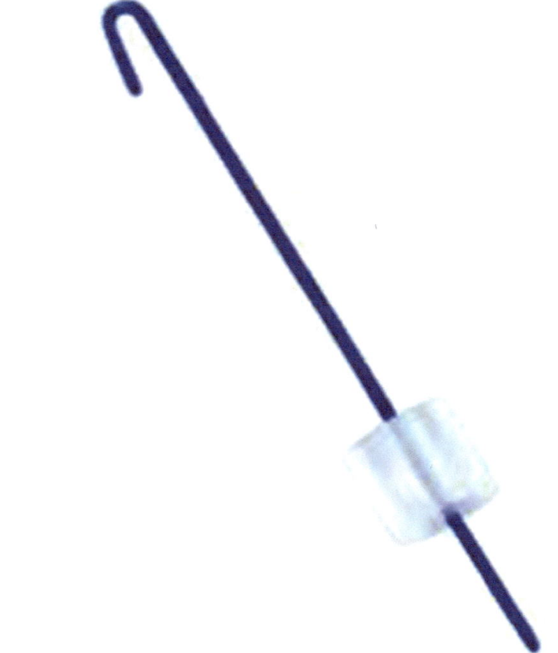

Fig. 14.4 Iris hook (blue) with a silicone stopper (transparent). The iris hook grasps the pupillary edge or the rhexis edge, and the silicone stopper fixates the hook. Indication: Small pupil or zonular lysis

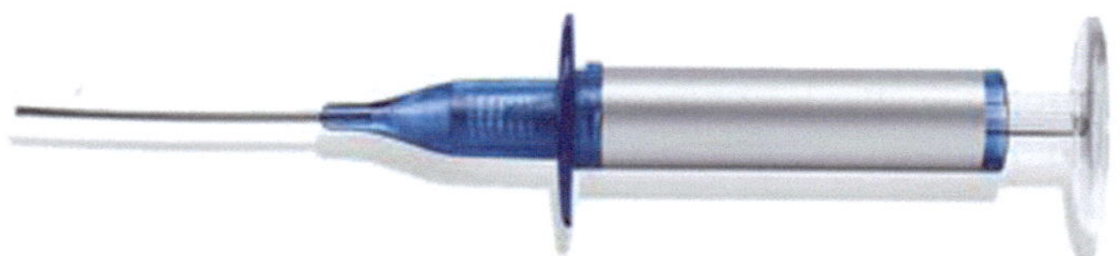

Fig. 14.5 Preloaded capsular tension ring. Indication: Zonular lysis, (Croma, Austria)

Individual steps.

(1) Rhexis.
(2) Phacoemulsification
(3) I/A.
(4) Implantation of capsular tension ring.
(5) Implantation of IOL in capsular bag.
(6) Maybe anterior vitrectomy.

The surgery step by step:

(1) **Rhexis**
(2) **Phacoemulsification**
(3) **I/A**

If you detect or suspect the zonular lysis under phacoemulsification, then continue with as little stress on the zonules as possible. Do not press with the phaco tip on the nucleus because pressure on the capsular bag increases the zonular lysis. Reduce also the height of the bottle as much as possible.

Tips and tricks:

If you have already implanted CTR before cortex removal, then try to remove the cortex by pulling cortex tangentially and not pulling centrally.

(4) **Implantation of capsular tension ring.**
(5) **Implantation of IOL in capsular bag.**

Two possible timings for implantation of capsular tension ring: (1) As soon as you notice the zonular lysis. The advantage is a stable capsular bag. The disadvantage of an early implantation is that the cortex is difficult to remove because the capsular tension ring presses against the cortex. (2) After removal of the cortex. Advantage: Easy removal of cortex (Fig. 14.6). We recommend to wait as long as possible with implantation of capsular tension ring. Inflate the capsular bag with viscoelastics (Viscoat®). Inject the capsular tension ring with an injector (Figs. 14.7 and 14.8). Be cautious that you place the tip in the capsular bag and not in the sulcus. If you have placed the CTR in the bag, the folds in posterior capsule starts flattening as the bag gets stretched.

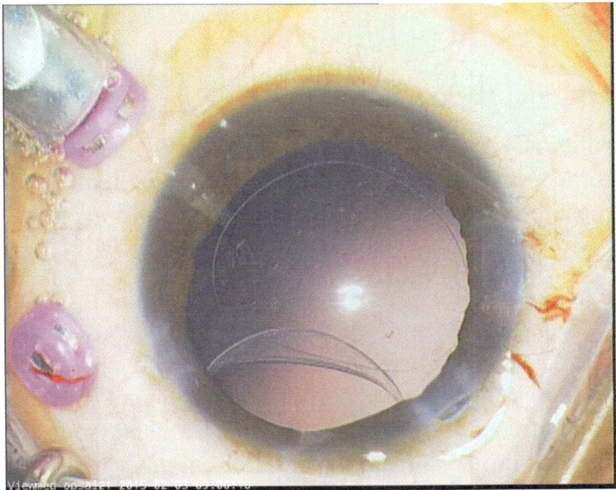

Fig. 14.6 Traumatic cataract with 1 quadrant zonular lysis

Fig. 14.7 Preloaded capsular tension ring in action

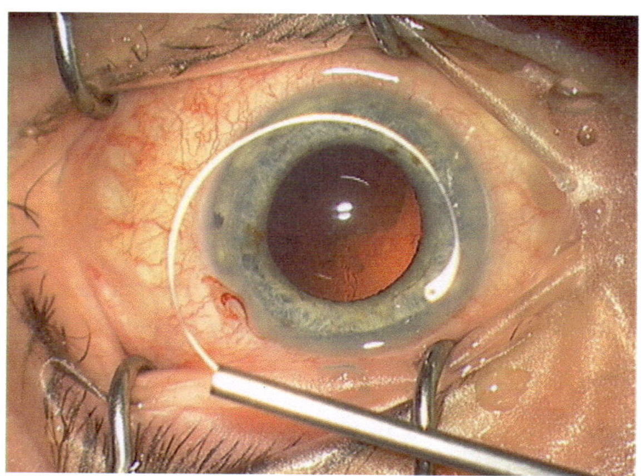

Fig. 14.8 After implantation of the capsular tension ring and the IOL, the lens capsule is fully inflated and a vitreous prolapse is impossible

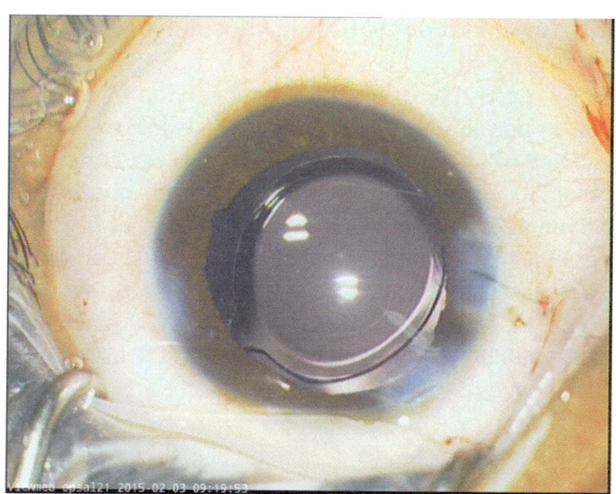

Tips and tricks:

Alternatively, you can implant the IOL so that one haptic presses against the zonular lysis and thereby fully inflating the lens capsule. It is important that the lens capsule is completely inflated in order to prevent vitreous prolapse.

(6) Maybe Anterior Vitrectomy

During cataract surgery, a peripheral vitreous prolapse may occur secondary to a zonular lysis. There is no posterior capsular rent (PCR) present. The vitreous prolapses through the area of zonular defect into the anterior chamber (Fig. 14.9). This vitreous prolapse can only be removed from pars plana (Fig. 14.9b). Stain the vitreous prolapse from the anterior chamber with triamcinolone to assess the extent of vitreous prolapse (video available).

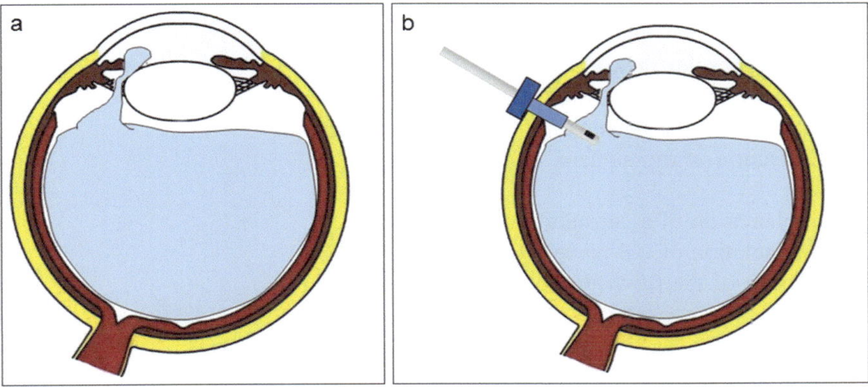

Fig. 14.9 **a** Vitreous prolapse secondary to zonular lysis. **b** The vitreous can only be removed from pars plana

14.3   Zonular Lysis of 1–2 Quadrants

If the nucleus is medium hard, then try to remove the nucleus with phacoemulsification. If the nucleus is, however, hard, then the risk is high that the complete lens with capsule drops into the vitreous cavity. Why? Because phacoemulsification causes additional stress on the zonules and may result in a dropped nucleus. In addition, if you increase the zonular lysis during phacoemulsification, then an in-the-bag implantation may not be possible. This technique can only be recommended, if a retinal backup is available.

Technically much easier and less risk full is a SICS (modified ECCE). The nucleus is luxated from the lens capsule and placed onto the iris and then extracted through a scleral incision. This technique causes minimal stress on the zonules and an IOL in-the-bag implantation is possible in most cases.

Instruments.

1. Calliper.
2. 15° knife.
3. 2.4 mm tunnel knife.
4. Crescent bevel-up knife.
5. Lens extraction hook (Geuder No: 32034, Germany); *alternative:* serrated lens loop.

Material.

(1)   Iris retractors
(2)   Capsular tension ring.
(3)   3-piece IOL or PMMA IOL.

Individual steps.

(1) Large capsular rhexis.
(2) Frown incision.
(3) Luxation of the nucleus into the anterior chamber.
(4) Extraction of the nucleus.
(5) I/A.
(6) Implantation of a capsular tension ring.
(7) Implantation of a 3-piece IOL.
(8) Closure of the frown incision and conjunctiva.

The surgery step by step:

1. Large capsular rhexis.
2. Frown incision.

In case of a small pupil insert iris hooks in order to obtain a large rhexis. Perform a large circular rhexis. If the lens capsule is very unstable, you can insert now the iris hooks into the rhexis margin (Fig. 14.10). Continue with the frown incision. Perform a limbal peritomy from 11 to 1 o'clock with Westcott scissors and cauterize the bleeding vessels. Then, mark an 8 mm wide incision with a calliper. The incision should be 1–1.5 mm behind the limbus. Continue with a frown incision with a 15° knife (50% scleral thickness). Then, dissect a scleral tunnel with the crescent angled bevel-up knife (Fig. 14.11).

3. Luxation of the nucleus into the anterior chamber.
4. Extraction of the nucleus.

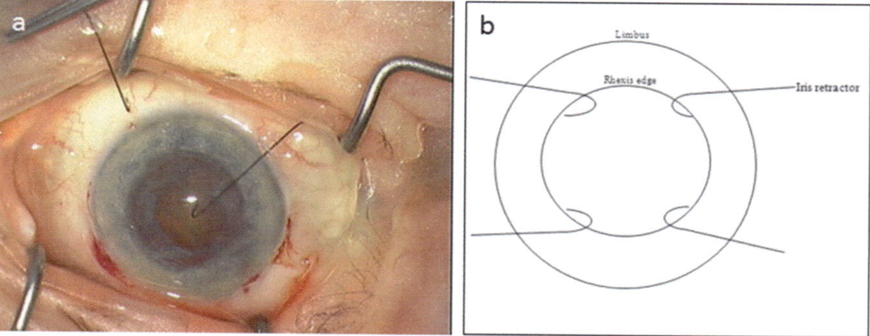

Fig. 14.10 (a) Iris hooks are placed in the rhexis edge. (b) Drawing of the implantation of iris hooks in the rhexis edge in case of a zonular lysis

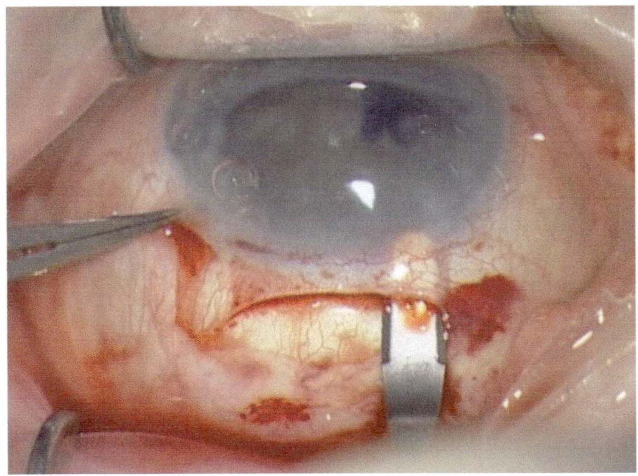

Fig. 14.11 Dissect a scleral flap for the frown incision. The incision is 8 mm wide

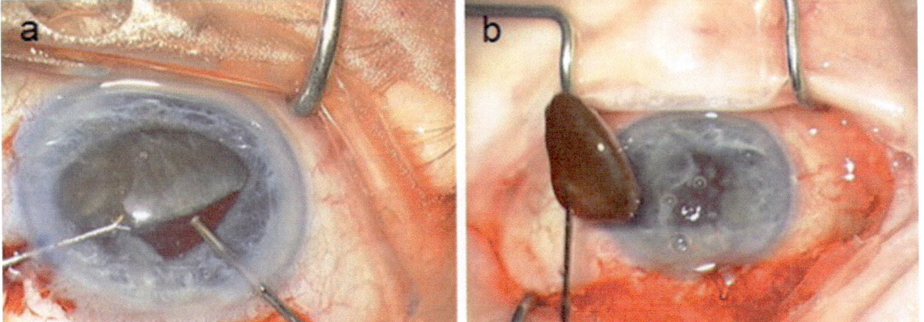

Fig. 14.12 (**a**) Elevate the nucleus with a nucleus manipulator (y-hook) and inject at once viscoelastic between nucleus and posterior lens capsule. **b** Extract the nucleus with a fish hook or a lens loop

Continue by luxating the nucleus bimanually with 2 manipulators (e.g. push–pull or Rosen chopper and viscoelastics cannula) into the anterior chamber (Fig. 14.12). Then use the lens extraction hook or a lens loop. Proceed by placing the tip of the vectis (lens hook, lens loop) behind the centre of the nucleus and then extract the nucleus with the lens hook (Fig. 14.12). If the nucleus gets stuck in the main incision, you have to extend it. After removal of the nucleus, you can express residual cortical material with viscoexpression.

5. I/A
6. Implantation of a capsular tension ring
7. Implantation of an iris-fixated IOL.

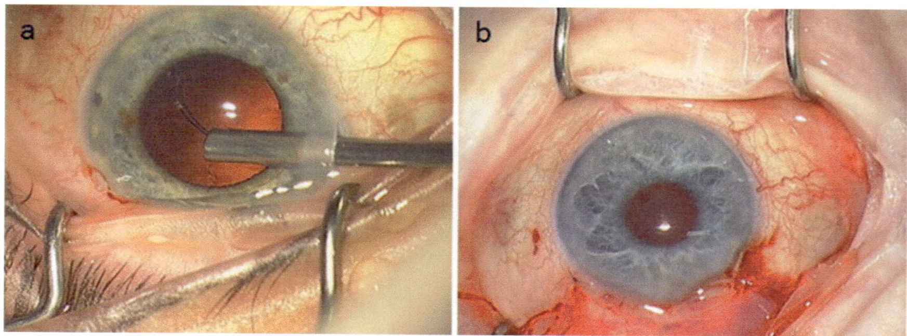

Fig. 14.13 (**a**) Inject a capsular tension ring to inflate the lens capsule and to prevent vitreous prolapsed. (**b**) Implant a 3-piece IOL or a PMMA IOL

Then continue with I/A and remove the cortex. This manoeuvre is of course difficult due to zonular lysis. Implant therefore at once or after I/A a capsular tension ring (Fig. 14.13). I recommend getting acquainted with the capsular tension ring before using it the first time. Then implant an IOL with or without injector into the lens capsule (Fig. 14.13).

Tips & tricks.

In case of zonular lysis, it is important to implant the IOL into the lens capsule and not into the sulcus because the IOL will luxate into the vitreous cavity if positioned in the sulcus.

Fig. 14.14 If the lens capsule is too unstable, then extract it with serrated jaws forceps (Alcon or Dorc)

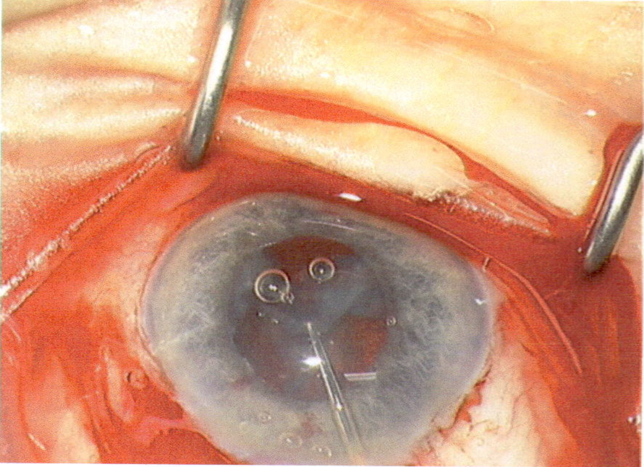

8. Closure of Frown Incision and Conjunctiva

Suture the frown incision with a Vicryl 8–0 cross-stitch and the conjunctiva with one Vicryl 8–0 interrupted stitch. Inject cefuroxime (Zinacef®) intracameral as endophthalmitis prophylaxis.

Tips & tricks.

Removal of lens capsule: In case of completely unstable lens capsule remove the lens capsule with forceps, for example a 20G or 23G serrated jaws forceps (Fig. 14.14). Now you have to implant a scleral or iris-fixated IOL.

14.4   Zonular Lysis of 2–3 Quadrants: ICCE

If 3 quadrants are affected, then it is advisable to remove the nucleus and the lens capsule with an ICCE procedure. The surgery is identical to the nucleus removal surgery in the previous chapter (SICS procedure). The only difference is that the frown incision is larger. A 9–10 mm frown incision is required. For the extraction of the nucleus, we recommend a serrated lens loop and not a fish hook because the nucleus is very unstable.

The surgery step by step:

1. **Insertion of 1–2 trocar cannulas**
2. **9–10 mm frown incision**

Start with insertion of 1–2trocar cannulas on the temporal side. Then continue with a limbal peritomy from 11 to 1 o′clock and then create a 9–10 mm scleral incision. For an ICCE, a large frown incision is required.

3. **Extraction of the nucleus**

Inject viscoelastics into the anterior chamber. Insert the vitreous cutter through the trocar cannula and elevate the nucleus at 12 o′clock. Then insert the serrated lens loop and place it behind the nucleus. Then extract the nucleus. The nucleus is removed together with the lens capsule in order to avoid loss of cortical fragments.

4. **Anterior vitrectomy**

Inspect the scleral incision for a vitreous prolapse and remove it with a Vannas scissors. Continue with an anterior vitrectomy from pars plana. The anterior vitreous can be visualized more easily with triamcinolone staining. The globe may be unstable due to the large frown incision. In this case, it is advisable to close the frown incision with a Vicryl 8–0 X-suture before continuing with anterior vitrectomy. Check with the index finger if the globe has normal tension.

5. **IOL implantation**

In case of a traumatic nucleus removal, we recommend a delayed IOL implantation. Otherwise, continue with a secondary IOL implantation. See chapter "Secondary IOL implantation techniques".

6. **Closure of frown incision with two X-sutures**

Close the frown incision with two Vicryl 8–0 X-sutures.

Summary: A large zonular lysis with hard nucleus is the most challenging case in cataract surgery. If you do not have retinal backup, then avoid a phacoemulsification. A phacoemulsification is very risk full. Extract the nucleus with SICS (modified ECCE), implant a capsular tension ring and implant the IOL inside the lens capsule. If the capsular support is too weak for an IOL implantation, it is advisable to remove the nucleus with the lens capsule (ICCE).

IOL Extraction Techniques, Iris Capture and Capsular Phimosis

All videos of this part be found in a playlist of my YouTube channel:
https://www.youtube.com/playlist?list=PL0dKYclPD7yMJRuQAIt9Dr7pOtuI0
Seex

Part V: IOL exchange
Part V: IOL refolding
Part V: IOL rolling
Part V: Bi-section of silicone IOL
Part V: iris capture

Extraction of an Acrylic IOL Through Cutting of IOL

15

Abstract

This chapter describes step-by-step the extraction of an acrylic IOL through cutting of IOL.

Keyword

IOL extraction

A delayed intraocular lens exchange is easier one month after surgery because the anterior and posterior capsule can be easily separated. This separation becomes more difficult with time but even one year an IOL extraction is possible. The most crucial point is the mobilization of the haptics. After one year, it may be surgically easier to cut the haptics with scissors and leave them in the lens capsule.

The surgical trick is to lift up the anterior rhexis with a 27G cannula and inject viscoelastics. Then you can continue with a regular viscoelastics cannula.

An alternative to an IOL extraction is the implantation of a piggy back IOL (addOn IOL from 1stQ, Germany). (video available)

Instruments

1. 15° paracentesis knife
2. 2.4 mm tunnel incision knife
3. Maybe: Iris spatula
4. Push–pull instrument or Sinskey hook (Fig. 15.1)
5. Capsulotomy scissors (Fig. 15.2)

Individual steps

(1) Paracentesis
(2) Injection of viscoelastic in capsular bag
(3) Mobilization of IOL

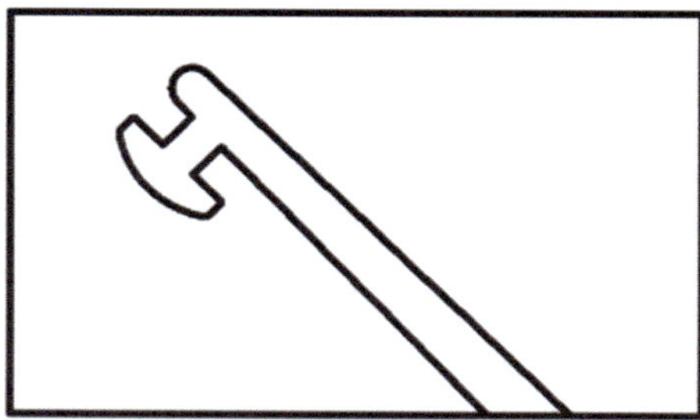

Fig. 15.1 Push–pull instrument, alternative Sinskey hook. Indication: Manipulator of nucleus, iris and IOL (Geuder 16175)

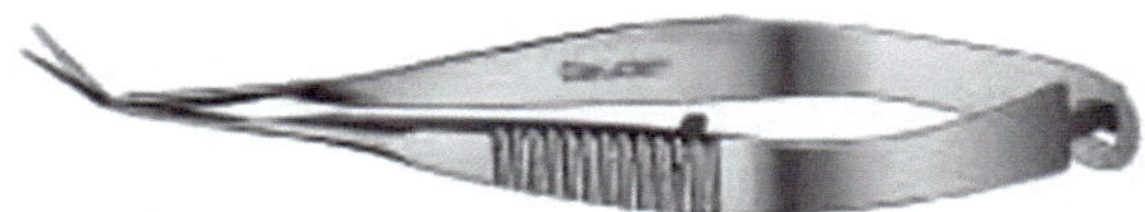

Fig. 15.2 Capsulotomy scissors. Indication: Cutting of an IOL (Geuder 19776)

(4) Rotation of IOL on iris
(5) Cutting of IOL
(6) Extraction of IOL
(7) Implantation of IOL

The surgery step by step

(1) Paracentesis

(2) Injection of viscoelastic in capsular bag

(3) Mobilization of IOL

Begin with a paracentesis at 10 o'clock and 2 o'clock and a main incision at 9 o'clock. Inject viscoelastic into the anterior chamber. Then inject viscoelastic between the anterior capsule and the IOL. This has to be done 360° (Figs. 15.3 and 15.4). Try cautiously to loosen the haptic with a push–pull manipulator or an iris spatula (Fig. 15.5). This manoeuvre is difficult at the haptics.

(4) Rotation of IOL on iris

(5) Cutting of IOL

If the IOL is mobilized, then rotate it outside the capsular bag (Fig. 15.6). Then luxate it with a rotational movement onto the iris (Fig. 15.7). The next step is the cutting of the IOL (Figs. 15.8, 15.9 and 15.10). Do not cut the IOL completely; leave 1–2 mm at the edge. Important regarding the cutting is that you begin to cut LEFT to the haptic (not right) (Fig. 15.11). From there, you cut the optic into two halves but leave 1–2 mm at the end.

Fig. 15.3 Preoperative status. A highly myopic patient, who was dissatisfied with his postoperative refraction of +1.0D

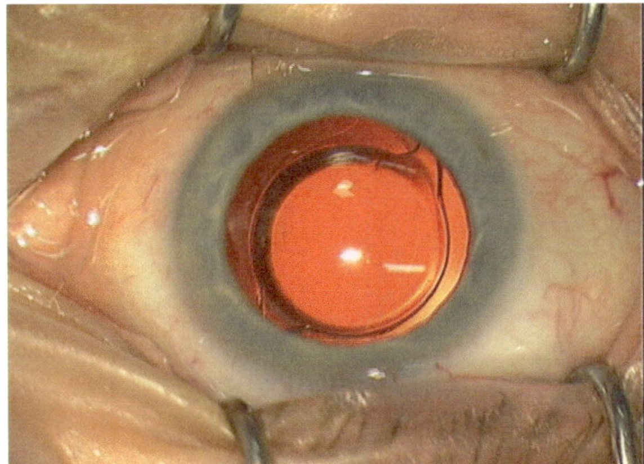

Fig. 15.4 Place the tip of the viscoelastic cannula between the anterior lens capsule and the IOL and inject viscoelastics in order to inflate the lens capsule

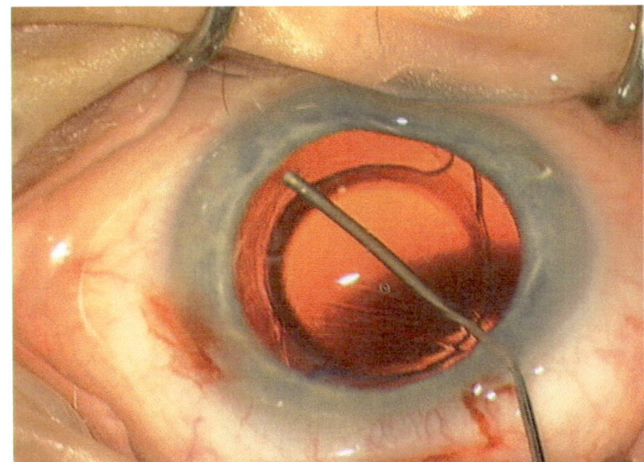

Fig. 15.5 Separate also the haptic from the lens capsule

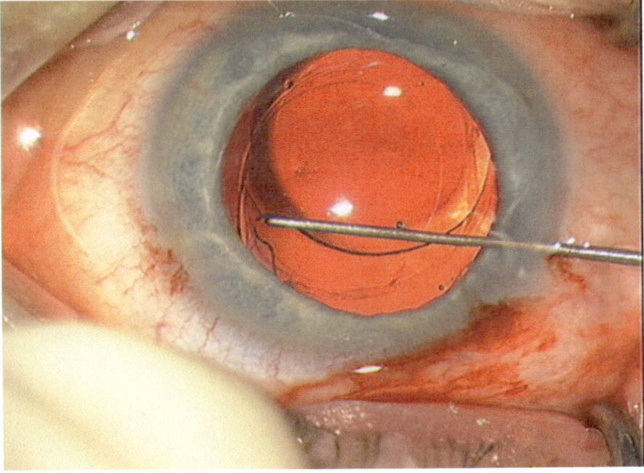

Fig. 15.6 Rotate the IOL out of the capsular bag with help of the push–pull. Inject viscoelastics behind the IOL to avoid a posterior capsular defect

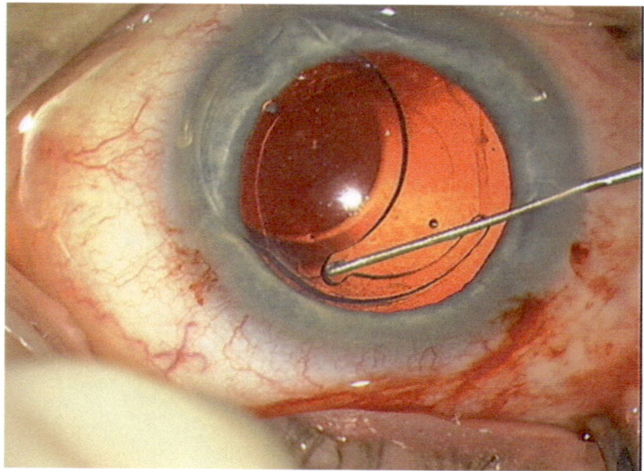

Fig. 15.7 Rotate a haptic towards the main incision

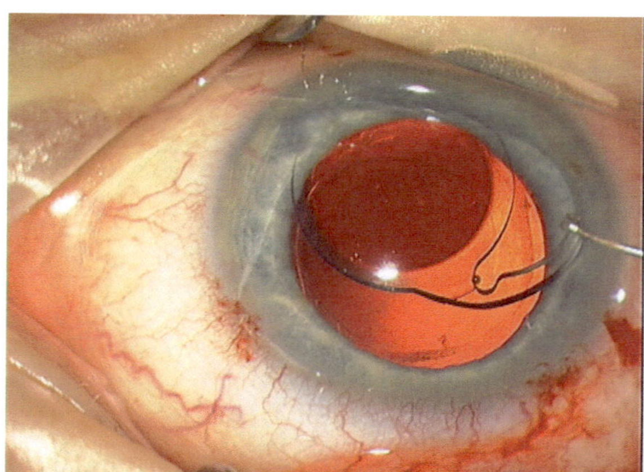

Fig. 15.8 Cut the IOL with the capsulotomy scissors

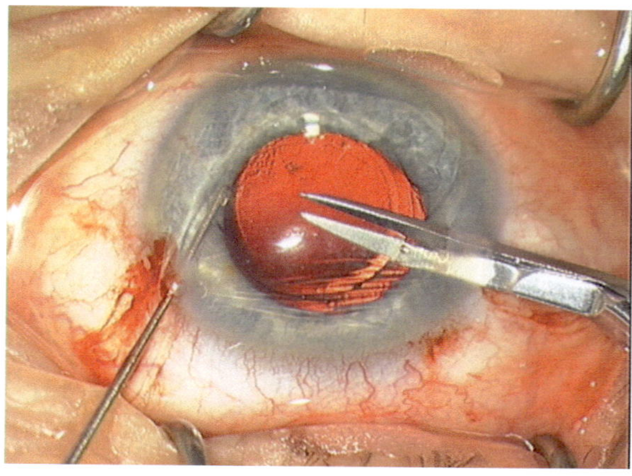

Fig. 15.9 Drawing how the IOL has to be cut. It is important to start the cutting on the left side (and not the right side) of the haptic

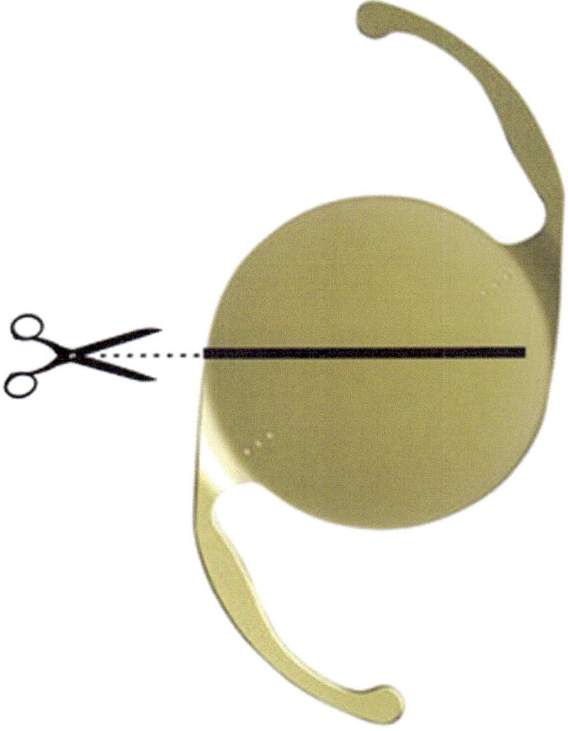

Fig. 15.10 If necessary, stabilize the IOL to avoid a damage of the endothelium

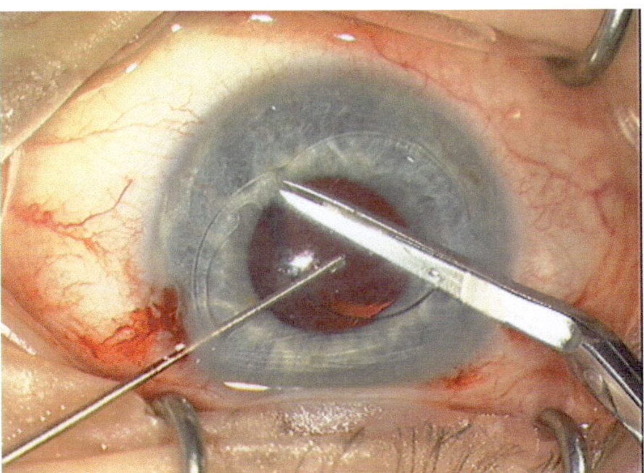

Fig. 15.11 Cut only 90% of the IOL. Then grasp the haptic with a surgical forceps

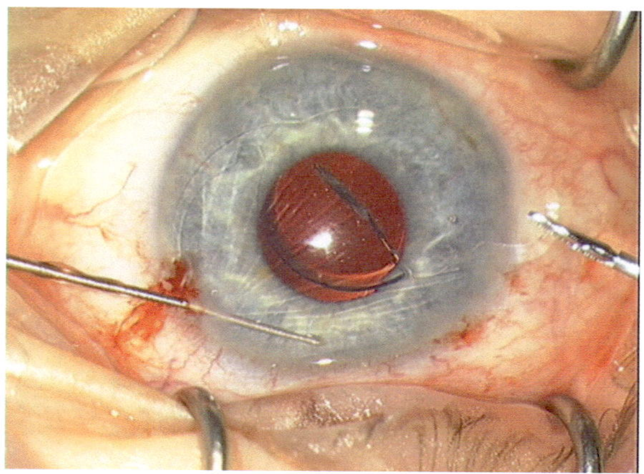

Fig. 15.12 Extract the first half of the IOL

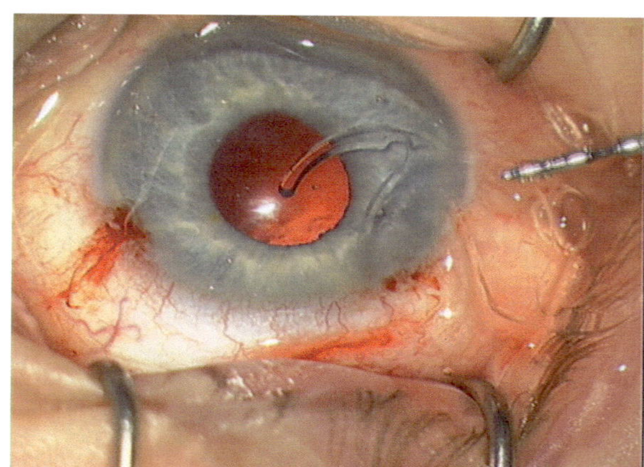

Fig. 15.13 Then extract the second half of the IOL

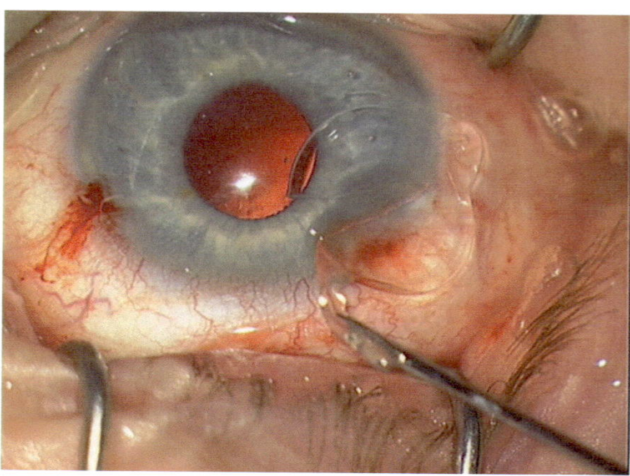

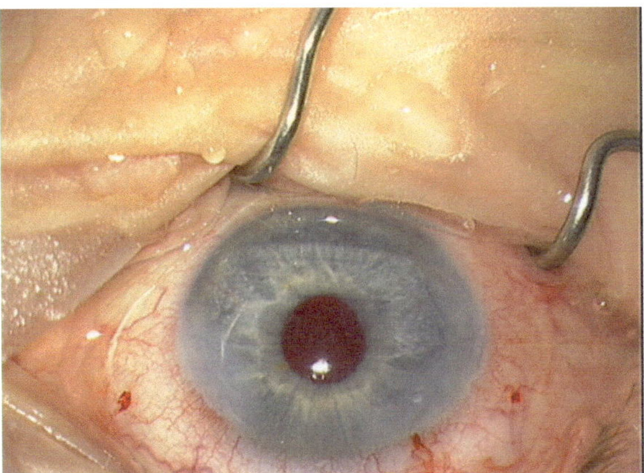

Fig. 15.14 Implant the new IOL into the bag

(6) Extraction of IOL

(7) Implantation of IOL

Draw the haptic through the main incision and then extract the first half of the optic, the second half of the optic follows automatically (Figs. 15.12 and 15.13). Implant finally the IOL and inject cefuroxime as endophthalmitis prophylaxis (Fig. 15.14).

Remark: The IOL extraction is easier if you cut the IOL in four quadrants.

Extraction of an Acrylic IOL Through IOL Refolding

16

Abstract

This chapter describes step-by-step the extraction of an IOL through refolding of the IOL.

Keywords

IOL extraction · IOL refolding

There are many reasons why an intraocular lens need to be explanted, e.g. damaged IOL or haptic after implantation, wrong IOL power, late optic calcification or other opacities, etc. PMMA IOL explantation requires large incision, but foldable IOL could be removed through small incision. For acrylic IOL, intraocular refolding is a good technique. Surgery lasts about 10–15 min and is performed in topical, local or general anaesthesia. (Video available)

Instruments

1. Viscoelastics
2. 15° knife
3. 3.0–3.2 mm phaco knife
4. Sinskey hook (push–pull)
5. Iris spatula
6. IOL implantation forceps (e.g. Geuder 31962)

Individual steps

1. Creating main incision and injection of OVD
2. Two side port incisions 80–90° from main incision
3. Small side port incision exactly 180° to main incision
4. Mobilization of IOL
5. Placing iris spatula under IOL and IOL implantation forceps over IOL optic

© The Author(s), under exclusive license to Springer Nature Switzerland AG 2022

U. Spandau and G. B. Scharioth, *Complications During and After Cataract Surgery*,

https://doi.org/10.1007/978-3-030-93531-3_16

6. Refolding of IOL
7. Explantation of IOL
8. Remove OVD and suture main incision if needed

The operation step by step

1. Creating main incision and injection of OVD
2. Two side port incisions 80–90° from main incision
3. Small side port incision exactly 180° to main incision

After creating the main incision, anterior camber is filled with OVD. Then two side port incisions are created 80–90° away from main incision. An additional small side port incision is created opposite to the main incision exactly at 180°.

4. Mobilization of IOL
5. Placing iris spatula under IOL and IOL implantation forceps over IOL optic
6. Refolding of IOL
7. Explantation of IOL

IOL is gently mobilized from capsular bag. Sometimes, this requires additional injection of OVD between the anterior and posterior capsule. Then place some additional OVD behind the IOL optic. Iris spatula is introduced through the opposite side port incision and placed behind the IOL. The implantation forceps is positioned on top of the IOL, and both instruments are pressed against each other (Fig. 16.1). The IOL starts to refold. After complete folding (Fig. 16.2), the forceps is released a bit to reduce friction, and the spatula is removed (Fig. 16.3). Now, implantation forceps is pressed again to fold the IOL completely. While turning the folded IOL 90°, it is explanted. It is important to ensure that anterior chamber stays deep and that is sufficiently filled with OVD to prevent contact to corneal endothelium while IOL is refolded and explanted. Explantation might need some pulling forces as the main incision is relatively tight for a refolded IOL with 6 mm optic diameter. If indicated now, a new IOL is implanted.

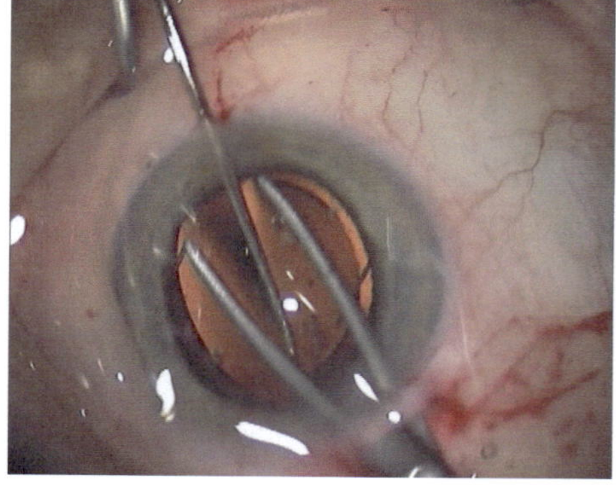

Fig. 16.1 Iris spatula is placed behind the IOL optic, and IOL implantation forceps is placed on top of the IOL, note both instruments are inserted from opposite incisions

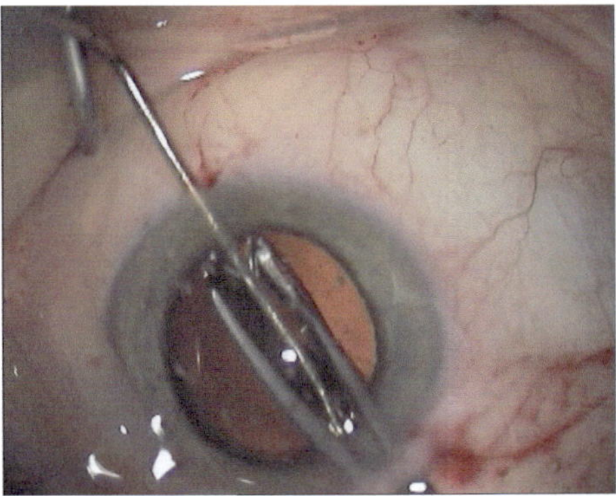

Fig. 16.2 IOL is intraocular refolded with pressure and counterpressure of both instruments

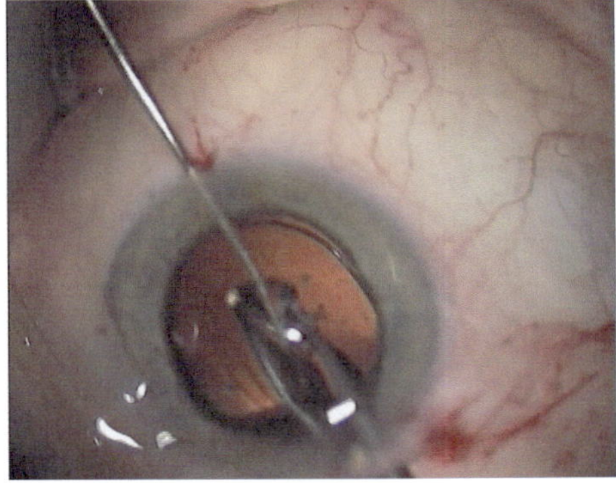

Fig. 16.3 Iris spatula is removed from behind the IOL, note IOL is turned 90° while explanted

8. Remove OVD and suture main incision if needed

Finally, OVD is removed from the anterior chamber, and incisions are hydrated and checked for leakage. They can be sutured if needed with 10/0 nylon.

Abstract

This chapter shows step-by-step the extraction of an IOL through Bi-secting of IOL.

Keywords

IOL extraction · Bi-secting of IOL

There are many reasons why an intraocular silicone lens needs to be explanted, e.g. damaged IOL or haptic after implantation, wrong IOL power, late optic calcification or persistent silicone oil adherence after vitreoretinal surgery, etc. Most techniques for explantation of silicone IOL are very difficult to perform because the silicone material is very slippery. We therefore favour IOL bi-secting technique. Surgery lasts about 10–15 min and is performed in topical, local or general anaesthesia (Video available).

Instruments

1. OVD
2. 15 deg knife
3. 3.0–3.2 main incision knife
4. Silicone lens bi-sector (e.g. G-32800 Geuder, Germany) (Fig. 17.1)
5. Sinskey hook
6. Suturing forceps (e.g. Castroviejo forceps).

Individual steps

1. Creating main incision and side port incision, injection of OVD
2. IOL mobilization
3. Haptics removal

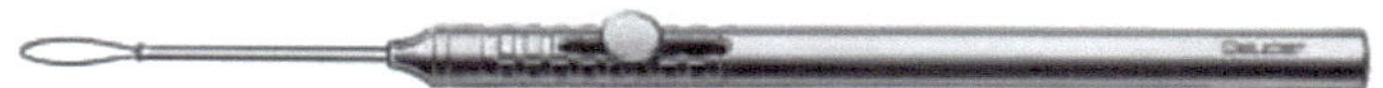

Fig. 17.1 Silicone lens bi-sector. Indication: for dividing implanted silicone lenses. Geuder, 32800

4. Placing the wire loop of the bi-sector around the IOL optic
5. Bi-secting the IOL
6. Explantation of the two IOL halves
7. Remove OVD.

The operation step by step:

1. Creating main incision and side port incision, injection of OVD
2. IOL mobilization
3. Haptics removal

After creating the main incision, anterior camber is filled with OVD (Figs. 17.2 and 17.3). Then two side port incisions are created 80–90° away from main incision. IOL is gently mobilized from capsular bag. Sometimes, this requires additional injection of OVD between the anterior and posterior capsule (Fig. 17.4). Then place some additional OVD behind the IOL optic. We prefer to cut the IOL haptic in case of a three-piece silicone IOL (Fig. 17.5). This could be done with a 20G endoscissors. Haptics are removed.

4. Placing the wire loop of the bi-sector around the IOL optic
5. Bi-secting the IOL

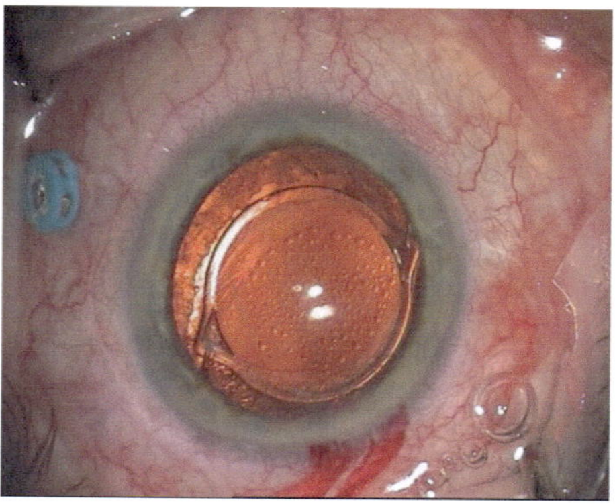

Fig. 17.2 Silicone IOL (SI60, AMO, USA) with massive silicone oil adherence after multiple vitreoretinal surgeries; several attempts to clean the IOL (e.g. with solvent solution F_6H_6, Fluoron, Germany) were unsuccessful

Fig. 17.3 Injection of OVD through main incision

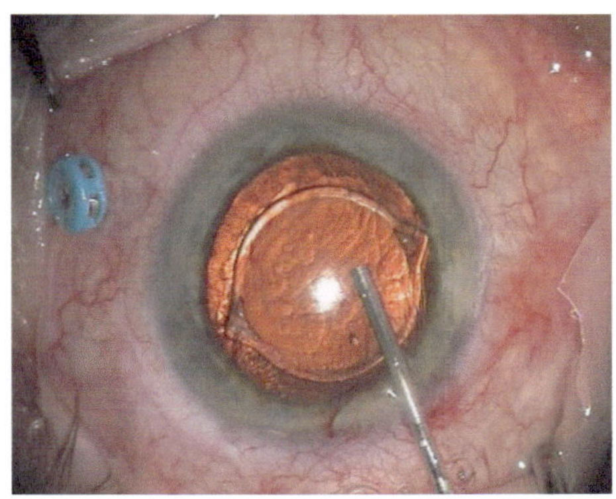

Fig. 17.4 IOL mobilization from capsular bag; haptic is placed on the anterior iris surface

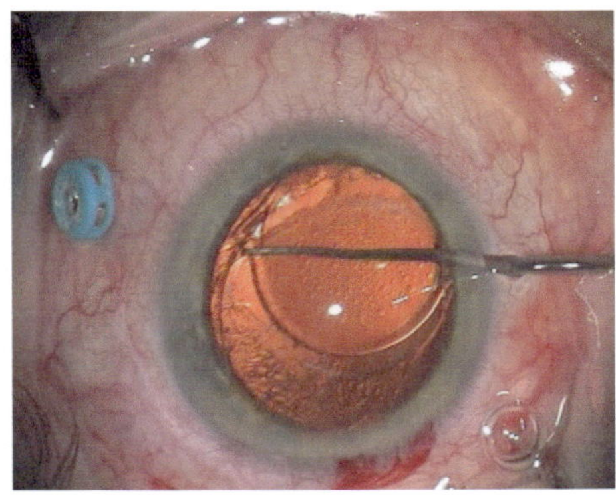

Fig. 17.5 IOL haptic is cut with a 20G endoscissors; second instrument is a curved Scharioth forceps (DORC, The Netherlands)

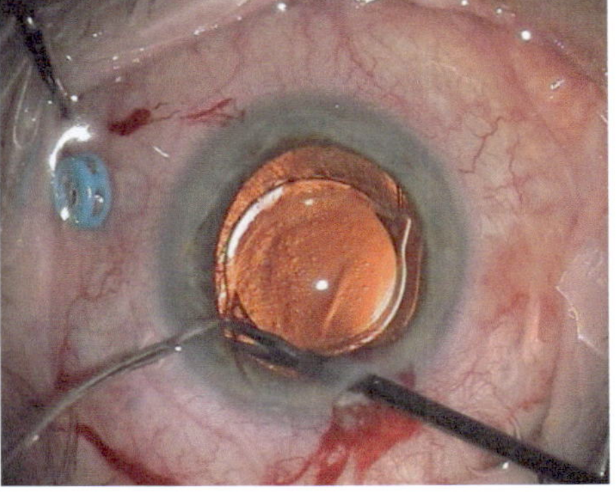

Fig. 17.6 IOL is slightly decentred, and wire loop of the bi-sector is placed over the IOL optic; second instrument is used to manipulate the IOL

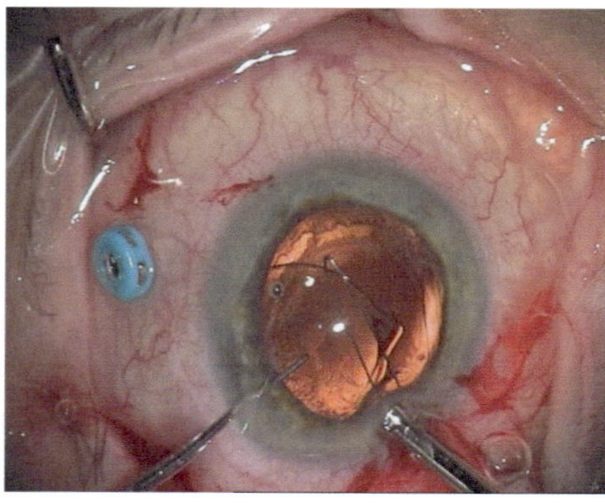

Fig. 17.7 IOL is recentered; wire loop is placed exactly over the middle of the optic

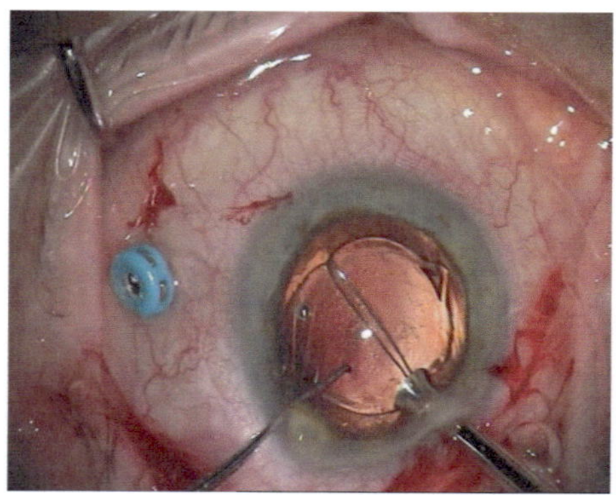

The bi-sector is inserted through the main incision, and the wire loop is externalized from the device (Fig. 17.6). IOL is gently decentred, and the wire loop is placed around the optic (Fig. 17.7). Sudden movement of the IOL pieces during bi-section could cause corneal endothelium damage. We place therefore a second instrument on top of the IOL optic (Fig. 17.8). While the wire loop is pulled back into the bi-sector, the optic is cut into two halves (Fig. 17.9). Bi-sector and Sinskey hook are removed.

6. Explantation of the two IOL halves
7. Remove OVD

IOL pieces are grasped with a toothed forceps (e.g. fine colibri forceps) and explanted (Figs. 17.10 and 17.11). If indicated now, a new IOL is implanted. Finally, OVD is removed from the anterior chamber, and incisions are hydrated and checked for leakage. They can be sutured if needed with 10–0 nylon.

Fig. 17.8 Wire loop of the bi-sector is pulled backwards; before the optic is cut, the IOL starts to fold; note second instrument is placed over the IOL to prevent uncontrolled movements of the IOL pieces

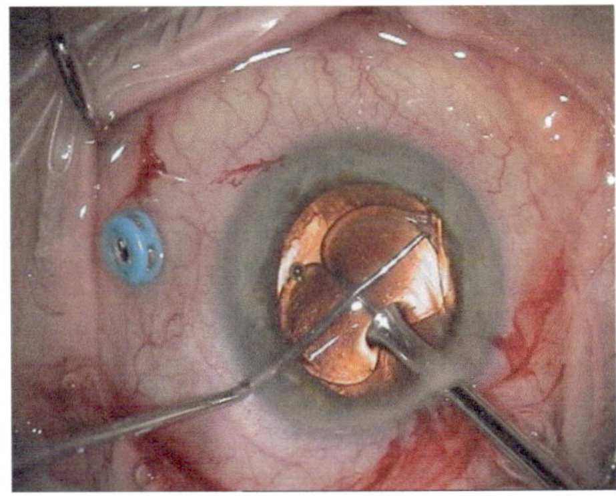

Fig. 17.9 IOL bi-section is completed, and wire loop is completely retracted; note the clear cut through the IOL optic

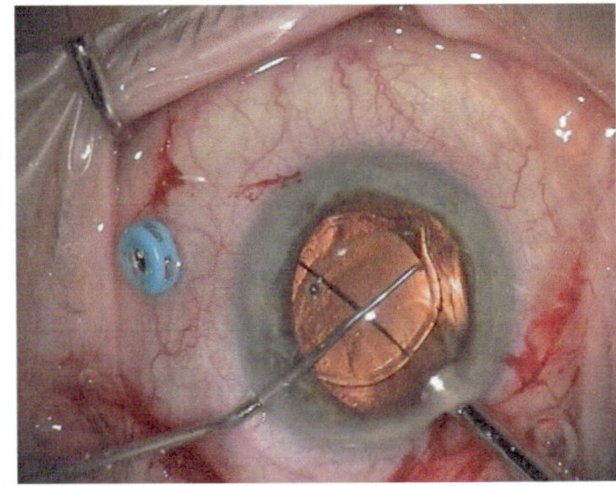

Fig. 17.10 First IOL piece is grasped with a toothed forceps and explanted

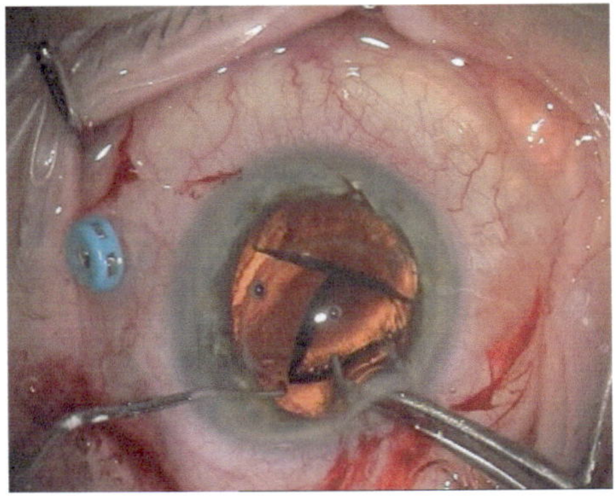

Fig. 17.11 Second IOL piece is grasped and removed

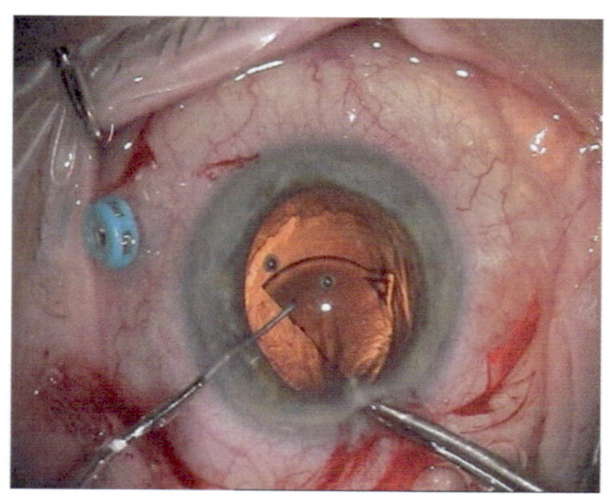

IOL Explantation with Intraocular Rolling

Abstract

This chapter shows step-by-step the extraction of an IOL though intraocular rolling. This technique is ingenious and simple.

Keywords

IOL extraction · Intraocular rolling · IOL rolling

Instruments

1. Tying forceps
2. Intraocular spatula
3. Sinskey hook
4. 15°knife
5. 2.8 mm main incision knife
6. OVD (e.g. HPMC 2.4%, Healon)

Individual steps

1. Paracentesis, main incision
2. Filling anterior chamber with OVD
3. Positioning of IOL into anterior chamber and externalization of one haptic
4. Insertion of spatula and grasping IOL with tying forceps
5. IOL rolling under the spatula
6. Explantation of rolled IOL

© The Author(s), under exclusive license to Springer Nature Switzerland AG 2022

187

U. Spandau and G. B. Scharioth, *Complications During and After Cataract Surgery*,
https://doi.org/10.1007/978-3-030-93531-3_18

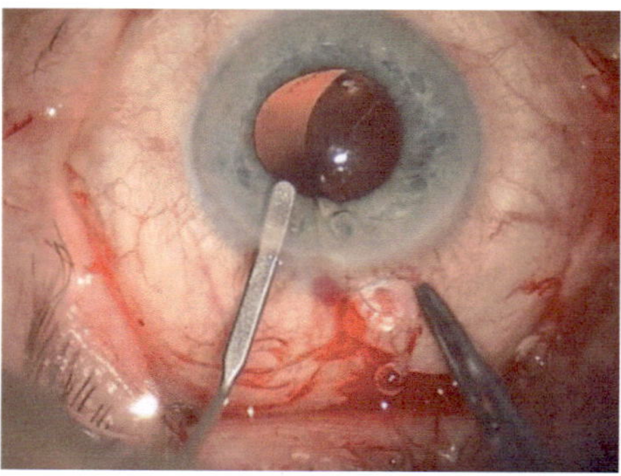

Fig. 18.1 IOL is positioned in anterior chamber, and one haptic is externalized; note spatula is inserted through paracentesis, and there is only a small distance between paracentesis and main incision

Fig. 18.2 IOL is grasped at optic side with tying forceps and surgical hand in maximum supination

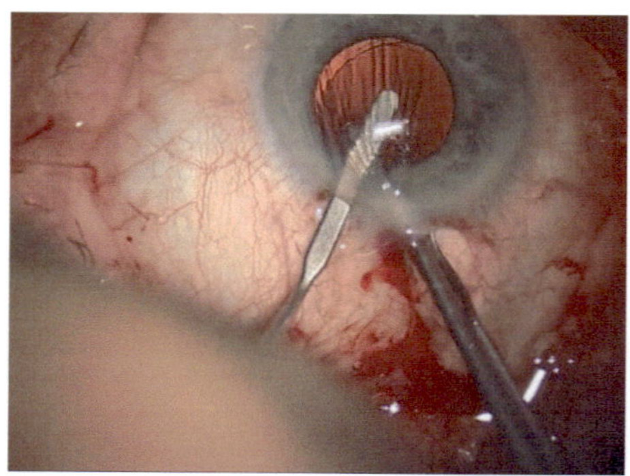

The Operation Step by Step (Figs. 18.1, 18.2, 18.3, 18.4, 18.5, 18.6, 18.7 and 18.8)

1. Paracentesis, main incision
2. Filling of anterior chamber with OVD and positioning of IOL into anterior chamber. Externalization of one haptic
3. Insertion of spatula through paracentesis and grasping the IOL optic with tying forceps near the edge. The operating hand must be in maximum supination. Try to perform this rotational manoeuvre dry before using it intraoperative
4. Now, IOL is rolled under the spatula while the hand is rotated almost 360°.
5. The rolled IOL is explanted through main incision.

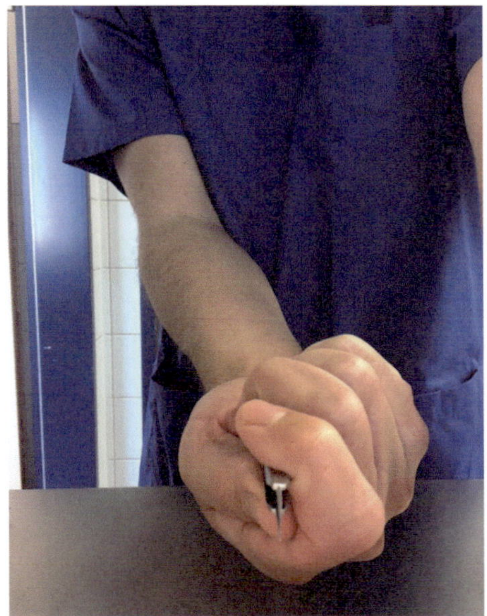

Fig. 18.3 Surgical hand in maximum supination

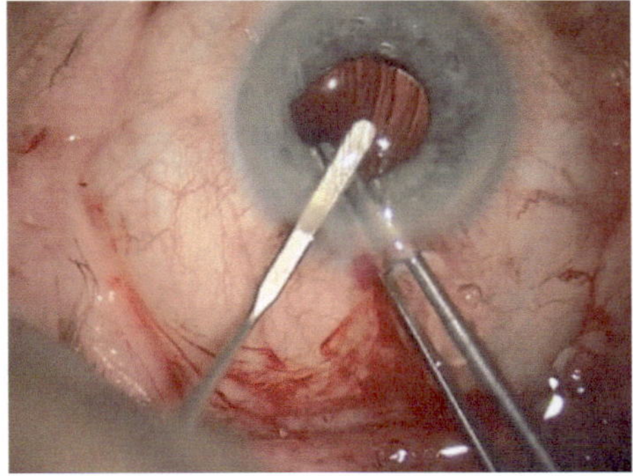

Fig. 18.4 While rotating the surgical hand, the IOL is rolled under the spatula

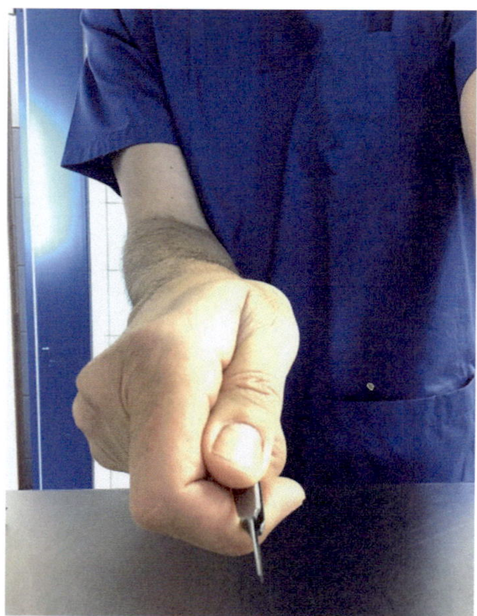

Fig. 18.5 Surgical hand in neutral position after 180° rotation

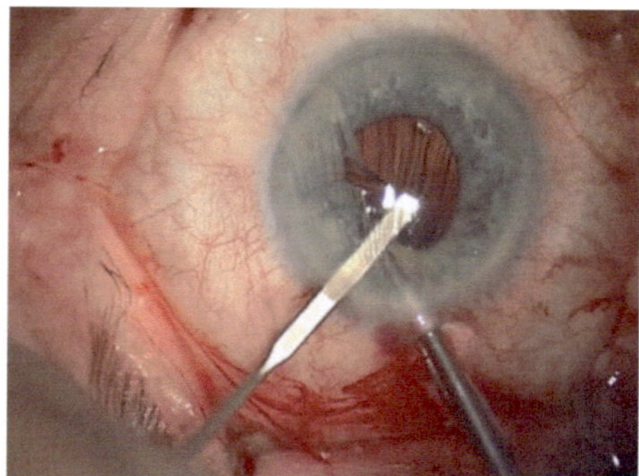

Fig. 18.6 IOL is rolled up completely

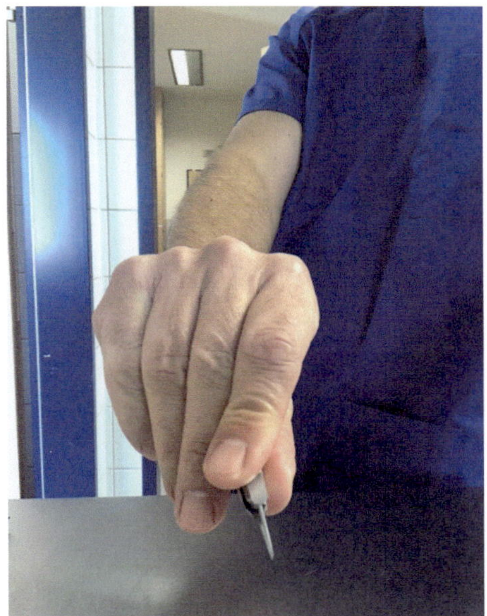

Fig. 18.7 Surgical hand after another 180° rotation in maximum pronation

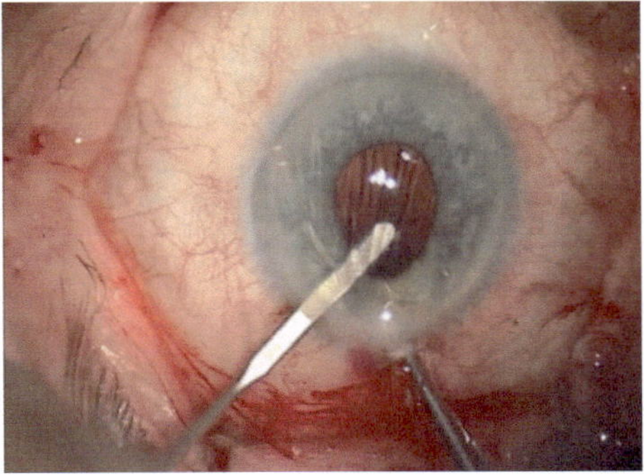

Fig. 18.8 Rolled IOL is explanted through main incision

Iris Capture by the IOL Optic

19

Abstract

This chapter explains step-by-step the surgical management of an iris capture of the IOL optic.

Keywords

Iris capture · Surgery · IOL capture

Figs. 19.1, 19.2, 19.3, 19.4 and 19.5.

An iris capture by the IOL optic causes a reduced mobility of the iris and pupil, dislocation of the IOL and may cause intraocular inflammation. We recommend removing an iris capture.

Instruments

1. Intravitreal scissors (Fig. 19.1), alternatively capsulotomy scissors (Fig. 19.2)
2. Maybe: Iris spatula.

Individual steps

(1) Removal of posterior synechiae
(2) Repositioning of IOL

The surgery step by step:

(1) Removal of posterior synechiae
(2) Repositioning of IOL

Inject viscoelastics into the anterior chamber. Try to loosen the posterior synechiae with the viscoelastic cannula or with an iris spatula (Figs. 19.3 and 19.4). If you do

© The Author(s), under exclusive license to Springer Nature Switzerland AG 2022
U. Spandau and G. B. Scharioth, *Complications During and After Cataract Surgery*,
https://doi.org/10.1007/978-3-030-93531-3_19

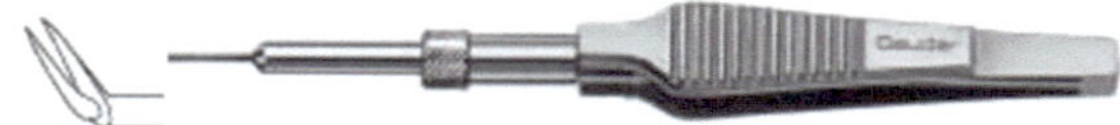

Fig. 19.1 Capsule scissors after Kampik. The instrument fits through a paracentesis. 22 gauge. Indication: Cutting of capsule or iris. Geuder 38,215

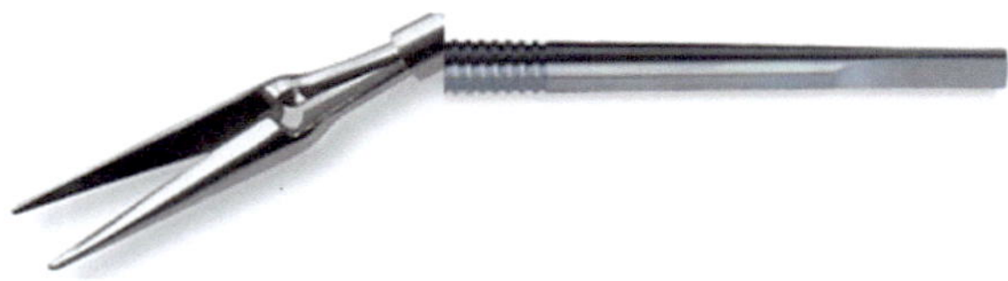

Fig. 19.2 Intravitreal scissors. 23 gauge. Indication: General cutting of tissue. DORC 1286.J06

Fig. 19.3 Long-standing iris capture. The left side of the IOL is located before the iris

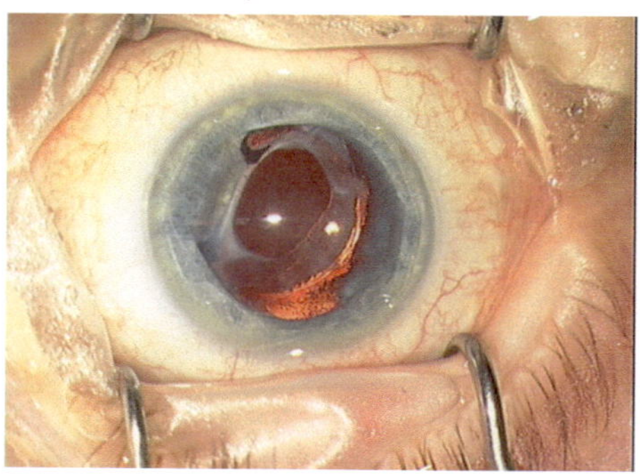

Fig. 19.4 Inject viscoelastics between IOL and iris

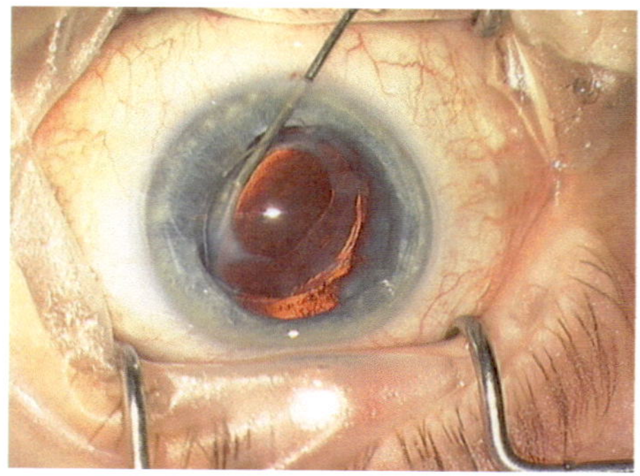

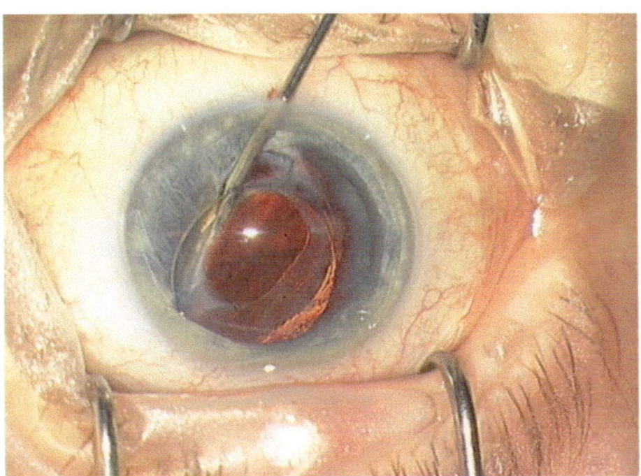

Fig. 19.5 Cut the iridal adhesion with intravitreal scissors, e.g. 23G straight intravitreal scissors. The advantage of intravitreal scissors or the capsule scissors of Kampik is that they fit through a paracentesis. Alternatively, regular capsulotomy scissors can be used but they require a main incision

not succeed, then cut the posterior synechiae as close as possible to the lens capsule with an intravitreal scissors. Constrict the pupil with Miochol to check if all synechiae have been removed (Fig. 19.5).

Pits & Pearls no. 18

If you discover an <u>IOL capture</u> within 1 week after surgery, then perform as follows: Attach a 27G cannula (grey cannula) onto a 2 ml syringe. Place patient behind the slit lamp. Drop topical anaesthesia + povidone iod. Perform a paracentesis and press the optic with the cannula behind the iris.

Peeling of Fibrosis in Capsular Phimosis

20

Abstract

This chapter explains step-by-step the peeling of fibrosis in capsular phimosis.

Keywords

Capsular phimosis · Surgery

Instruments

1. Endoforceps
2. Sinskey hook
3. 15° knife
4. OVD (e.g. HPMC 2.4%, Healon).

Individual steps

1. Paracentesis, main incision
2. Filling anterior chamber with OVD
3. Mobilizing, grasping and removal of fibrosis
4. Additional steps (e.g. aspiration of secondary cataract, ILO exchange).

The Operation Step by Step (Figs. 20.1, 20.2, 20.3, 20.4, 20.5, and 20.6).

1. Paracentesis
2. Filling of anterior chamber with OVD
3. Using an endgripping endoforceps the edge of fibrosis is mobilized and carefully pulled from the capsular bag. One should prevent excessive traction and damage to zonules. If needed, a second instrument could be used to enhance separation and reduce tractional forces to capsular bag and zonules
4. Stiff and strongly attached parts of fibrosis could be excised with endoscissors.

Fig. 20.1 Excessive capsular fibrosis with capsular bag phimosis

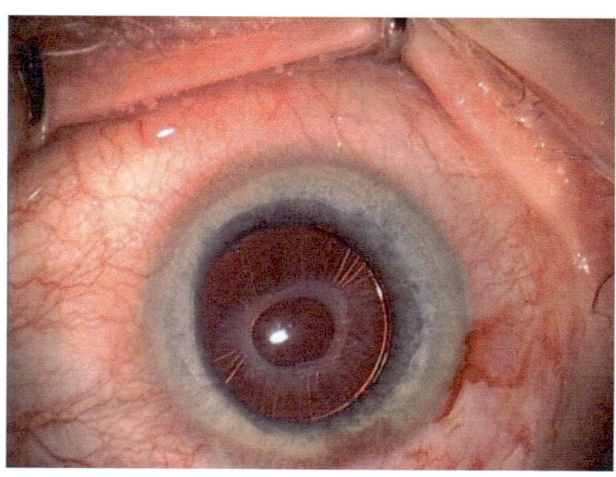

Fig. 20.2 Endgripping forceps is used to mobilize and grasp fibrosed ring

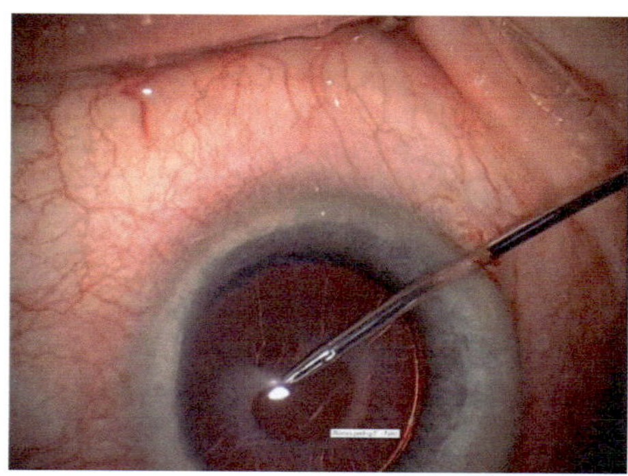

Fig. 20.3 Fibrosed tissue is pulled carefully from capsular bag

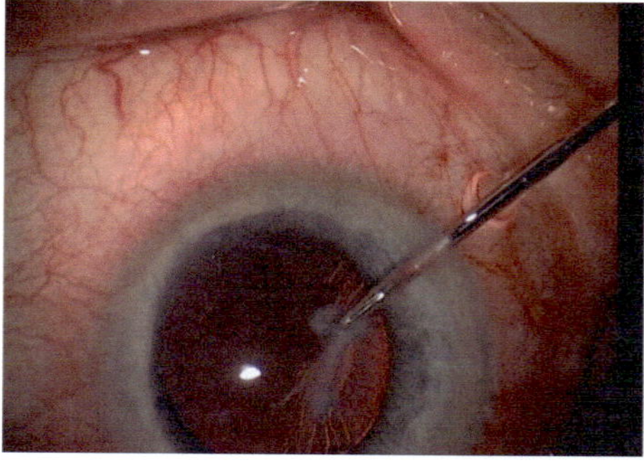

Fig. 20.4 Second instrument is used to enhance separation and reduce tractional forces to capsular bag and zonules

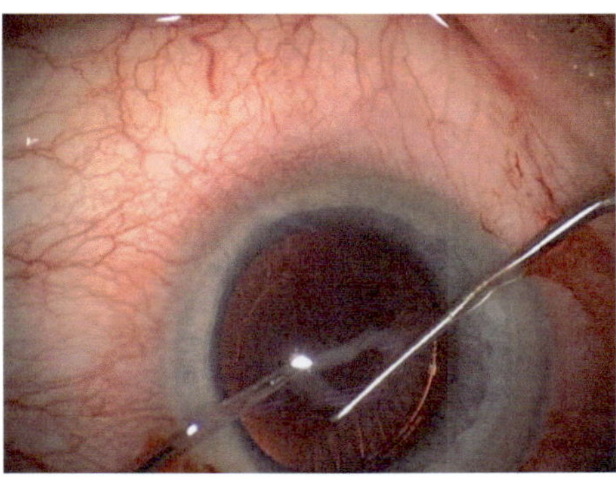

Fig. 20.5 Remaining fibrosed tissue that could not be peeled is excised with endoscissors

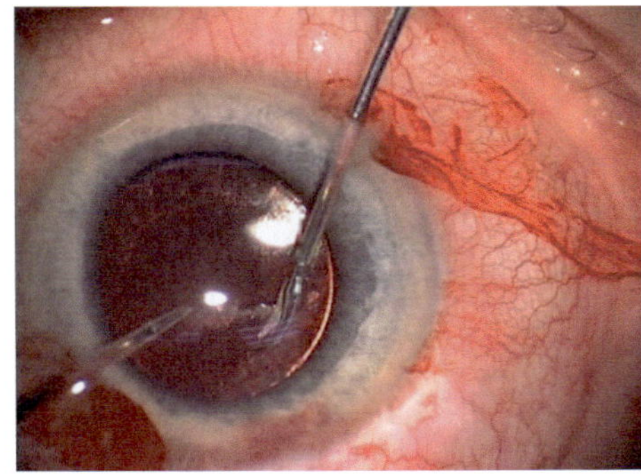

Fig. 20.6 Final situation with relaxed capsular rhexis margins, clear visual axis and well-positioned IOL

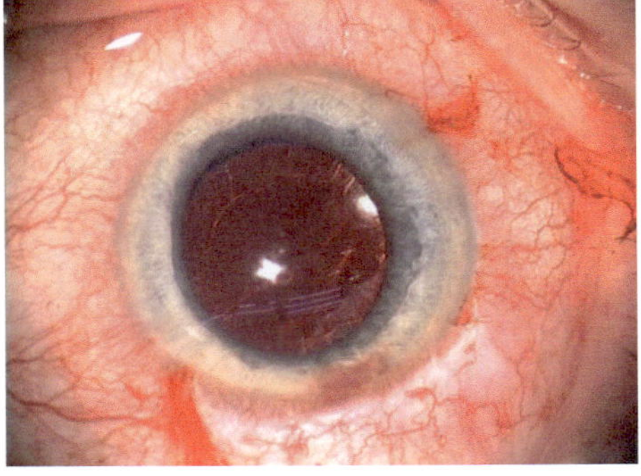

Secondary IOL Implantation Techniques

All videos of this part be found in a playlist of my YouTube channel:
https://www.youtube.com/playlist?list=PL0dKYclPD7yMJRuQAIt9Dr7pOtuI0
Seex

Part VI: Surgical management of anterior dislocated IOL from pars plana
Part VI: Sulcus implantation for dummies
Part VI: IOL extraction and iris claw IOL implantation
Part VI: Subluxated IOL and Artisan IOL implantation, operated with one trocar
Part VI: Intrascleral PCIOL fixation (Scharioth)
Part VI: Intrascleral fixation with DORC forceps 1
Part VI: Intrascleral fixation with DORC forceps 1
Part VI: Yamane technique
Part VI: Scleral fixation of IOL
Part VI: IOL refixation with Hoffmann technique
Part VI: Fixation of an IOL to iris with suture
Part VI: Fixation of an IOL-in-the-bag with suture to iris, an elegant and simple technique

IOL Implantation in the Sulcus

21

Contents

Abstract

This chapter explains step-by-step the implantation of an IOL into the sulcus.

Keywords

Sulcus · Sulcus implantation · IOL implantation

21.1 Introduction

After a posterior capsular rupture, some surgeons prefer to implant an IOL and others prefer to leave the eye aphakic. The implanted IOL may dislocate after surgery and require a reposition (Fig. 21.1). The aphakic eye needs an IOL implantation. If the anterior capsule is intact, then a sulcus implantation can be performed. If the anterior capsule is defect or absent, then a scleral/intrascleral or iris-fixated IOL implantation must be performed. See treatment algorithm in Fig. 21.2.

Remark: All videos of this chapter can be watched in a playlist of my YouTube channel:

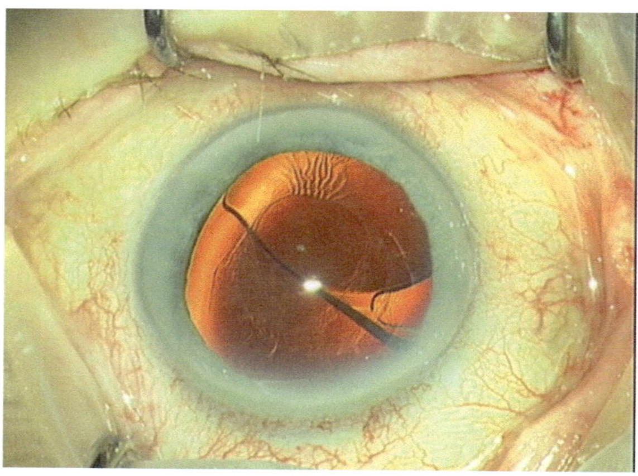

Fig. 21.1 Decentred IOL 1 week after an uneventful cataract surgery

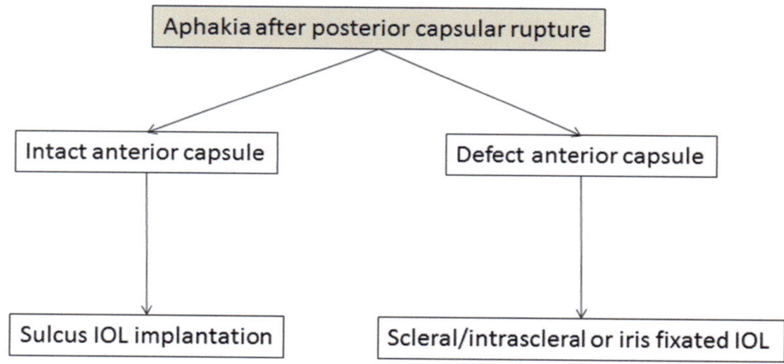

Fig. 21.2 Our treatment algorithm for aphakia or dislocated IOL after posterior capsular rupture

https://www.youtube.com/playlist?list=PL0dKYclPD7yMJRuQAIt9Dr7pOtuI0Seex

Assessment and surgical planning:

The crucial point is whether the anterior capsule is intact or not. If it is intact, then an IOL can be implanted into the sulcus. If the anterior lens capsule is absent, then a complicated scleral/intrascleral or iris-fixated implantation must be performed. Try to get a preoperative assessment at the slit lamp. In many cases, however, the lens capsule cannot be fully assessed. In this case, the assessment must be done on the surgical table (Figs. 21.3, 21.4, 21.5 and 21.6). If you do the assessment in the OR, then you must be prepared for both surgical options: Sulcus IOL or scleral/intrascleral/iris-fixated IOL implantation.

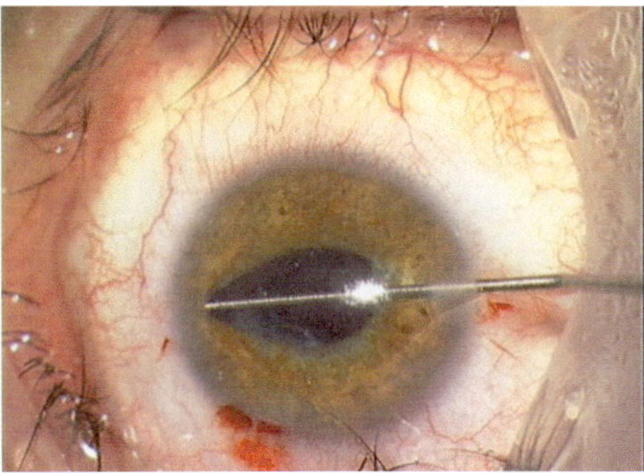

Fig. 21.3 Examination of the lens capsule of an aphakic eye. The examination is performed with a push–pull instrument (Sinskey hook), which allows an easy manipulation of the iris

Fig. 21.4 Posterior capsule is defective. The inferior anterior capsule is not broad but intact

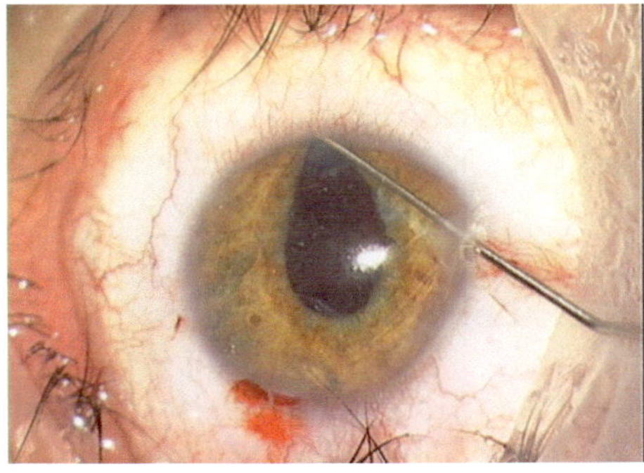

Fig. 21.5 Nasal anterior capsule is intact

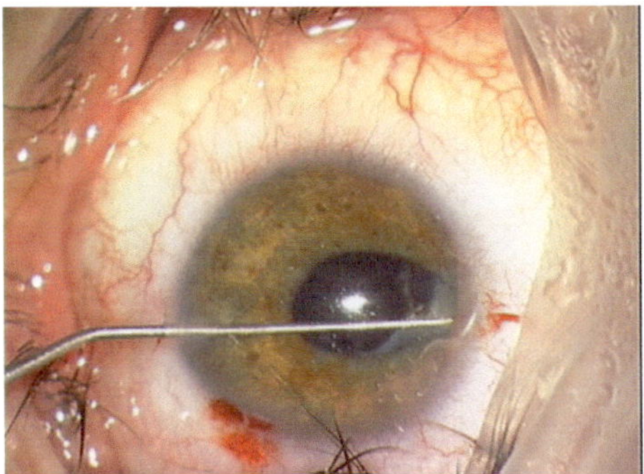

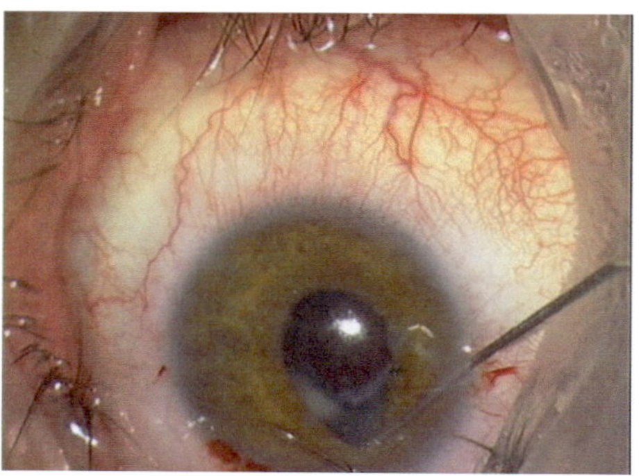

Fig. 21.6 Superior anterior capsule is broad and intact

Anatomy of sulcus:

The IOL is implanted in the sulcus (Fig. 21.7). The sulcus is located between the anterior capsule and the iris. In contrast to an in-the-bag implantation, a sulcus IOL is mobile. If you want to prevent this movement, you can fixate the IOL in the rhexis. The IOL optic is captured behind the anterior rhexis, and the haptics are located in the sulcus, a so-called optic-in, haptic-out implantation (Fig. 21.8). This IOL capture can only be done in a fresh rhexi and not in a fibrosed rhexis.

21.2   Correct IOL Choice

If you plan a sulcus IOL implantation, you must choose a 3-piece IOL. A 1-piece IOL is not suitable for sulcus implantation because the thick haptics cause iris chaffing (Fig. 21.9).

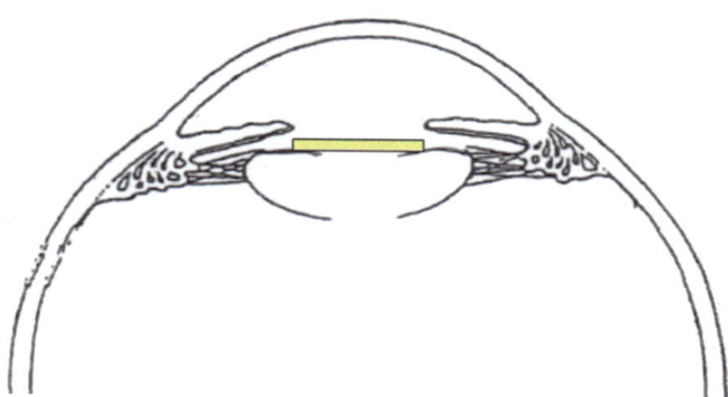

Fig. 21.7 Drawing of the anatomy of a sulcus-fixated IOL. The IOL is located between the iris and the anterior capsule

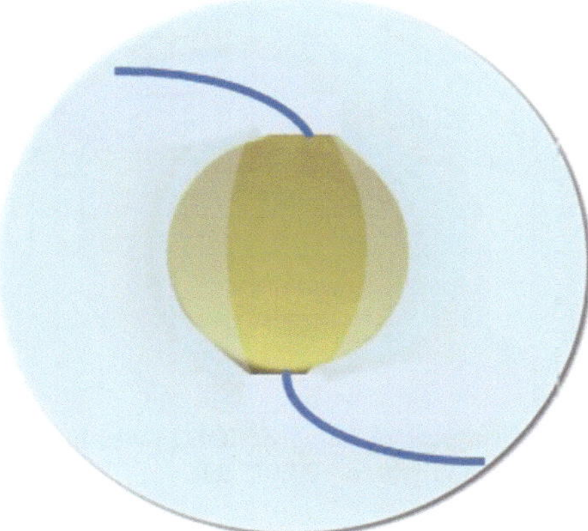

Fig. 21.8 Drawing of an IOL capture. The 3-piece IOL is implanted in the sulcus and then the IOL is buttonholed behind the rhexis. The haptics are located in the sulcus, and the IOL is located behind the anterior capsule. The rhexis becomes an almond formed shape

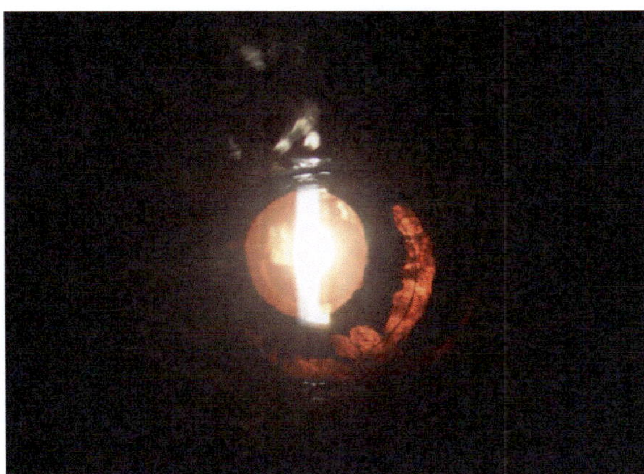

Fig. 21.9 Iris depigmentation secondary to implantation of a 1-piece IOL into the sulcus (iris chaffing)

If the IOL is not located in the bag, calculations for the IOL should take into consideration the effective lens position of the optic within the eye. The general rule is: The more anterior the IOL, the less diopter. An anterior chamber lens has less diopter than an in-the-bag IOL. If the IOL is completely in the sulcus, the optic will be more anterior and the power should be decreased by 0.5D. Intrascleral-fixated IOL's end up having the same power calculations as in-the-bag placement. Retropupillar-fixated iris-claw IOL's have approximately 2D less than in-the-bag IOL's (Figs. 21.10, 21.11, 21.12, 21.13 and 21.14).

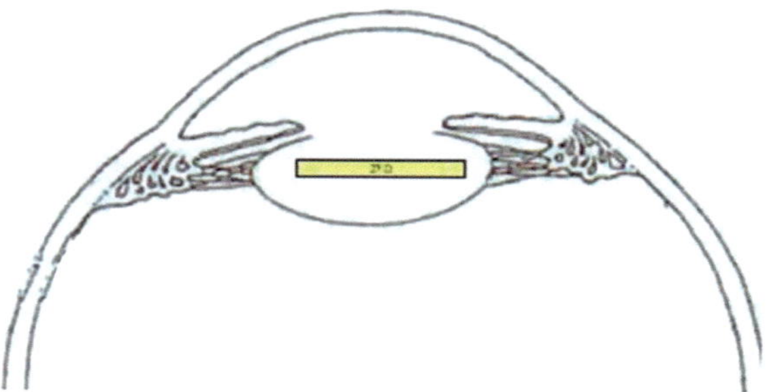

Fig. 21.10 Drawings for the surgical planning of IOL power in case of a complication. The normal case is an in-the-bag location with a +23.0D IOL

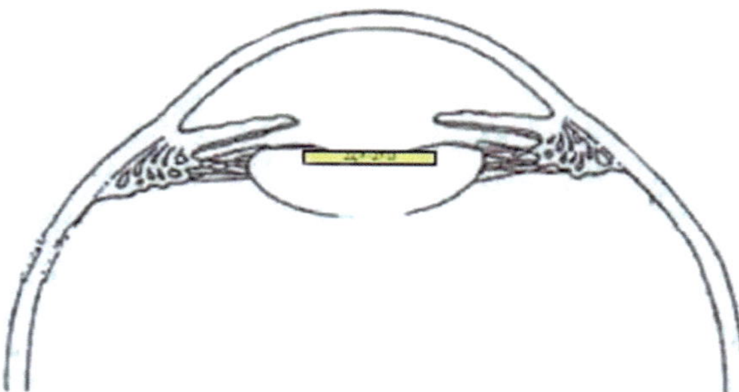

Fig. 21.11 Lens capture after posterior capsular defect. The IOL power is between 22.5D and 23.0D

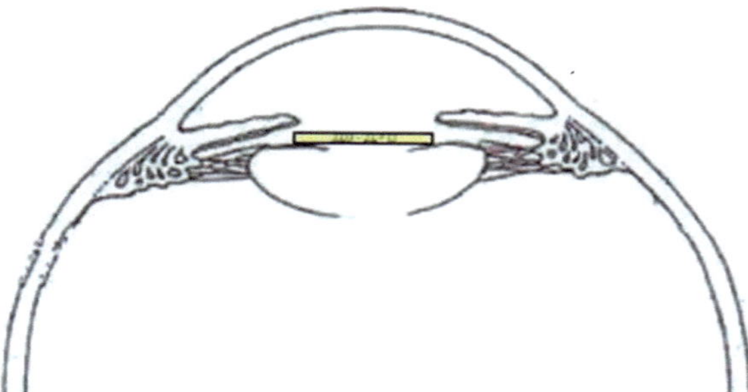

Fig. 21.12 Sulcus implantation. The IOL power is between 22.0 and 22.5D

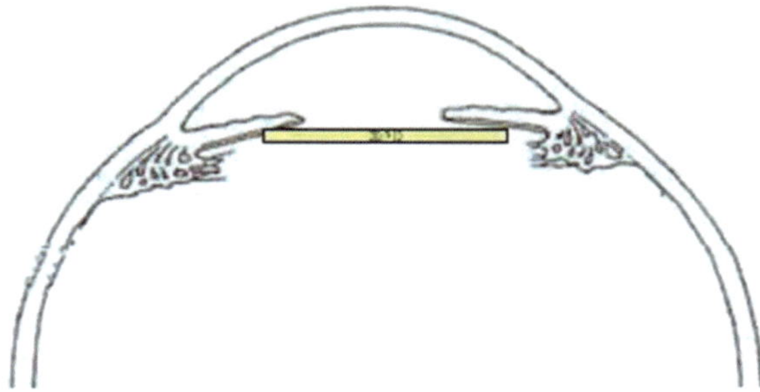

Fig. 21.13 Retropupillar iris-fixated IOL. The IOL power is approximately 20.5D

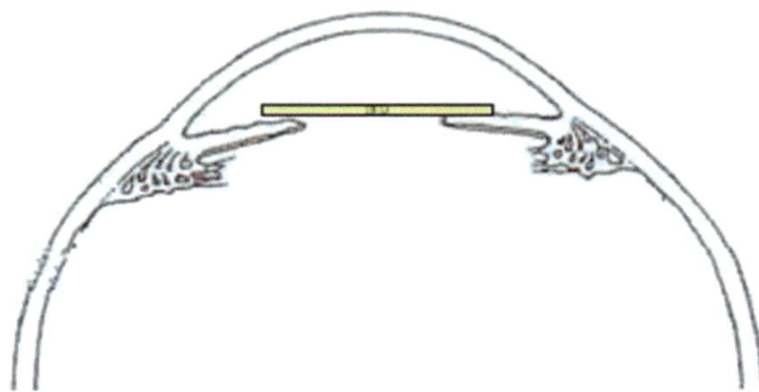

Fig. 21.14 Antepupillar iris-fixated IOL. The IOL power is approximately 18.0D

21.3   Anaesthesia

The usual anaesthesia nowadays for phacoemulsification is topical anaesthesia (e.g. Tetracaine drops) and in addition intracameral anaesthesia (e.g. Xylocain 1%). For complication management or a secondary IOL implantation, we recommend peribulbar anaesthesia. We use a blunt cannula which has a low risk for a globe perforation (BD, 25G or 27G retrobulbar cannula, Atkinson).

21.4   Sulcus Implantation with Intact Anterior Capsule

Instruments

1. Iris hooks
2. Sinskey hook
3. Maybe: Vitreous cutter.

IOL choice

Three-piece IOL.

(Remark: A 1-piece IOL cannot be used because it causes iris chaffing).

Dye

Maybe: Triamcinolone.

Individual steps

(1) Viscoelastics into the anterior chamber
(2) Insert iris hooks
(3) Triamcinolone into the anterior chamber
(4) Anterior vitrectomy
(5) IOL implantation
(6) IOL capture
(7) Remove iris hooks.

The surgery step by step:

1. Viscoelastics behind the IOL
2. Insert iris hooks

Inject viscoelastics into the anterior chamber. Insert iris hooks to visualize the complete anterior capsule. Examine now the anterior capsule with the push–pull instrument (Sinskey hook). Is the rhexis intact, is there a zonular lysis? If the anterior lens capsule is intact, you can proceed with sulcus implantation.

3. Triamcinolone in the anterior chamber
4. Anterior vitrectomy

Inject triamcinolone into the anterior chamber and remove a possible vitreous prolapse. Then proceed with an anterior vitrectomy. I recommend performing the vitrectomy from pars plana in order to remove as much anterior vitreous as possible. Insert a trocar 3.5 mm behind the limbus and remove the anterior vitreous from pars plana.

5. IOL implantation
6. IOL capture
7. Remove iris hooks

Inject the IOL and place the leading haptic on the iris. Then rotate the trailing haptic into the anterior chamber and also onto the iris. If you have clear view to the anterior capsule, you can continue to rotate first one haptic and then the second haptic into the sulcus. Two paracentesis at an angle of about 90 degrees to the haptics. If the haptics are located at 12 and 6 o'clock, then place the paracentesis at 3 and 9 o'clock. Take two Sinskey hooks (alternatively spatula), one Sinskey hook

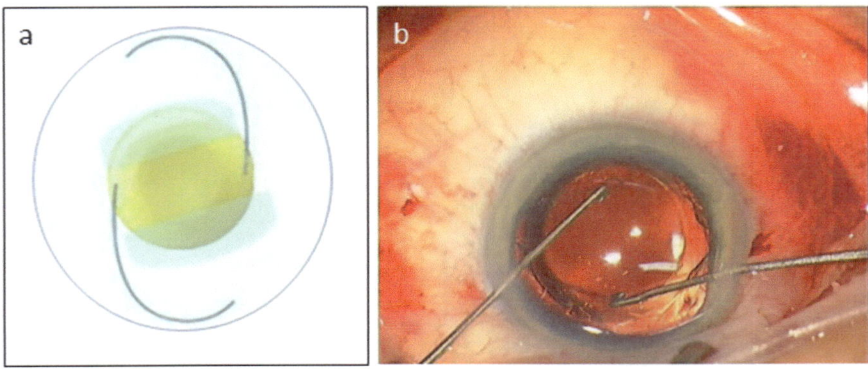

Fig. 21.15 **a** Drawing of a lens capture. The posterior capsule is defective. The IOL is placed in the sulcus and the optic is buttonholed behind the rhexis. The haptics remain in the sulcus. The round rhexis takes an almond shape. **b** Lens capture manoeuvre. Work bimanually with two Sinskey hooks or iris spatulas and press the optic at one side behind the rhexis while stabilizing the optic at the other side. Then the same manoeuvre at the other side

presses one side of the IOL behind the anterior capsule, while the other Sinskey hook stabilizes the IOL (Fig. 21.15). Then the same manoeuvre on the other side. Then examine with the push–pull instruments whether the rhexis margins are located before the IOL. When properly performed, the rhexis takes an oval shape (Fig. 21.15).

21.5 Sulcus Implantation with Defect Anterior Capsule

Sulcus implantation becomes difficult when a rift is present. A haptic may dislocate through the rift resulting in a dislocation of the complete IOL.

We start with the same procedure. Insert four iris hooks and examine the anterior capsule. Where is the rift located? If the rift is located at 6 o'clock, then you must place the haptics in a diagonal way (Fig. 21.16). It may, however, happen that a haptic rotates during the postoperative course towards 6 o'clock and the IOL dislocates.

The IOL is safer, if the rift is located at 3 or 9 o'clock. In this case, the IOL can be placed in the 12 and 6 o'clock position. A dislocation in the postoperative course is very unlikely (Fig. 21.17).

Two case reports illustrate the surgical spectrum:

Case 1: An 82-year-old female patient with a dislocated IOL (Fig. 21.18). She was cataract operated for 15 years ago. An examination with the push–pull instrument demonstrates that the IOL is located in the sulcus (Fig. 21.19). A lens capture is performed, but the superior part of the anterior capsule tilts back due to superior

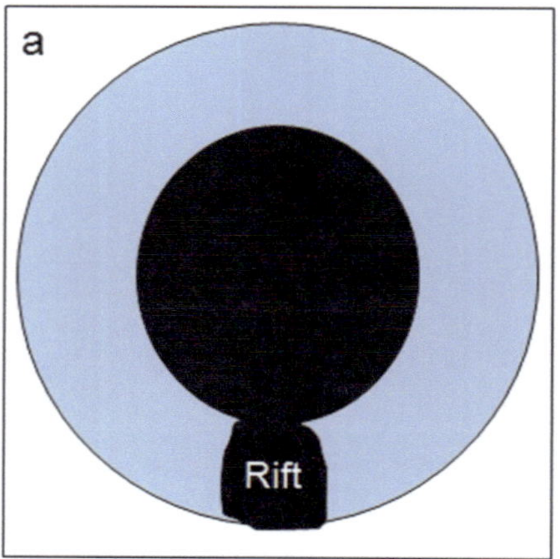
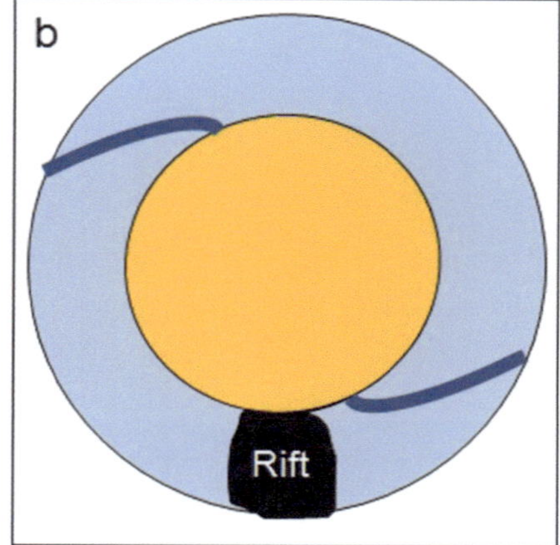

Fig. 21.16 **a** A rift at 6 o'clock. **b** Place the haptics in a diagonal position away from the 6 o'clock rift

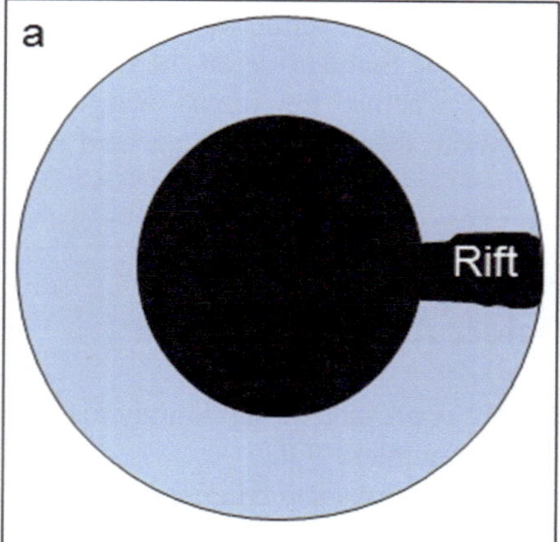
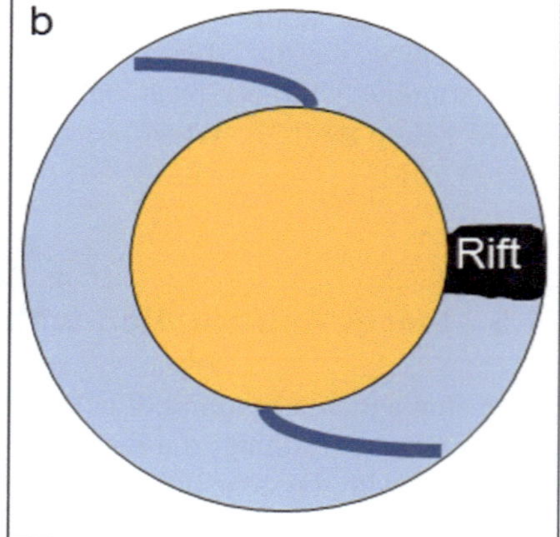

Fig. 21.17 **a** A rift at 3 or 9 o'clock. **b** Place the IOL with the haptics in the 6 and 12 o'clock position. Principle is to place the haptics away from the rift and at a maximum distance possible from the rift

zonular lysis (Fig. 21.20). Therefore, the IOL in the bag is extracted (Fig. 21.21) and an iris-fixated IOL implanted. Alternatively, an intrascleral fixation can be performed.

Case 2: A 24-year-old male patient presents with a five-year-old traumatic cataract (Fig. 21.22). The natural lens cannot be identified, only a central fibrosis and iris pigmentation can be seen. The central fibrosis is removed with a capsulorhexis

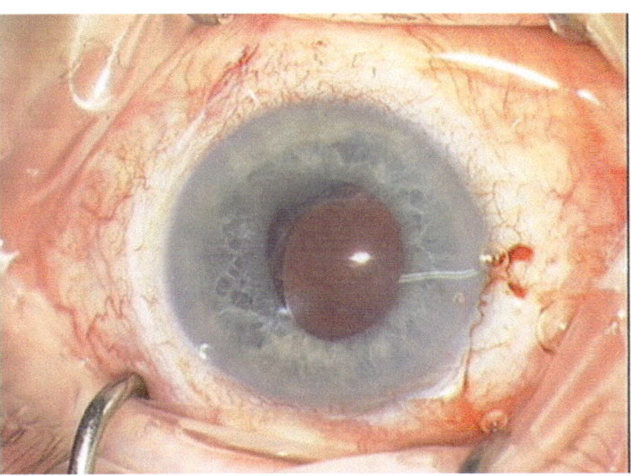

Fig. 21.18 Decentred IOL. The cataract surgery was performed a long time ago

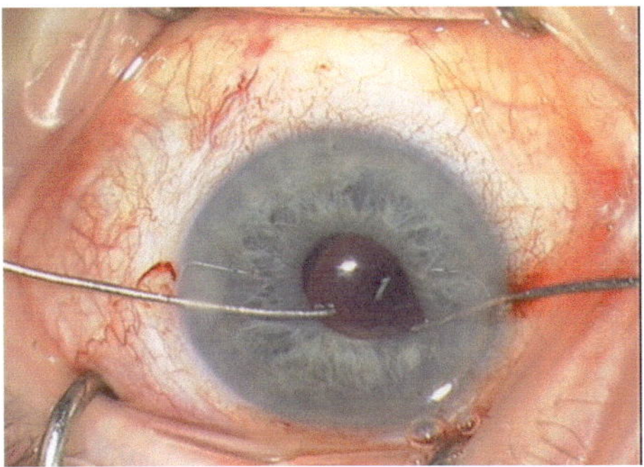

Fig. 21.19 Examination with two push–pull instruments does not deliver sufficient information about the status of the anterior capsule

forceps and a round rhexis is cut with a vitrector (200 cuts/min) (Fig. 21.23). A three-piece IOL is implanted in the sulcus. An examination on the first postoperative day showed an inferiorly dislocated IOL (Fig. 21.24). The cause of the decentration was an undetected inferior zonular lysis. The patient was reoperated. The IOL was then buttonholed into the anterior rhexis (lens capture manoeuvre) (Fig. 21.25). Postoperatively the IOL was centred without a tilt.

Remark; See our treatment algorithm for sulcus implantation and defect zonules (Fig. 21.26).

Summary

In case of aphakia or dislocated IOL after a complicated cataract surgery, assess first the status of the anterior lens capsule. If the anterior capsule is intact, then a sulcus implantation is possible. Remark: Choose a 3-piece IOL because a 1-piece IOL causes iris chaffing.

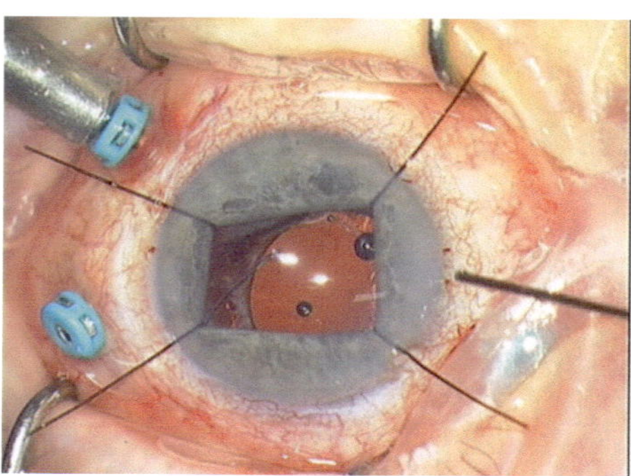

Fig. 21.20 Therefore, iris retractors are inserted. The anterior capsule is intact. The rhexis is enlarged with the vitreous cutter and the optic buttonholed into the rhexis. After this manoeuvre, the complete bag-IOL complex tilted backwards. The cause is a superior zonular lysis. Now, three main techniques are possible: (1) Fixation of the bag (Hoffmann technique), (2) removal of bag and intrascleral implantation (Scharioth technique) or (3) IOL explantation and iris-claw IOL implantation

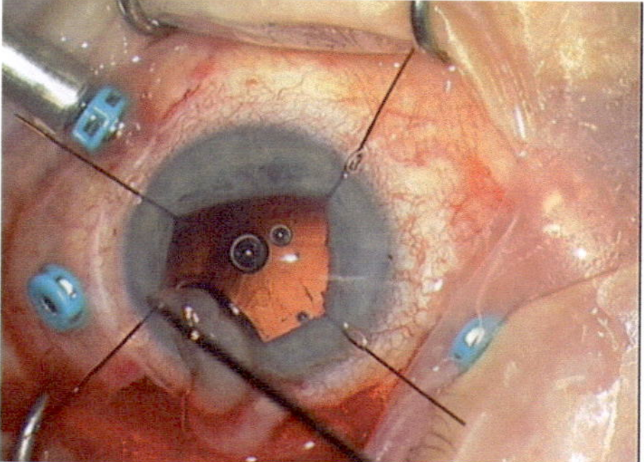

Fig. 21.21 IOL was removed and an iris-fixated IOL implanted

Fig. 21.22 Traumatic cataract of a young African patient

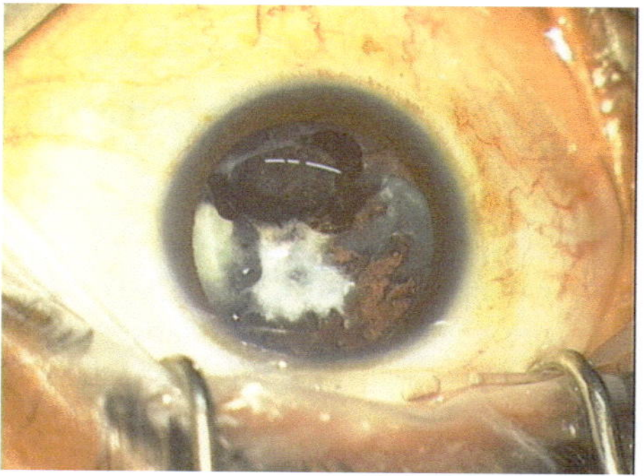

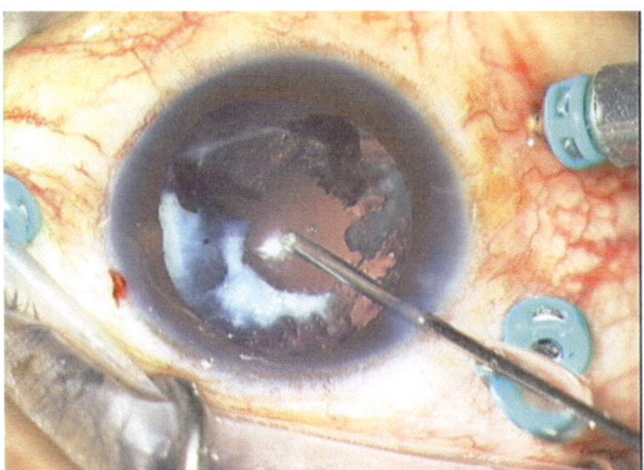

Fig. 21.23 The anterior capsule was stained with vision blue. Then a rhexis was performed with help of a capsulorhexis forceps and a capsulotomy scissors (Geuder). Then an anterior vitrectomy was performed and finally an IOL implanted in the sulcus

Fig. 21.24 At the first postoperative day, the IOL was inferiorly dislocated. The reason was an undetected inferior zonular lysis

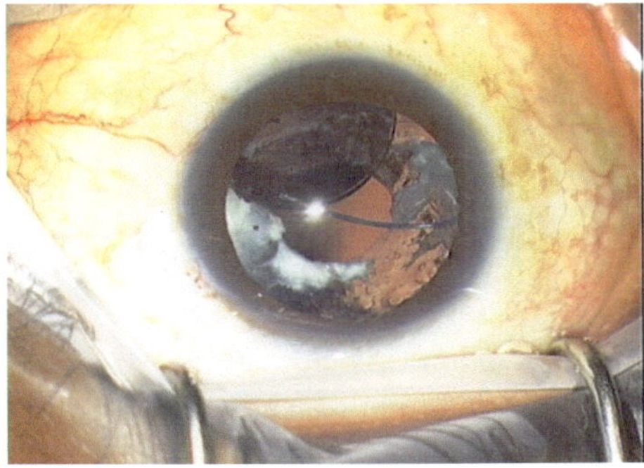

Fig. 21.25 In a second surgery, the same IOL was repositioned. The optic was buttonholed, and the haptics remain in the sulcus (lens capture)

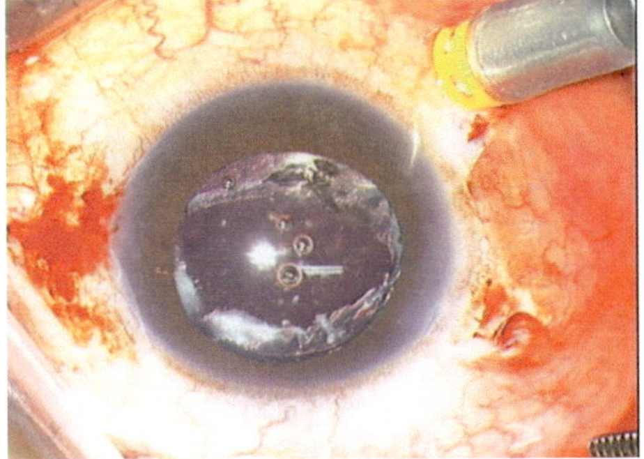

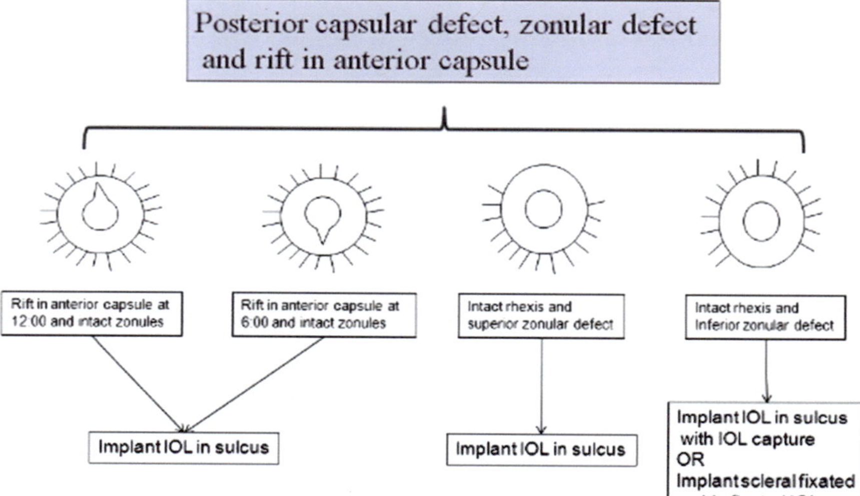

Fig. 21.26 Treatment algorithm in case of posterior capsule defect, rift in anterior capsule and defect zonules

In case of an <u>absent</u> lens capsule, there are four main possibilities to fixate the IOL into the posterior chamber.

1. Iris fixation (iris-claw IOL).
2. Scleral suturing of haptics (3-piece or 1-piece IOL).
3. Intrascleral fixation of IOL (Scharioth technique).
4. Intrascleral fixation of IOL (Yamane technique).

In case of an IOL-in-the-bag dislocation, there are two options to fixate the IOL into the posterior chamber.

1. Fixation of IOL in the bag (Hoffmann technique)
2. Suture of IOL bag complex to iris.

These surgeries can be performed with a phacoemulsification machine and the insertion of one or two trocars at pars plana. All surgical methods are described in the following chapters.

Iris-Claw IOL Implantation

22

Contents

Abstract

The iris claw IOL is called Artisan or Verisyse IOL. This IOL is implanted sutureless into the iris tissue. The retropupillar implantation of an iris claw IOL is explained step-by-step.

Keywords

Iris claw IOL · Artisan · Verisyse · Retropupillar

The most popular secondary IOL implantation technique is the intrascleral IOL implantation, and here, the Yamane technique is especially popular. Common are also the scleral and the iris-claw implantation technique. Less common but very elegant is the refixation of the IOL in the bag with the Hoffmann technique. Another technique which is still in use today is iris suturing of the IOL. All techniques will be demonstrated in this chapter. See treatment algorithm, Fig. 22.1.

The benefits of an iris-claw IOL implantation are a short surgical time, a sutureless implantation, an excellent centration without risk of tilting and a short learning curve (approx. 5 surgeries). The disadvantage is that the IOL is fixated into the iris tissue and a too traumatic implantation may lead to an inflammation. This postoperative inflammation with cellular proliferation of the IOL is induced by macrophages. This occurs, however, only in the learning curve. In addition, sufficient iris tissue is required for implantation. See next chapter.

© The Author(s), under exclusive license to Springer Nature Switzerland AG 2022

U. Spandau and G. B. Scharioth, *Complications During and After Cataract Surgery*,
https://doi.org/10.1007/978-3-030-93531-3_22

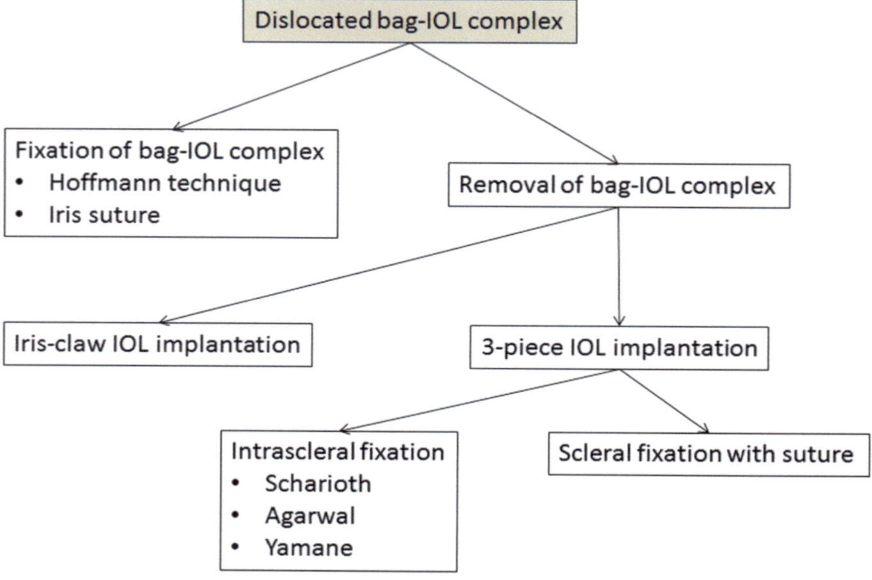

Fig. 22.1 Our treatment algorithm for dislocated bag-IOL complex

The advantages of the intrascleral IOL fixation (Scharioth technique) are a sutureless implantation, an excellent centration of the IOL with a low inflammation risk and less problems with the ciliary body in comparison to scleral fixation. The disadvantage is a longer learning curve (10–15 surgeries), possible tilting and dislocation.

The advantages of scleral fixation are a relatively short learning curve (5–10 operations). The disadvantages are a possible lens tilt (unstable position of the lens), discomfort with the ciliary body (due to the haptic), and (depending on the technique) discomfort due to the knot.

The first author (USA) performs almost exclusively the iris-claw IOL implantation technique because the surgical time is short (15–20 min). The IOL is always centrated and a dislocation is very rare. The second author (GS) is the inventor of the intrascleral technique, and he performs always this technique.

The benefits of an iris-claw IOL (Artisan) implantation are a short surgical time, a sutureless implantation, an excellent centration without risk of tilting and a short learning curve (approx. 5 surgeries). The surgical time is approximately 15 min. A redislocation happens seldom, maybe one patient per year. The disadvantage is that the IOL is fixated into the iris tissue and a too traumatic implantation may lead to an inflammation. This postoperative inflammation with cellular proliferation of the IOL is induced by macrophages. This occurs, however, only in the learning curve. If you combine the Artisan implantation with a complete PPV, then a pseudophacodonesis may occur. If the Artisan implantation, however, is only combined with an anterior vitrectomy, then the risk for a pseudophacodonesis is low.

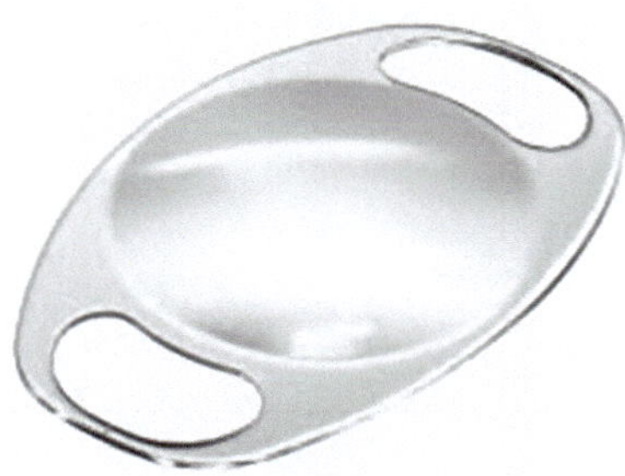

Fig. 22.2 Iris-claw IOL (Artisan®, Ophtec and Verisyse®, AMO)

In addition, sufficient iris tissue is required for implantation, e.g. an implantation in case of aniridia is not possible.

We will demonstrate the implantation of an iris-claw IOL (Verisyse®, Abbott and Artisan®, Opthec) (Fig. 22.2). The iris-claw IOL can be implanted before the pupil or behind the pupil. If you implant the IOL retropupillary, then it has to be done "upside down" (= on the back) because the haptics are bent upwards.

We will demonstrate the retropupillary method, which is easy to learn. We recommend starting with an aphakic eye which underwent an anterior vitrectomy. The pupil should be constricted before surgery. We recommend retrobulbar anaesthesia.

There are different A-constants for antepupillar and retropupillar IOL implantations; the A-constant for retropupillar implantation is 116.9.

The most difficult part of the surgery is the dissection of a scleral tunnel, which is the same as for the SICS technique (modified ECCE). We prefer a scleral tunnel to a corneal tunnel in order to reduce astigmatism; this tunnel is 6 mm wide. Why? Because the iris-claw IOL is 6 mm wide and because the extracted IOL is also 6 mm wide. What may happen if the tunnel is 8 mm wide? The wider the tunnel, the more you risk a choroidal detachment. In the beginning, we recommend starting with a 6 mm limbal tunnel. If you feel safe with the technique, you can continue with a scleral tunnel.

How many trocars? We use usually only two trocars without a viewing system. We perform only an anterior vitrectomy and no core vitrectomy. A core vitrectomy increases the risk for pseudophacodonesis.

22.1 Special Instruments for Iris-Claw IOL Implantation

Instruments for iris-fixated IOL

The required instruments for the implantation of an iris-fixated IOL can be acquired from the company (Verisyse®, Abbott and Artisan®, Opthec):

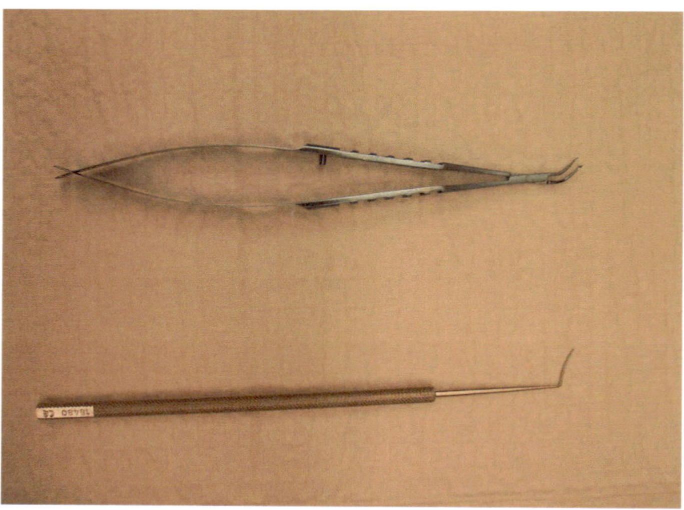

Fig. 22.3 Two instruments are required for the implantation of an Artisan IOL. 1) An IOL implantation forceps (AMO), 2) an enclavation spatula from Sekundo (Geuder) for implantation of an iris-claw IOL. Alternative: Iris spatula or anterior chamber cannula

IOL implantation forceps (Fig. 22.3).

Indication: Holds the Artisan (Verisyse IOL) during implantation. A very important instrument.

Enclavation spatula (Fig. 22.3).

Indication: Retropupillar fixation of IOL claws in iris tissue. This spatula is thin so that only a little iris tissue is enclavated. Sekundo enclavation spatula, Geuder-32724.

Caliper (Fig. 22.4).

Indication: Marking of main incision and sclerotomy. The main incision for the implantation of an iris-fixated PMMA IOL is 6 mm wide. Caliper by Castroviejo, Geuder 19,135.

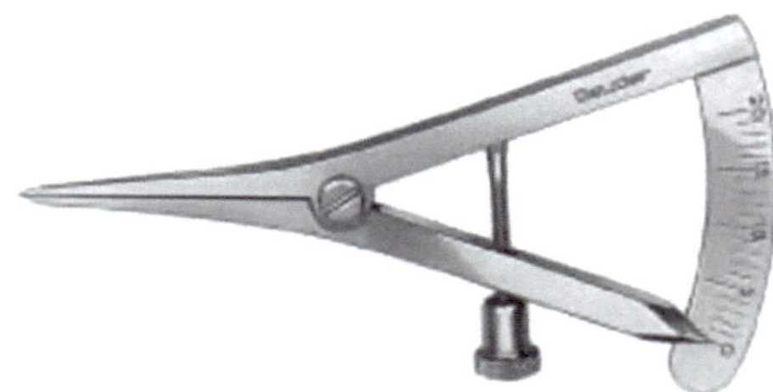

Fig. 22.4 Useful is also a Castroviejo's caliper. Indication: Frown incision (Geuder)

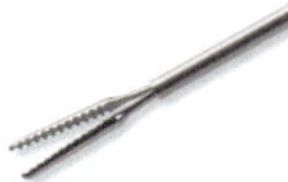

Fig. 22.5 23G intravitreal serrated jaws forceps (DORC). Indication: Extraction of the subluxated IOL from the anterior chamber

Serrated jaw forceps (Fig. 22.5).

Indication: Extraction of subluxated IOL with lens capsule. 20G or 23G. DORC. 1286.C06.

22.2 Iris-Claw IOL Implantation Surgery

Instruments

1. Crescent bevel up knife
2. 15° knife
3. 2.4 mm tunnel knife
4. Caliper
5. IOL implantation forceps (AMO)
6. Enclavation spatula
7. 20G or 23G serrated jaw forceps.

Material

Acetylcholine (Miochol).
Iris-claw IOL (Artisan®, Verisyse®)
Maybe: Triamcinolone.

Individual steps

(1) **Two 23G trocars**
(2) **Paracentesis at 3 and 9 o'clock**
(3) **Limbal main incision / scleral frown incision**
(4) **Extraction of an anterior dislocated IOL**
(5) **Anterior vitrectomy**
(6) **Injection of Miochol**
(7) **Implantation of iris-fixated IOL (upside down)**
(8) **Enclavation of iris-fixated IOL**
(9) **Closure of the frown incision and conjunctiva.**

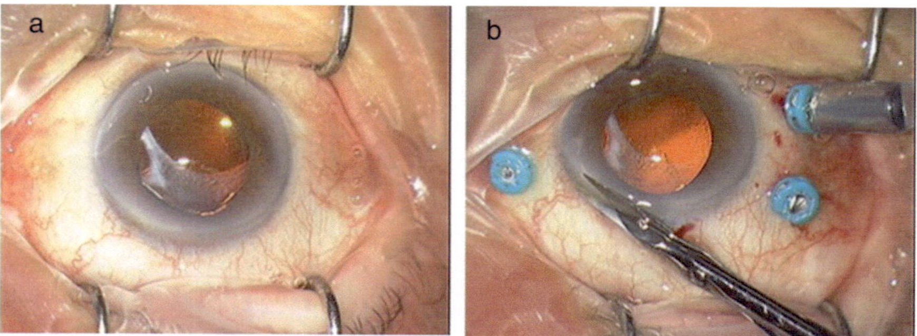

Fig. 22.6 **a** Anterior dislocated bag-IOL complex secondary to zonular lysis. **b** Open the conjunctiva along the limbus from 11 o'clock to 1 o'clock with the Vannas scissors (limbal peritomy)

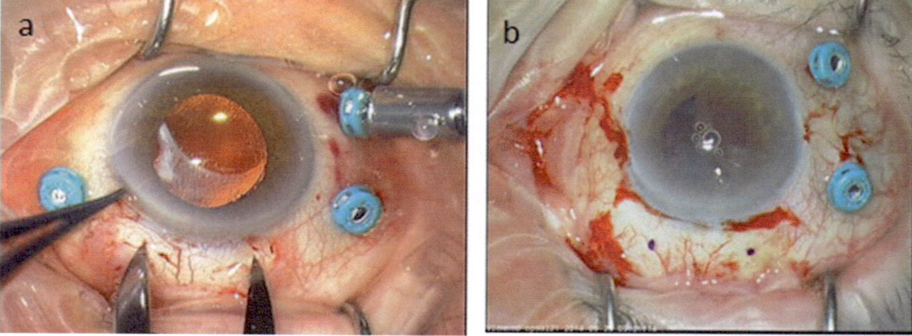

Fig. 22.7 **a** Mark a 6 mm broad scleral incision with the caliper. The incision is approximately 1.5 mm behind the limbus. **b** Mark the frown incision with a marker pen

The surgery step by step: Figs. 22.6, 22.7, 22.8, 22.9, 22.10, 22.11, 22.12, 22.13 and 22.14.

(1) **Two 23G trocars**
(2) **Paracentesis at 3 and 9 o'clock**

Insert two trocars at the temporal side. Continue with a short paracentesis at 3 o'clock and 9 o'clock. The paracentesis is short so that you can reach the peripheral iris with the enclavation spatula.

Note: The location of the IOL is determined by the position of the frown incision. If the claws are located at 3 o'clock and 9 o'clock, then the frown incision must be located at 12 o'clock. In case of an iris defect at 3 o'clock or a filtration

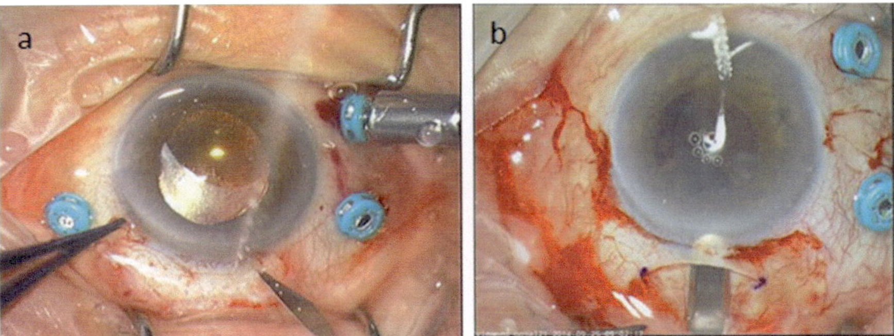

Fig. 22.8 **a** 50% scleral thickness incision with the 15 deg knife is performed. **b** Dissect a scleral tunnel with the bevel up crescent knife. If the knife is visible through the sclera, then you have the correct depth

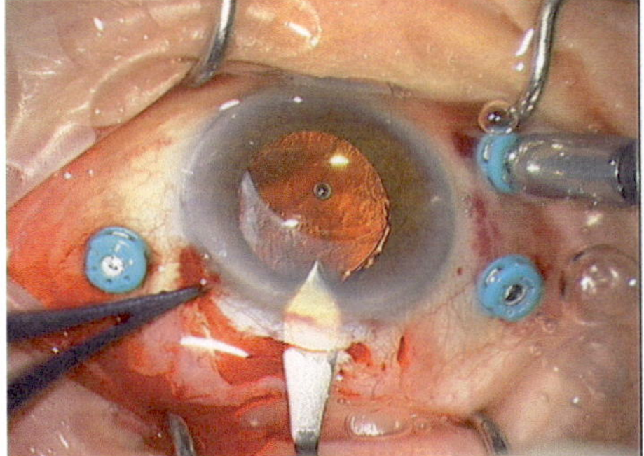

Fig. 22.9 Then open the anterior chamber in the clear cornea with a 2.4 mm blade

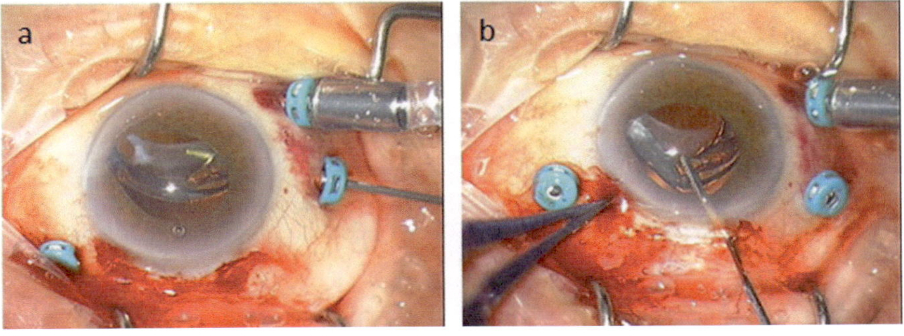

Fig. 22.10 **a** Prolapse the IOL at 12 o'clock up to the pupillary plane in order to access it with the forceps. **b** Then remove the IOL with the serrated jaws forceps

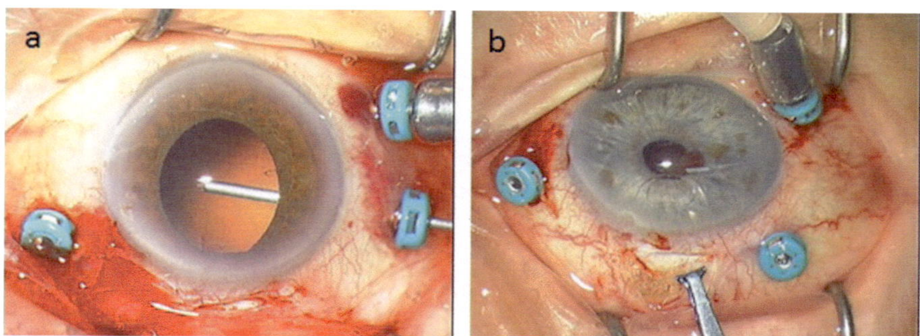

Fig. 22.11 **a** Perform an anterior vitrectomy. **b** Turn the iris-claw IOL upside down for implantation and implant it with the IOL implantation forceps (AMO)

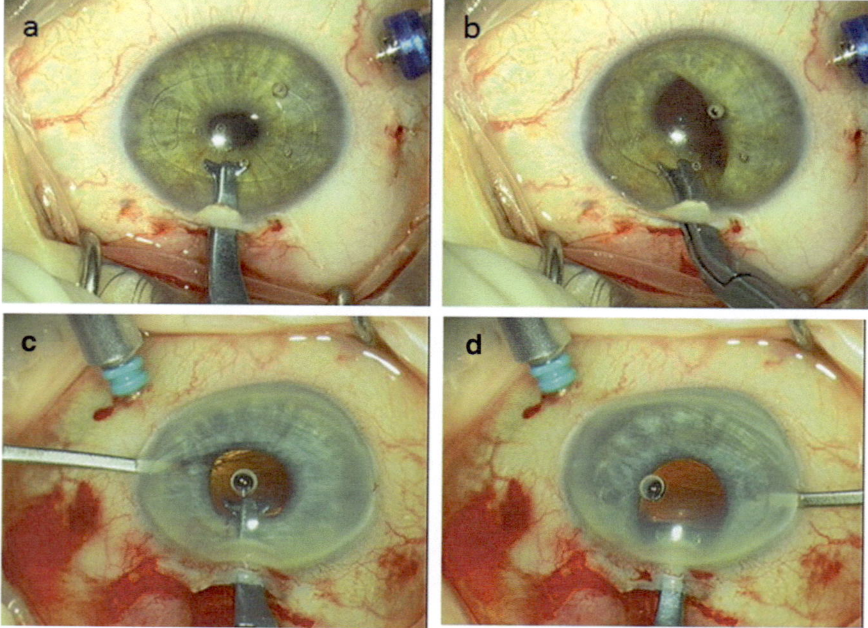

Fig. 22.12 **a** Centrate the IOL and fixate it with the IOL implantation forceps (AMO). **b** Tilt the IOL behind the iris on one side. **c** Tilt the IOL behind the iris on the other side and then press the iris tissue with the Sekundo enclavation spatula (Geuder) (no Sinskey hook instrument) behind the claws. **d** Switch hands and perform the same manoeuvre on the other side

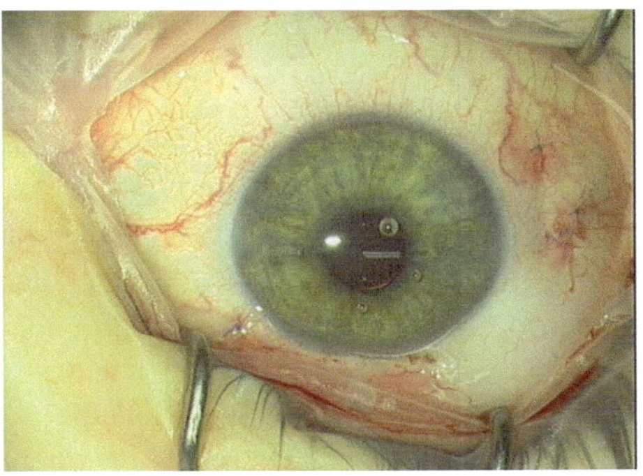

Fig. 22.13 Note the enclavated iris tissue at 3 and 9 o'clock

bleb at 12 o'clock, you must choose the position of the IOL and frown incision accordingly.

(3) Limbal main incision/Scleral frown incision

Continue with the frown incision. Perform a limbal peritomy from 11 to 1 o'clock with Westcott scissors and cauterize the bleeding vessels (Fig. 22.6). Then mark a 6-mm-wide incision (not wider!) with a caliper (Fig. 22.7). The arc of the incision should be approximately 1–2 mm behind the limbus. Dissect a 50% scleral thickness deep frown incision with a 15° knife (Fig. 22.8a). Then dissect a scleral tunnel with the crescent angled bevel up knife (Fig. 22.8b) and open finally the anterior chamber with a 2.4 mm blade (Fig. 22.9). Note: Enter the anterior chamber with the 2.4 mm blade in the clear cornea in order to avoid an intracameral bleeding and also to create a valve at the inner lip of the tunnel.

(4) Extraction of an anterior dislocated IOL

The extraction is easier, if the eye is not vitrectomized and the IOL is located behind the iris. Close the infusion line during extraction. Inject viscoelastics (Viscoat®) into the anterior chamber and then behind the IOL and elevate then the IOL a little bit up at 12 o'clock so that the optic edge or a haptic is visible (Fig. 22.10a). Grasp the IOL ideally at the haptic with the serrated jaw forceps and extract the IOL with the lens capsule (Fig. 22.10b). Often, some fibrotic parts of the lens capsule remain in the anterior chamber. Remove them with viscoexpression, e.g. inject viscoelastics behind them into the anterior chamber and then press on the posterior scleral lip of the scleral tunnel; the fragment will leave the anterior chamber passively.

Reopen the infusion line and continue with an anterior vitrectomy from pars plana.

(5) Anterior vitrectomy
(6) Injection of Miochol

(7) **Implantation of iris-fixated IOL (upside down)**

Continue with an anterior vitrectomy (Fig. 22.11a). Move the tip of the vitreous cutter along the pupillary edge. The opening of the vitreous cutter points towards the optic disc. The next step is pupil constriction. Before implantation of an iris-claw IOL, the pupil must be constricted. Inject first acetylchloline (Miochol®) and then viscoelastics (Viscoat®) to maintain anterior chamber. Using an IOL forceps (AMO), place the IOL *upside down* onto the iris (Fig. 22.11b). Then rotate the IOL so that the claws are located in the 3 and 9 o′clock position. Check the paracentesis with the Sekundo spatula. The view must be free in the area of the claws, remove blood if present. *Remark*: For retropupillar implantation, the Artisan IOL is implanted upside down. Otherwise, a basal iridectomy is required.

(8) **Enclavation of iris-fixated IOL**

Instrumentation:
Dominant hand: IOL implantation forceps (Abbott).
Non-dominant hand: Enclavation spatula.

Close the infusion line during IOL implantation. Centrate the IOL with a manipulator (e.g. push–pull) inside the anterior chamber. Grasp the IOL at the superior edge with the IOL implantation forceps (Abbott) (Fig. 22.12a). Flip the IOL to the right (Fig. 22.12b) so that half of the IOL is behind the iris and then to flip it to the left so that the IOL is completely behind the iris. Hold the IOL now in the middle of the pupil. Do not move it to the left or right.

Take then the enclavation spatula in your left hand. Lift the IOL a little bit up, so that the iris claws make an elevated impression behind the iris tissue. Then insert the spatula in the 3 o'clock paracentesis and clamp the iris tissue between the iris claws (Fig. 22.12c). Then the hands for the implantation forceps have to be switched. This manoeuvre should be practised preoperatively. Then take the enclavation spatula in your right hand and perform the same manoeuvre at 9 o'clock (Fig. 22.12d). Remove finally the implantation forceps and open the infusion line to achieve normotension. A retropupillary implantation requires no iridectomy.

(9) **Closure of the frown incision and conjunctiva**

Suture the frown incision with a Vicryl 8–0 cross stitch and the conjunctiva with a Vicryl 8–0 interrupted stitch (Fig. 22.13).

Postoperative treatment: Combined Dexamethasone-Gentamicin drops 3 × daily for three weeks. No mydriatics. If you want to do a dilated fundus exam later, it is absolutely safe to dilate with an iris-claw IOL in place.

22.3 Complications

Complete iris-claw IOL dislocation: The complete dislocation of an iris-claw IOL is very unusual. It may happen postoperatively secondary to a trauma. *See video*: Completely luxated iris-claw IOL after retropupillar fixation.

Remark: All videos of this chapter can be watched in a playlist of my YouTube channel:

https://www.youtube.com/playlist?list=PL0dKYclPD7yMJRuQAIt9Dr7pOtuI0Seex

Partial dislocation of an iris-claw IOL: Perform a corneal 2,4 mm main incision. Elevate the IOL up pars plana and place the dislocated part of the IOL onto the iris and then fixate the loose side.

See video: An easy technique to reposition a luxated Artisan (Verisyse) IOL: https://www.youtube.com/watch?v=FhguhNRBPQY&t=117s

Postoperative inflammation due to traumatic surgery, which occurs only in the learning phase. Do not enclavate too much iris tissue. It may cause ocular pain. In order to avoid this side effect, use the thin enclavation spatula by Sekundo from Geuder.

22.4 FAQ

Is an iris-claw implantation after trauma possible?

If the eye underwent a traumatic surgery due to a difficult cataract surgery with loss of the lens capsule, we would prefer a delayed implantation. We would implant the iris-claw IOL after approximately one month in order to obtain an uninflamed iris.

Why do you implant the Artisan IOL upside down?

The design of the Artisan IOL is convex; the haptics bend downwards. This makes them difficult to enclavate into the iris tissue. If you implant the Artisan IOL upside down, then the haptics are bent upwards and the enclavation is much easier.

Is an iridectomy necessary?

No, not in case of an upside-down implantation.

Yes, in case of a non-upside-down implantation. Why? Because the IOL with the haptics have a convex shape. If you enclavate the IOL non-upside down, then a pupillary block will occur. In the upside-down position, however, the IOL has a concave shape preventing a pupillary block.

Is a core vitrectomy necessary?

A core vitrectomy increases the risk of a pseudophacodonesis. We perform therefore only an anterior vitrectomy.

Pupil dilatation before surgery?

Only 1–2 drops tropicamide. Do not dilate maximally because you need a small pupil for implantation.

Is it possible to perform this surgery in two sessions?

Yes, of course. You may in one session extract the IOL and perform an anterior vitrectomy and then in a second session implant an Artisan IOL. The advantage of two sessions is that the pupil can be constricted preoperatively with pilocarpine and that you work with a non-inflammed iris.

I am a beginner, what is the best eye to start with?

An aphakic eye with small pupil and removed anterior vitreous.

How do you treat a macular edema secondary to pseudophakia?

With topical eye drops, by posterior subtenon triamcinolone injection or with intravitreal triamcinolone injection.

Is a treatment with Ozurdex possible?

No. The Ozurdex pellet will enter the anterior chamber and cause a corneal damage. An Ozurdex injection is contraindicated in eyes with aphakia and aphakic Verisyse IOL's.

Remark: The surgical technique of scleral fixation is demonstrated in a later chapter of this book.

Intrascleral IOL Implantation (Scharioth Technique)

23

Contents

Abstract

The intrascleral IOL implantation is very popular. The haptics of an IOL are fixated sutureless into the sclera. This technique was invented by Prof Scharioth. In this chapter Prof Scharioth explains step-by-step his original technique.

Keywords

Intrascleral IOL implantation · Scharioth technique

This sutureless technique for fixation of a posterior chamber intraocular lens is using permanent incarceration of the haptics in a scleral tunnel parallel to the limbus. The intrascleral haptic fixation technique is the best choice for aniridia or eyes with damaged iris.

A standard three-piece IOL suitable for sulcus fixation should be used for this technique. An implantation with injector through the main incision is possible. For PCIOL calculation the SRK-T formula and the same A-constant as for in-the-bag implantation is recommended. Surgery lasts about 30 min and is performed in local or general anaesthesia (Videos available).

Fig. 23.1 Scharioth forceps for intrascleral IOL fixation, straight and curved. Indication: intrascleral insertion of IOL. DORC 1286.SFD

Fig. 23.2 Sinskey hook, indication: manipulation of IOL. Geuder: 16167

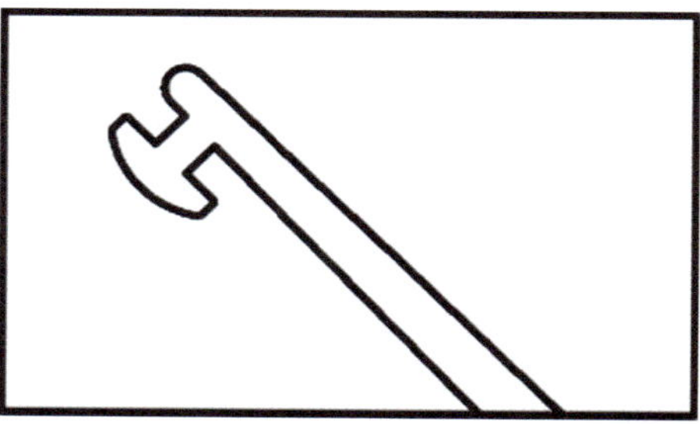

23.1   Standard Instruments for Intrascleral IOL Implantation

(1) Scharioth IOL Scleral Fixation Set 2 × 25G forceps, straight and curved. Indication: Intrascleral insertion of IOL. DORC 1286.SFD (Fig. 23.1).
(2) Sinskey hook. Indication: Manipulation of IOL. Geuder: 16167 (Fig. 23.2).

23.2   Intrascleral IOL Implantation Surgery

Instruments

(1) Anterior chamber maintainer or pars plana infusion
(2) Vitrector
(3) Scharioth IOL fixation forceps set
(4) 23G cannula
(5) 15° knife
(6) 2.8 mm main incision knife
(7) Sinskey hook.

Individual steps

1. Insertion of permanent infusion
2. Superior and inferior limbal peritomy
3. Ciliary sulcus sclerotomies and limbus-parallel intrascleral tunnel
4. Paracentesis at 3 and 9 o'clock, main incision
5. Deep anterior vitrectomy
6. Insertion of IOL
7. Haptic externalization and intrascleral fixation
8. Close conjunctiva, remove infusion.

The surgery step by step

1. Insertion of permanent infusion
2. Superior and inferior limbal peritomy
3. Ciliary sulcus sclerotomies and limbus-parallel intrascleral tunnel

After peritomy, the eye is stabilized either by pars plana infusion (i.e. 25G) or by anterior chamber maintainer. We try to prevent any diathermy of episcleral vessels to reduce the risk for scleral atrophy. Two straight sclerotomies ab externo are prepared with a sharp 23G cannula or 23G MVR blade about 1.5 mm postlimbal exactly 180° from each other and directed towards the centre of the globe (Fig. 23.3). A toric marker could be used to mark exactly 180° or the cannula is placed over the centre of the cornea to estimate position of the second sclerotomy (Figs. 23.4 and 23.5).

Then new cannulas are used to create a limbus-parallel tunnel at about 50% of scleral thickness, starting from inside the ciliary sulcus sclerotomies and ending with externalization of the cannula after 2.0–3.0 mm (Figs. 23.6 and 23.7).

4. Paracentesis at 3 and 9 o'clock, main incision
5. Deep anterior vitrectomy
6. Insertion of IOL

It is very important that the intraocular pressure is maintained during this step to prevent collapse and dislocation of the haptic out of the corneal incision. A standard 3-piece IOL with a haptic design fitting to the diameter of ciliary sulcus is implanted with an injector, and the tailing haptic is fixated in the corneal incision. Some might prefer to place the leading haptic on top of iris. But the leading haptic could also be directed immediately in the posterior chamber. In case of a large corneal incision (e.g. after ECCE/ICCE or explantation of a dislocated IOL), the IOL could be implanted with a forceps. This might be also easier for the first cases.

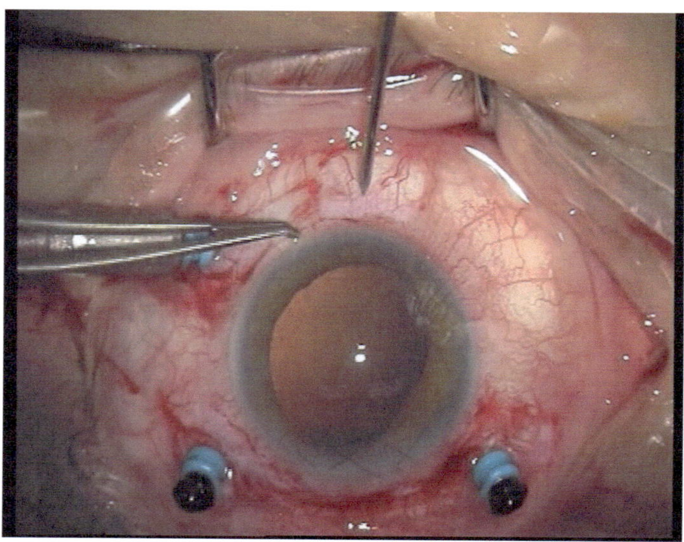

Fig. 23.3 After peritomy, a ciliary sulcus sclerotomy 1.5–2.0 mm postlimbal is created with a straight sharp 23G cannula

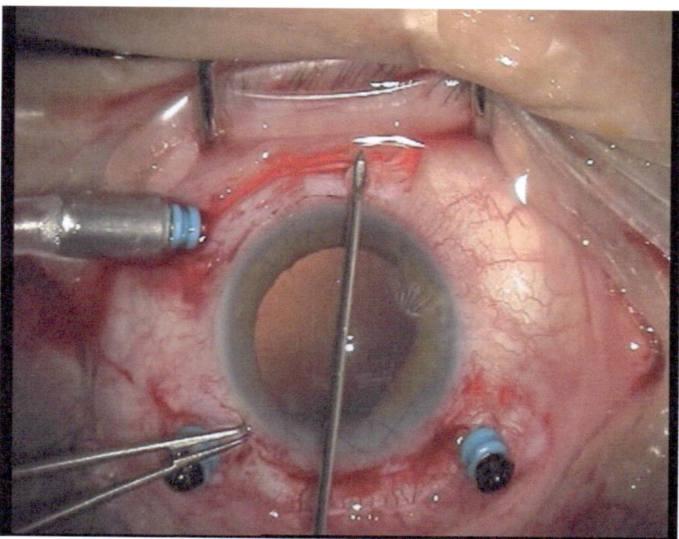

Fig. 23.4 Marking 180°, alternatively a toric marker could be used; continuous infusion via pars plana or as anterior chamber maintainer via side port incision is installed

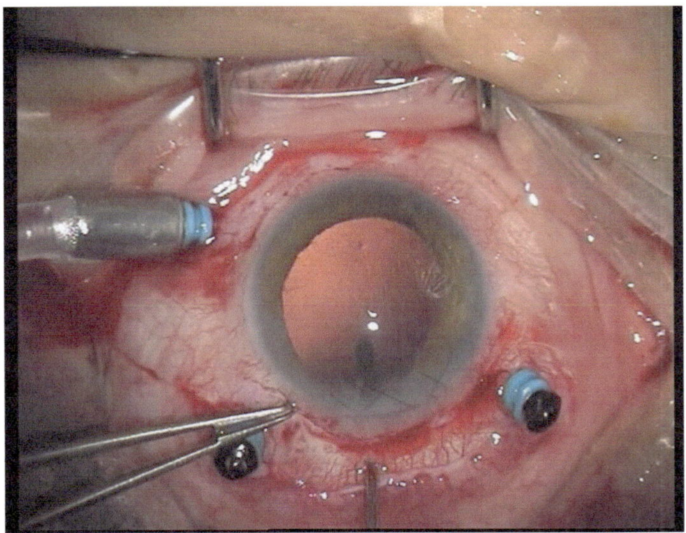

Fig. 23.5 Second ciliary sulcus sclerotomy is performed with straight sharp 23G cannula

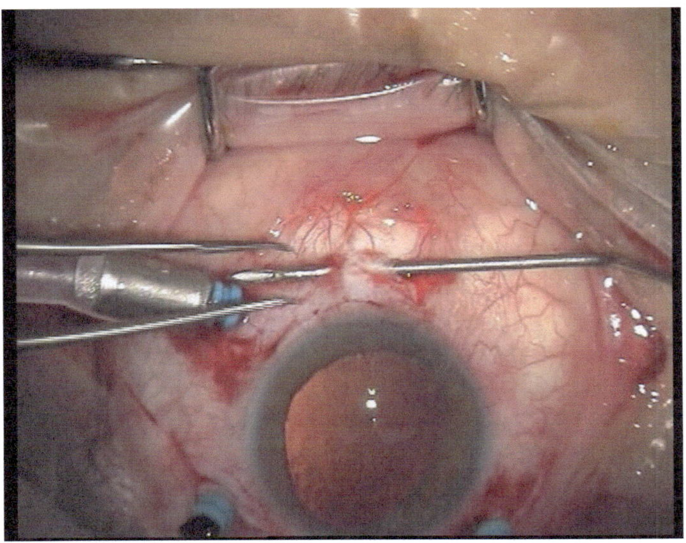

Fig. 23.6 Starting from the ciliary sclerotomy, a limbus-parallel intrascleral tunnel is created with a bended sharp 23G cannula, the tip of this cannula is externalized after 2–3 mm

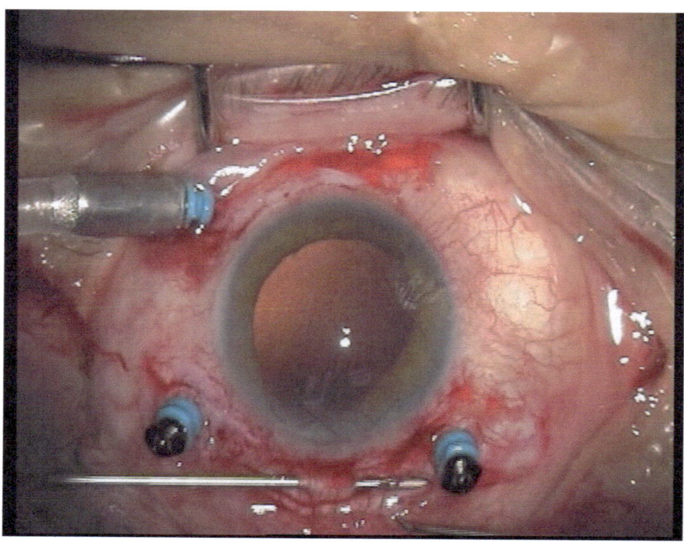

Fig. 23.7 Similar an intrascleral tunnel is created from the opposite sclerotomy, both tunnels are directed counterclockwise

7. Haptic externalization and intrascleral fixation

The leading haptic is then grasped at its tip with a special straight 25G forceps (Fig. 23.8) (Scharioth IOL fixation forceps), pulled through the sclerotomy and left externalized (Figs. 23.9 and 23.10). It is very important to grasp the very tip of the haptic to prevent damage to the haptic. For intraocular manipulations (hand shake technique), it is useful to use two intraocular forceps (e.g. straight and curved Scharioth forceps). With the curved Scharioth forceps, then the haptic is grasped at its tip, pushed a little back into the vitreous cavity, introduced into the intrascleral tunnel and pushed through (Figs. 23.11 and 23.12). Then the haptic is released (Fig. 23.13), the forceps is turned, closed and pulled back leaving the haptic in the sclera (pushing technique). Alternatively, you can introduce the Scharioth forceps from the distal end of the intrascleral tunnel until it becomes visible in the sclerotomy, then the haptic tip is grasped and pulled in the scleral tunnel (pulling technique). The same manoeuvres are performed with the tailing haptic. The ends of the haptic are left in the tunnel to prevent foreign body sensation, erosion of the conjunctiva and to reduce the risk for inflammation. The IOL should be well centred and without tilt (Figs. 23.14 and 23.15). If needed IOL, could be centred ab interno with a Sinskey hook.

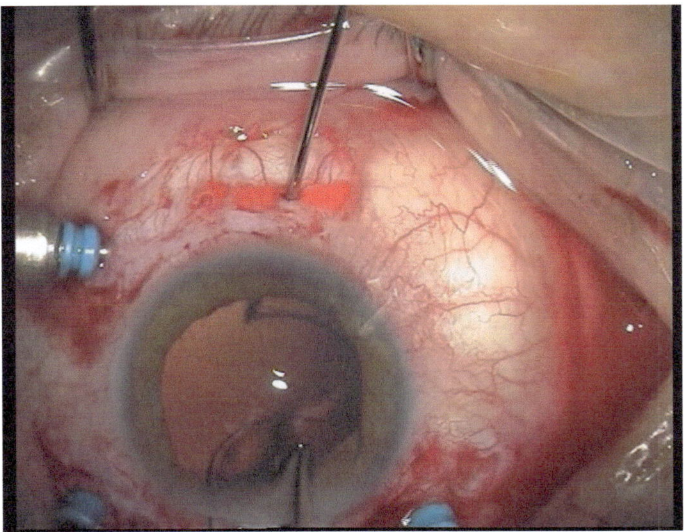

Fig. 23.8 IOL is inserted through main incision and held with a forceps while the leading haptic is grasped at its tip with the straight 25G Scharioth forceps; alternatively, the IOL could be injected through cartridge. If one feels more secure, the leading haptic could be placed first on the iris surface

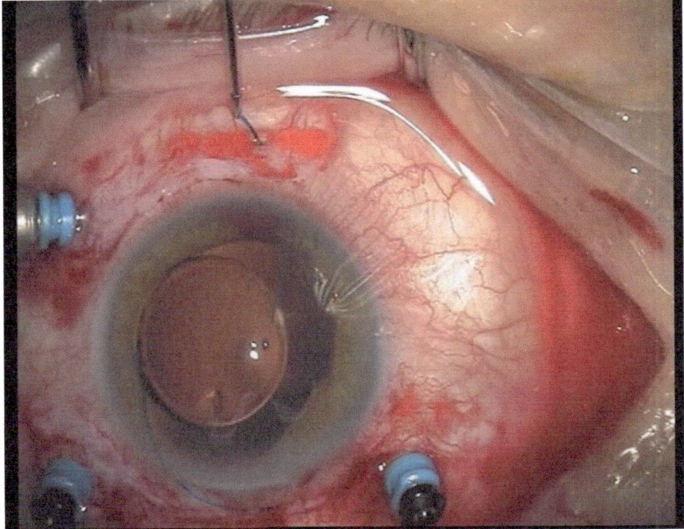

Fig. 23.9 Leading haptic is externalized via ciliary sulcus sclerotomy, trailing haptic is fixed in the main incision, continuous infusion is on

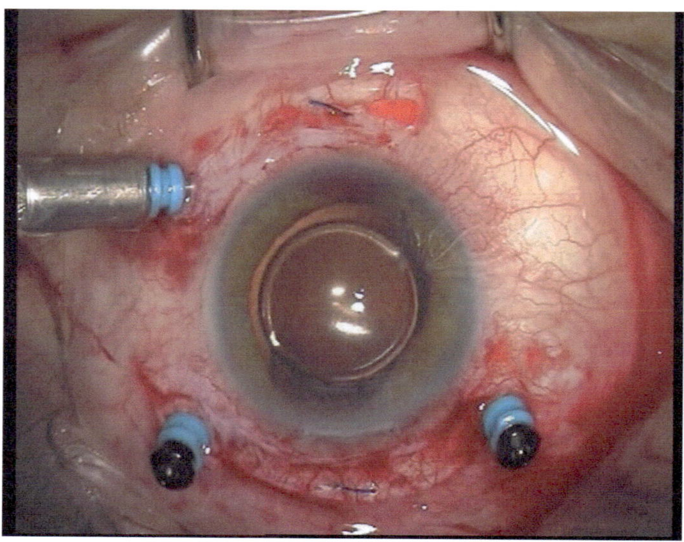

Fig. 23.10 Trailing haptic is inserted, grasped at its tip with straight Scharioth forceps and externalized via second ciliary sulcus sclerotomy

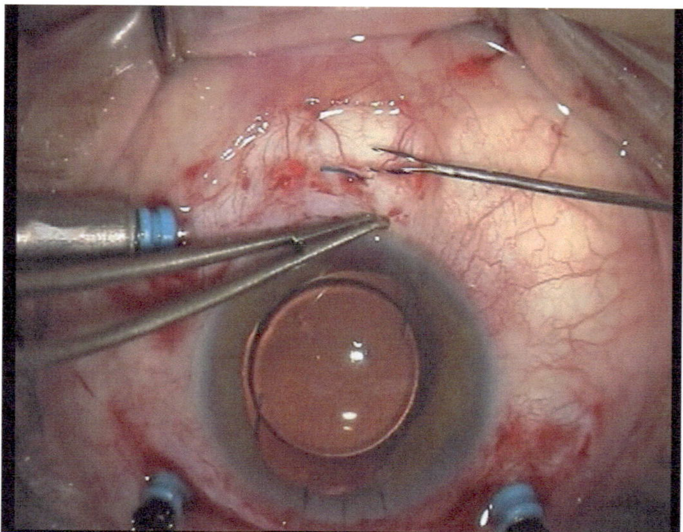

Fig. 23.11 Externalized haptic is grasped at its tip with curved Scharioth forceps, then pushed back into the sclerotomy and inserted into the intrascleral tunnel

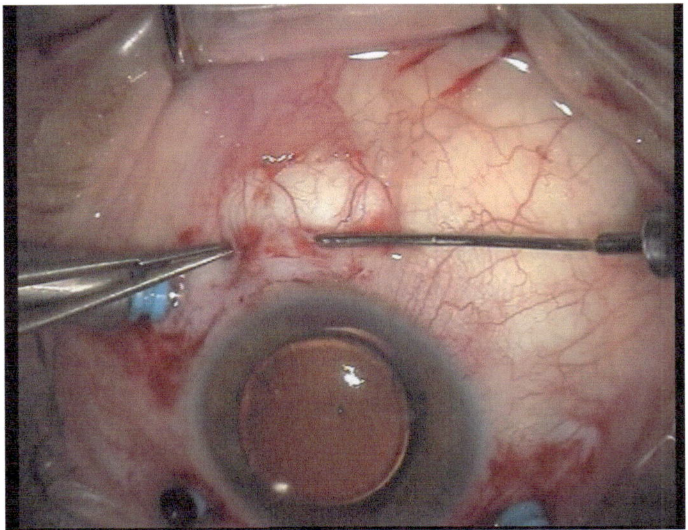

Fig. 23.12 Haptic is pushed through the intrascleral tunnel and externalized on the opposite site

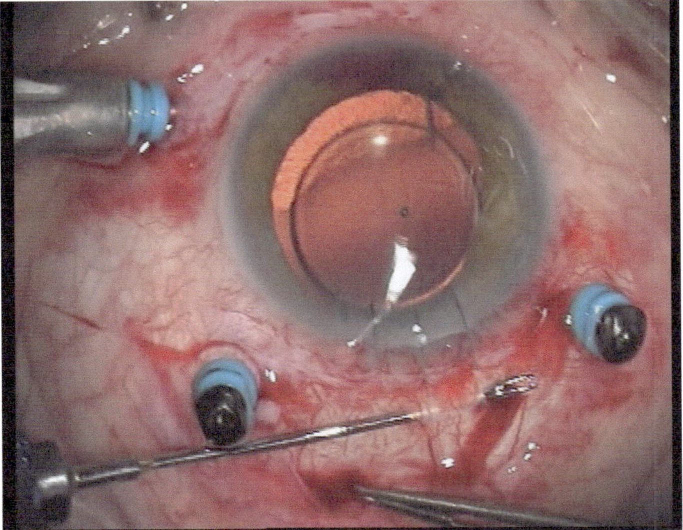

Fig. 23.13 Second haptic is introduced into the intrascleral tunnel, then the forceps is opened, turned and retracted

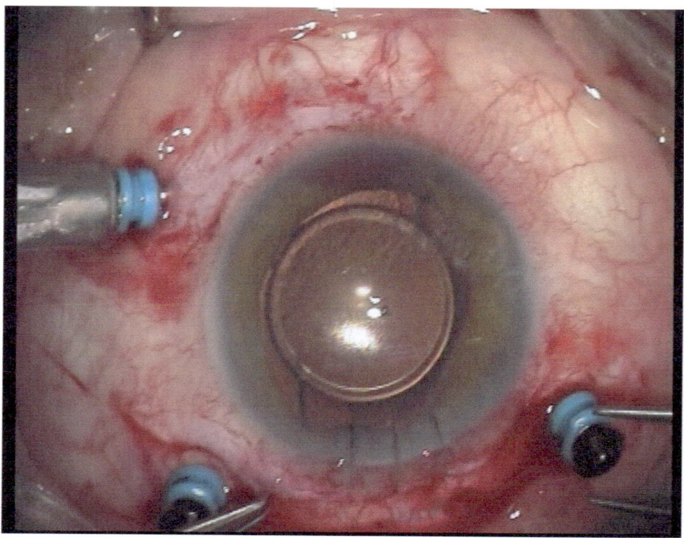

Fig. 23.14 Both haptics are implanted, note that the haptic is completely buried intrascleral, IOL is well centred without tilting, finally trocars are removed, incisions are checked for leakage and sutured if needed

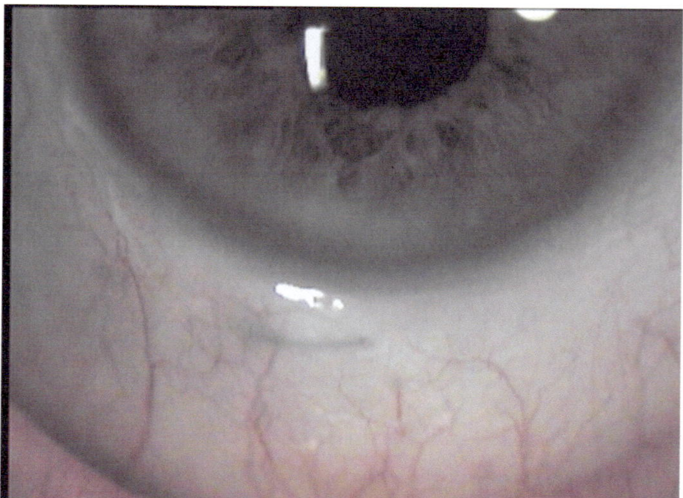

Fig. 23.15 Five-year post-OP. The blue haptic at 6 o'clock is intrasclerally located. After five-year follow-up, the IOL is centred, and there is no sign of inflammation, erosion or dislocation of the haptics

8. Close conjunctiva, remove infusion

Some young patients with floppy iris showed postoperative recurrent iris capture which disappeared after NdYAG laser iridotomy. If this condition is anticipated (e.g. extreme deepening of the AC during hydration of the side port incisions), an intraoperatively iridectomy with the vitreous cutter is helpful. The sclerotomies are checked for leakage and if necessary sutured with absorbable suture (e.g. Vicryl 8–0). Finally, the infusion is removed, corneal incisions are hydrated and conjunctiva is closed.

Pits and Pearls no. 20

<u>Intrascleral IOL fixation:</u>

(1) It is very important to perform sclerotomies symmetrically 180^c from each other and about the same distance to the limbus to prevent decentration or tilt. If surgeon is not satisfied with IOL position, minimal adjustment could be performed intraoperatively by positioning the IOL with the help of Sinskey hook. In case of major misplacement, new sclerotomies should be created.
(2) IOL haptic has to be fully covered by sclera. Subconjunctival placement will cause conjunctival erosion and other complications.
(3) In case of haptic dislocation in the early postoperative period, intrascleral fixation can be repeated. We have not seen late dislocations.

Intrascleral IOL Fixation with Flanged Haptics (Yamane Technique)

24

Abstract

The intrascleral IOL implantation is very popular nowadays. The Yamane technique is the most popular intrascleral technique. In this chapter the Yamane technique is described step-by-step.

Keywords

Yamane · Intrascleral IOL fixation

Instruments

1. Anterior chamber maintainer or pars plana infusion
2. Vitrector
3. Intraocular forceps (e.g. Scharioth IOL fixation forceps)
4. 26-G or 30-G cannula
5. 15° knife
6. 2.8 mm main incision knife
7. Cautery (e.g. single use Kirwan cautery (Kirwan Surgical Products (ksp.com))).

IOL selection

We use J&J AR40e or Alcon MA60

Individual steps

1. Insertion of permanent infusion
2. Paracentesis
3. Vitrectomy
4. Insertion of IOL
5. Transconjunctival ciliary sulcus sclerotomy with cannula
6. IOL haptic insertion into cannula and externalization

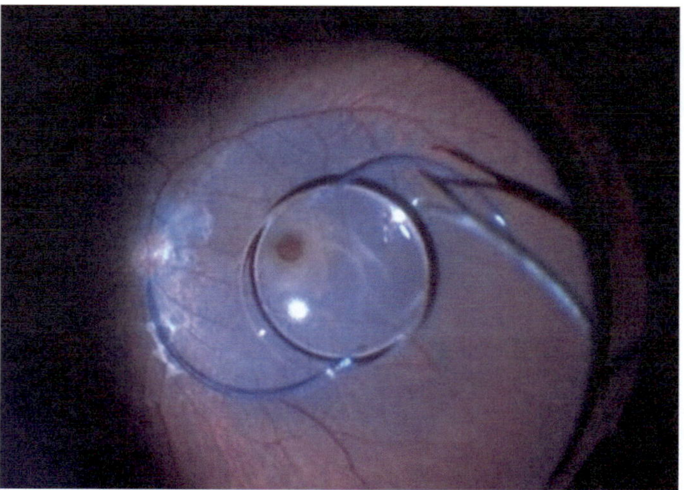

Fig. 24.1 Completely dislocated IOL

7. Cautery of haptic end
8. Intrascleral positioning of flanged haptic.

The operation step by step (Figs. 24.1, 24.2, 24.3, 24.4, 24.5, 24.6, 24.7, 24.8, 24.9, 24.10, 24.11, 24.12 and 24.13)

1. Insertion of a permanent infusion
2. Paracentesis, main incision
3. Insertion of three-piece IOL

   One should test before that the IOL haptic fits into the cannula lumen

4. A 26-G (or 27G) cannula is transconjunctivally inserted 1.5 to 2.0 mm postlimbal while creating an intrascleral tunnel clockwise and then introduced into the posterior camber
5. The leading haptic is then grasp with intraocular forceps and pushed into the lumen of the cannula. Then cannula is carefully withdrawn and the haptic is pulled out.
6. Same is performed exactly 180° from this sclerotomy
7. Haptic is grasped with a tying forceps 1 mm from the tip and a flanged end is created by melting with a cautery. The tip of the cautery should not come in contact with the haptic itself
8. Haptic is pushed backwards so that the tip is plane with scleral surface. Conjunctiva is massaged, and the second haptic is handled same way
9. Finally, the infusion is removed, and corneal incisions are hydrated.

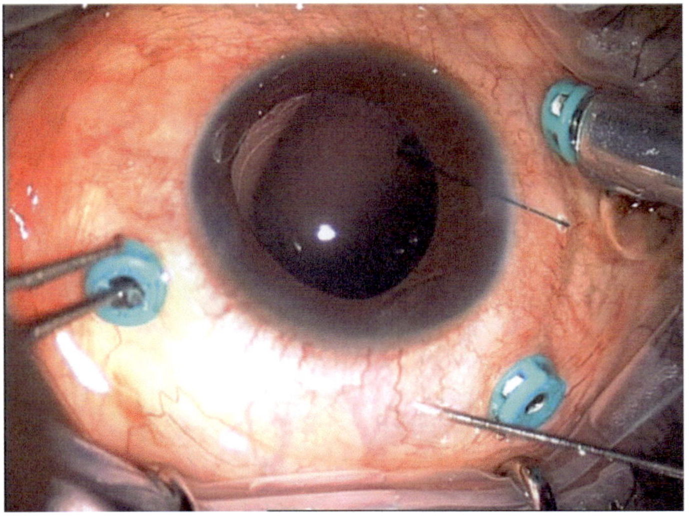

Fig. 24.2 Pars plana vitrectomy performed and IOL lifted into anterior segment. One IOL haptic is fixed into a paracentesis

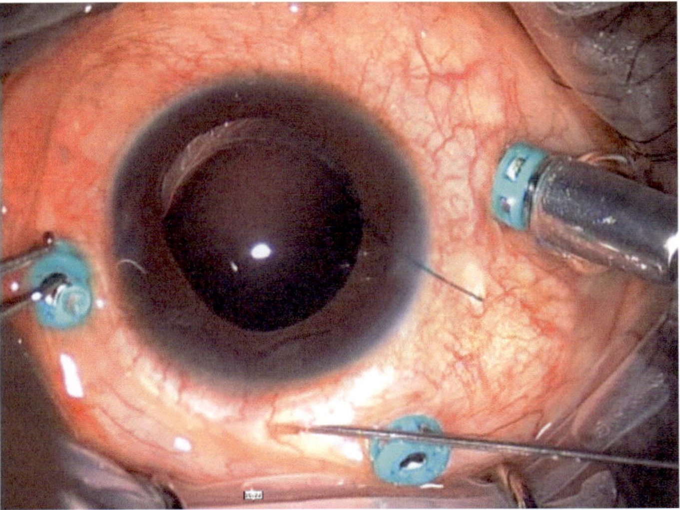

Fig. 24.3 Cannula is transconjunctivally inserted to create a limbus-parallel tunnel clockwise 1.5–2.0 mm postlimbal

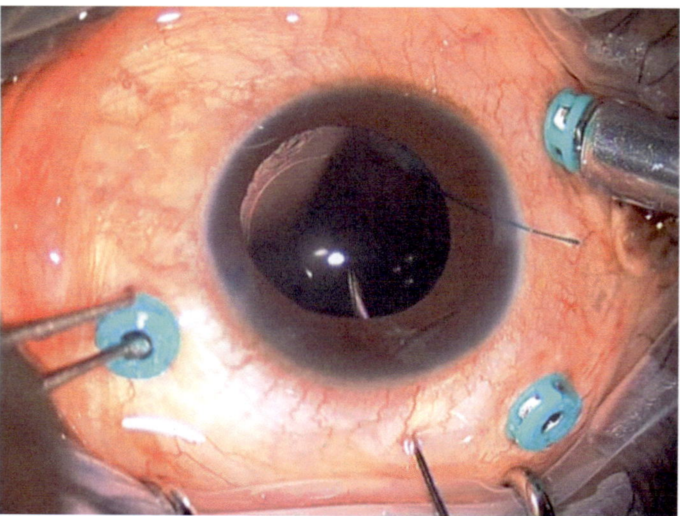

Fig. 24.4 Cannula is then pushed into the vitreous cavity and left in place

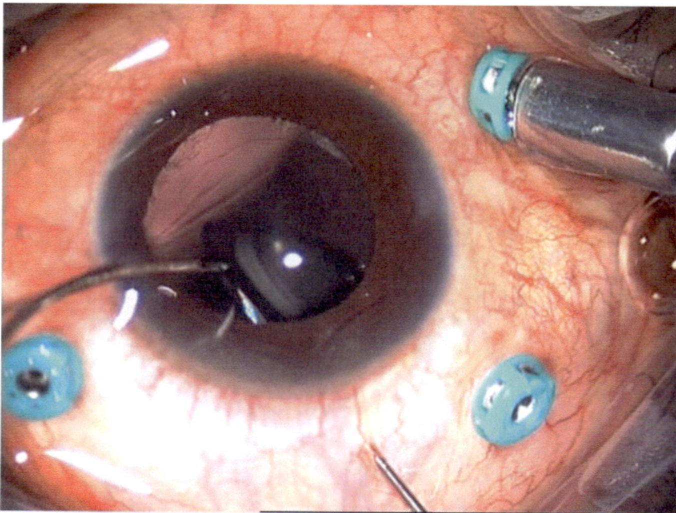

Fig. 24.5 Intraocular forceps is used to grasp the haptic and then to introduce the haptic into the lumen of the cannula

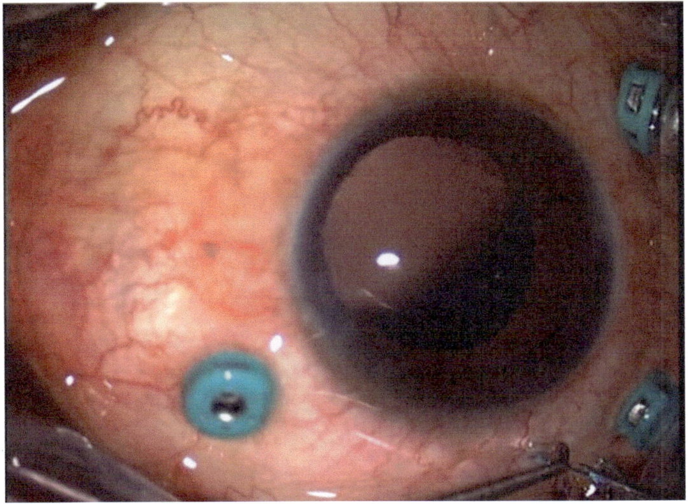

Fig. 24.6 Cannula is withdrawn and haptic is temporally externalized

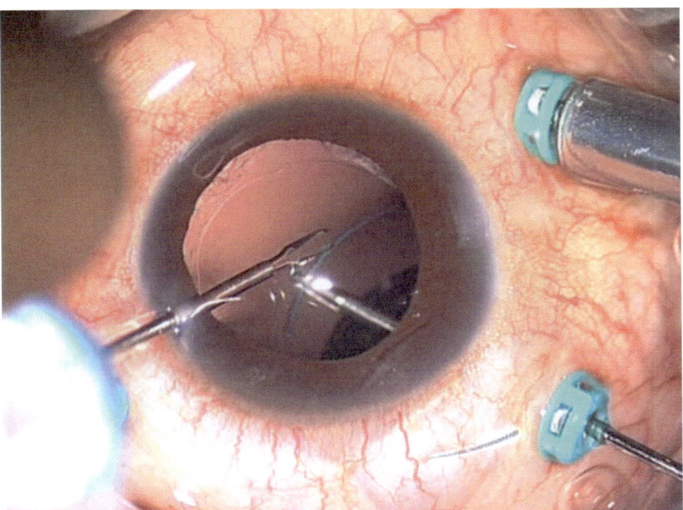

Fig. 24.7 Hand shake manoeuvre to manipulate the IOL haptic

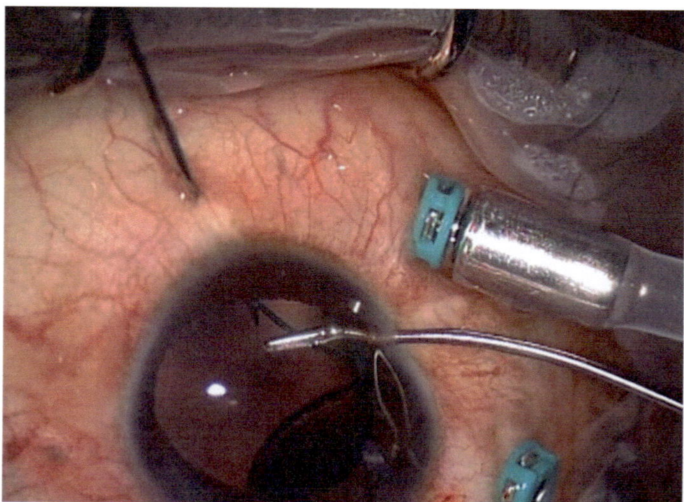

Fig. 24.8 After cannula is inserted 180° opposite to the first sclerotomy, the haptic is inserted into the lumen of the cannula

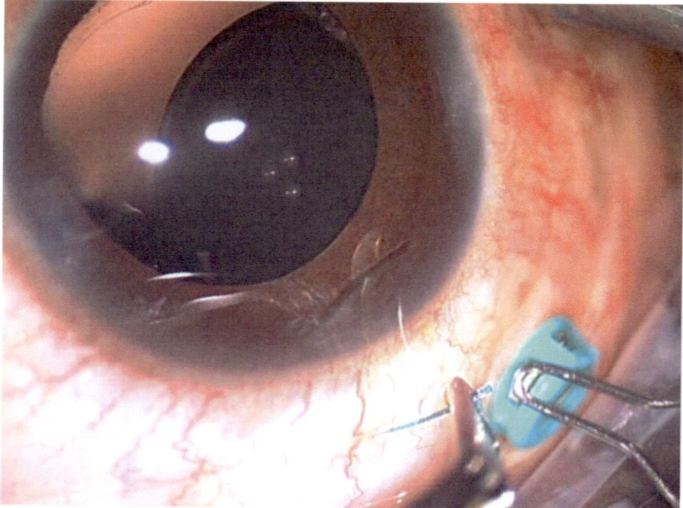

Fig. 24.9 IOL haptic is grasped around 1 mm form distal end. Then with a cautery, a flanged end is created by melting. Direct contact between IOL haptic and cautery should be prevented

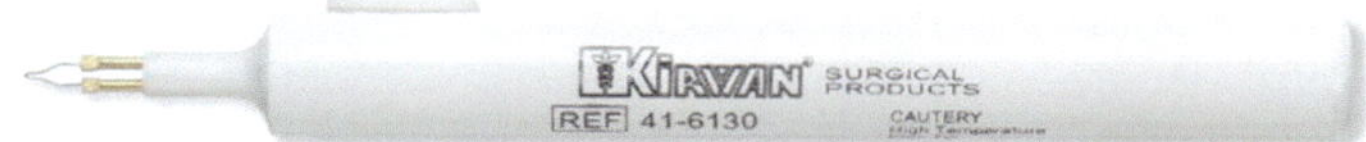

Fig. 24.10 Single use cautery (Kirwan cautery 41-6120 low temperature or 41-6130 high temperature)

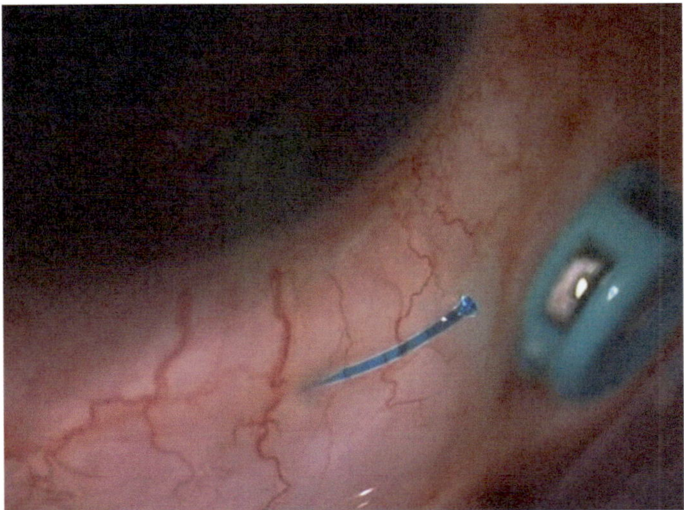

Fig. 24.11 IOL haptic with flanged haptic after cautery

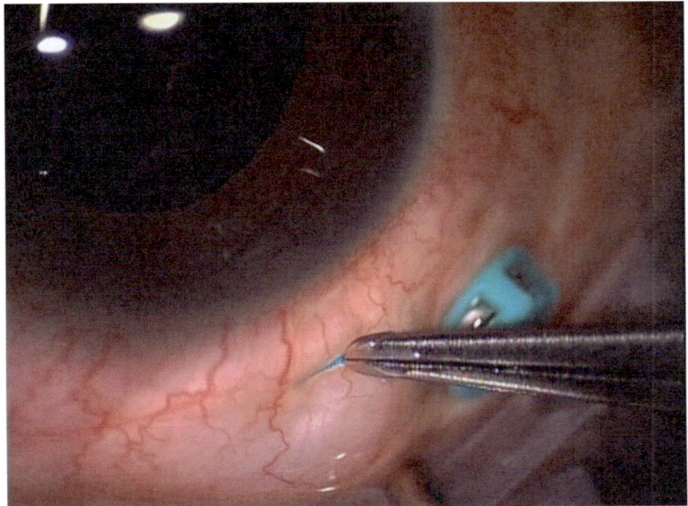

Fig. 24.12 Haptic is pushed back into sclera and covered with tenon and conjunctiva

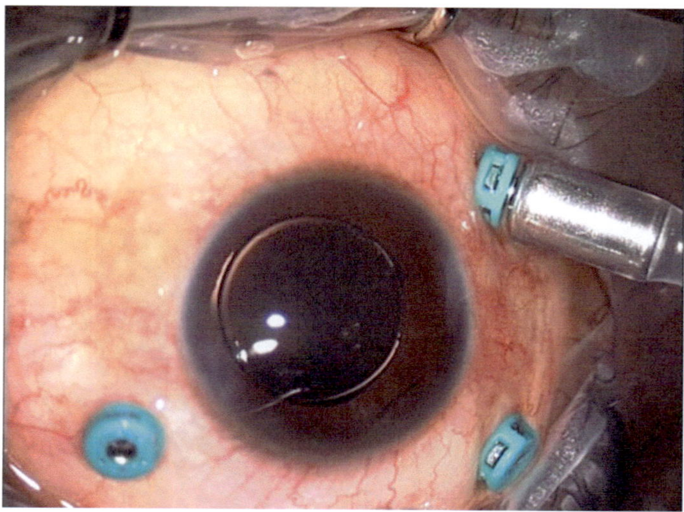

Fig. 24.13 Final situation with well-centred IOL and covered IOL haptics

Scleral IOL Fixation

25

Abstract

An IOL can be fixated with scleral sutures. This chapter explains step-by-step the scleral fixation of an IOL.

Keywords

Scleral IOL fixation

This surgery is usually performed due to a dislocated IOL (Fig. 25.1). The IOL is recovered, and the same IOL is sutured to the sclera. The suture is fastened to the haptic and then to the sclera. If you use the same IOL, then externalize the haptics at the sclerotomies and suture the haptics. If you do not use the same IOL, then implant a 3-piece IOL. You can either: (1) implant the IOL, externalize the haptics through the sclerotomies and fasten the sutures to the haptics or (2) fasten the sutures to the IOL and then implant the IOL. For the sclera, there are many different suture techniques. (Videos available).

Sutures for scleral-fixated IOL

(1) 2 curved needles. Alcon. Polypropylene, blue monofilament, double armed. 8,065.307.601.

Indication: Scleral fixation of a dislocated IOL.

OR

(2) 1 needle straight, 1 curved needle. Alcon. Polypropylene, blue monofilament, double armed. 8,065,304,901.

Indication: Secondary implantation and scleral fixation of an IOL secondary to aphakia.

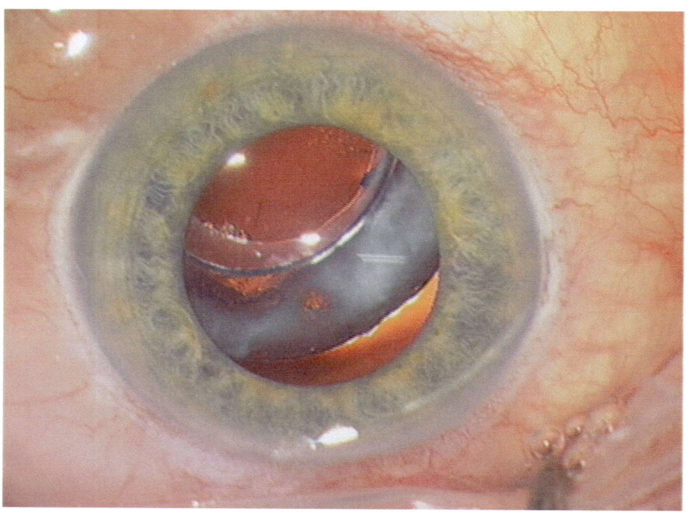

Fig. 25.1 Anteriorly dislocated bag-IOL complex. With courtesy of the Kaden Verlag

Instruments

1. 2× intravitreal forceps, e.g. serrated jaws forceps
2. Polypropylene 10–0 suture with curved needle (i.e. Alcon. Polypropylene, blue monofilament, double armed. 8,065,307,601).

Individual steps

1. Focal peritomy at 3 and 9 o'clock
2. Two sclerotomies (1.5 mm posterior to the limbus) at 3 and 9 o'clock
3. Extraction of a haptic at 3 o'clock, place a suture onto the haptic and push it back into the eye; the same procedure at 9 o'clock.
4. Suture the haptic suture in a snake shape to the sclera
5. Close the conjunctiva, removal of the trocars.

Operation step by step:

1. Focal peritomy at 3 and 9 o'clock
2. Two sclerotomies (1.5 mm posterior to the limbus) at 3 and 9 o'clock

Open the conjunctiva at 3 and 9 o'clock to make space for one sclerotomy and a scleral suture, i.e. approximately from 2 to 4 o'clock and from 8 to 10 o'clock. Then, cauterize the bleeding vessels.

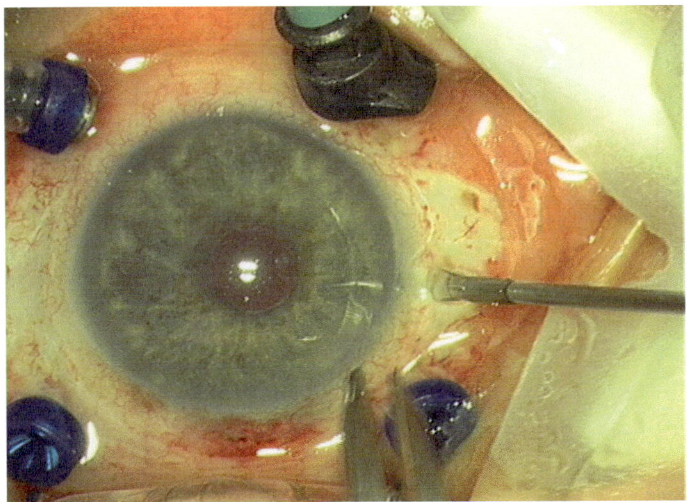

Fig. 25.2 Perform a focal peritomy at 3 and 9 o'clock. Perform then a sclerotomy 1.5 mm behind the limbus with the V-lance. With courtesy of the Kaden Verlag

3. Two sclerotomies (1.5 mm posterior to the limbus) at 3 and 9 o'clock
4. Extraction of a haptic at 3 o'clock, place a suture onto the haptic and push it back into the eye; the same procedure at 9 o'clock.

In case of a 3-piece IOL, fasten the suture in the middle of the haptic and in case of an 1-piece IOL at the end of the haptic.

In the area of the sulcus, 1.5 mm posterior to the limbus, perform an approximately 1.3 mm sclerotomy (Fig. 25.2). The sclerotomy must be perpendicular (i.e. approximately 90° to the sclera), in order not to harm the anterior chamber. Via the sclerotomy at 3 o'clock, grasp a haptic with an Eckardt forceps (Fig. 25.3), and pull it out of the eye. Cut a polypropylene 10–0 suture with two curved needles in two halves. Then, suture one half (suture) to the haptic (Fig. 25.4), and insert the haptic back into the eye. Perform the same manoeuvre at the 9 o'clock sclerotomy. After the haptic has been pushed back, centre the IOL by pulling carefully on both sutures.

5. Suture the haptic suture in a snake shape to the sclera

Different techniques are now possible. You can place five U-shaped in a shape snake to the sclera and then cut off the suture without a knot. A knot can cause a disturbing foreign body sensation to the patient (Fig. 25.5). Alternatively, you can prepare a scleral flap, fasten the suture to the sclera and place the knot under the scleral flap.

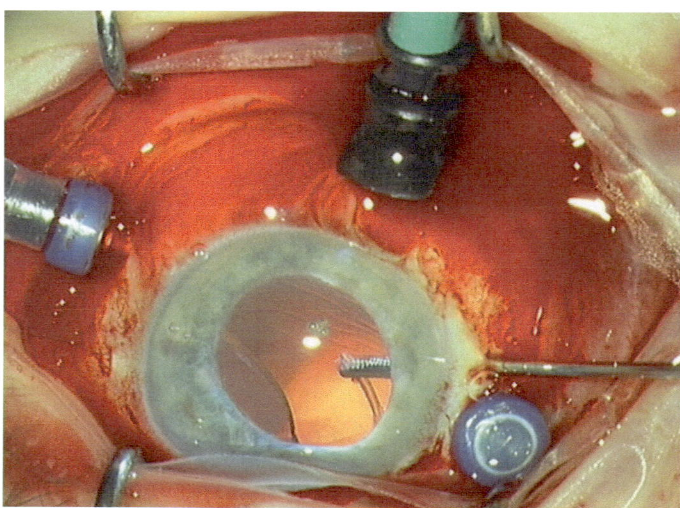

Fig. 25.3 Insert the intravitreal forceps through the sclerotomy, grasp the tip of the haptic, and pull it through the sclerotomy. With courtesy of the Kaden Verlag

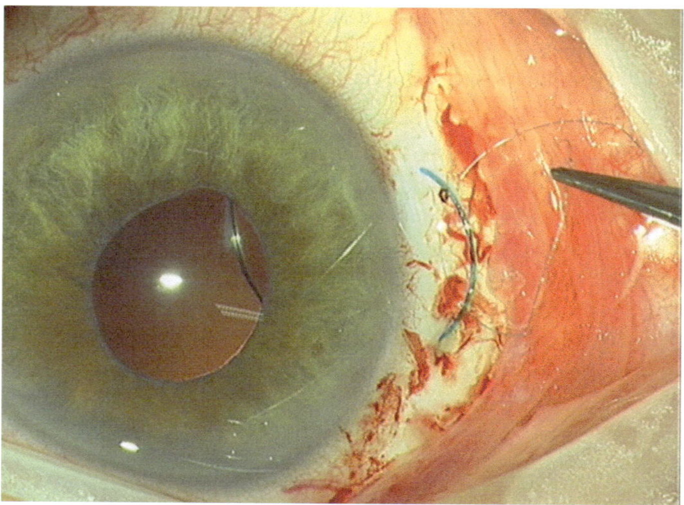

Fig. 25.4 Knot a polypropylene 10–0 suture (2 curved needles) to the haptic, and reinsert the haptic into the eye. Perform the same manoeuvre at the other side. With courtesy of the Kaden Verlag

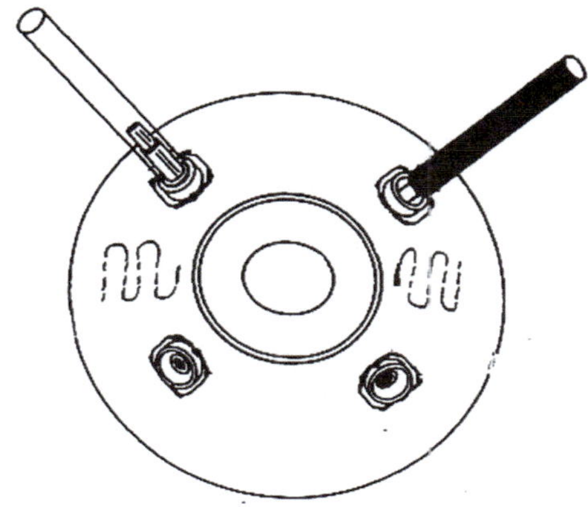

Fig. 25.5 Then, perform a snake formed suture on each side; four rounds are sufficient; a knot is not necessary

6. Close the conjunctiva, removal of the trocars

The conjunctiva is closed with a Vicryl 8-0 interrupted stitch. The sclerotomies do not need to be sutured.

Abstract

The Hoffmann technique is very similar to the scleral fixation technique with the difference that the sutures are placed in scleral pockets. The scleral pockets prevent ocular irritation. The Hoffmann technique is explained step-by-step.

Keywords

Scleral fixation · Hoffmann technique

This suture fixation technique is using reverse scleral pockets without conjunctival opening to reduce surgical trauma. The technique could be used for transscleral suture fixation of a PCIOL, subluxated fibrosed capsular bag-IOL complex or modified capsular tension ring. Surgery lasts about 30 min and is performed in local or general anaesthesia.

Remark: All videos of this chapter be seen in a playlist of my youtube channel:

https://www.youtube.com/playlist?list=PL0dKYclPD7yMJRuQAIt9Dr7pOtuI0
Seex

Instruments

1. Anterior chamber maintainer or OVD
2. Double armed polypropylene suture (9–0 or 10–0) with long needle (Alcon. Polypropylene. 8,065,304,901)
3. 15 deg knife
4. Mini crescent knife (e.g. Mini glaucoma knife, DORC, The Netherlands or Ultra sharp scleral pocket knife 1.0 mm, Alcon Grieshaber, USA)
5. Sharp 27G needle and/or endoforceps (e.g. Scharioth IOL fixation forceps set 1286.SFD, DORC Int., The Netherlands)
6. Push–pull instrument (Sinskey hook).

Individual steps

1. Insertion of permanent infusion or injection of OVD
2. Partial thickness paralimbal incision
3. Scleral pocket dissection
4. Transscleral suture placement through scleral pockets with double armed suture
5. Externalization of suture from scleral pockets towards cornea
6. Tying and knotting the suture
7. Burring the suture ends in scleral pocket
8. Remove infusion and/or OVD.

The surgery step by step:

1. Insertion of permanent infusion or injection of OVD
2. Partial thickness paralimbal incision
3. Scleral pocket dissection.

After creating a paracentesis, the eye is stabilized either by anterior chamber maintainer or OVD filling of anterior chamber. Two partial thickness paralimbal incisions approximately 2.0–3.0 mm wide are made inside the clear cornea using a 15° straight knife or a guarded blade with 0.3 mm incision depth at the desired fixation site (Fig. 26.1). This is usually repeated for a second fixation site. This is exactly 180° in case of transscleral fixation of a PCIOL or a capsular bag, but not in case of a modified capsular tension ring (Cionni 2L CTR, Morcher, Germany). Starting from these incisions, scleral pockets are dissected posteriorly at this depth using mini crescent knife (Fig. 26.2). This scleral pocket has to be at least 2.5–3.0 mm long to facilitate later externalization of the sutures.

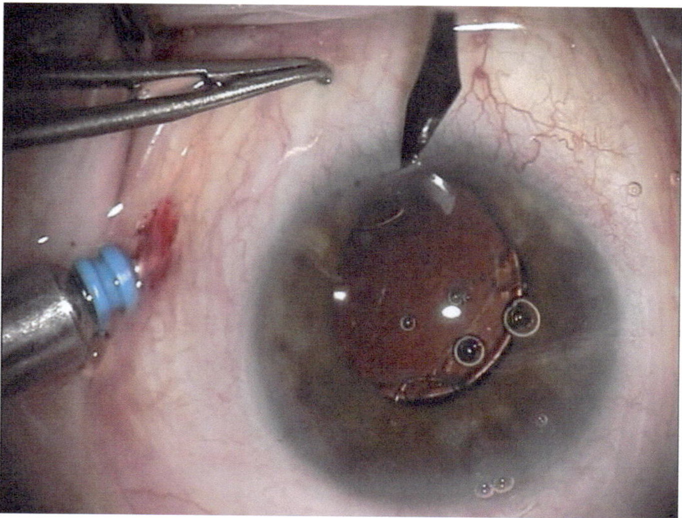

Fig. 26.1 Creating a 2.0–3.0 wide limbusparallel incision with 15° knife or 0.3 mm guarded blade

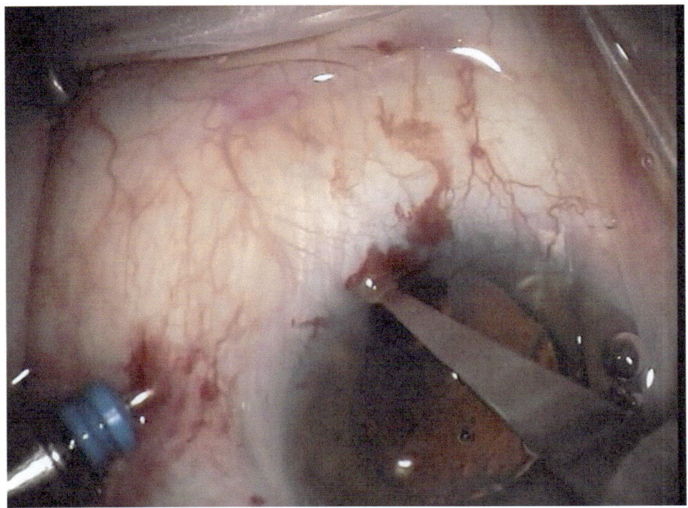

Fig. 26.2 Posteriorly directed dissection of scleral pocket with mini crescent knife

4. Transscleral suture placement through scleral pockets with double armed suture
5. Externalization of suture from scleral pockets towards cornea.

Side port incisions are made almost opposite to these scleral pockets, and the needle of the double armed 9–0 or 10–0 polypropylene suture is introduced through the side port incision. The first needle is then stitched through the ciliary sulcus, sclera and conjunctiva ab interno in the area of the scleral pocket (Fig. 26.3). If iris is moving, needle should be placed a bit more posterior to prevent damage to the iris root and postoperative UGH syndrome.

The second needle of the double armed suture is then placed through the side port incision with special care that no corneal tissue is caught. Then, the needle is placed through the peripheral fibrosed capsular bag catching the IOL haptic or even better a capsular tension ring in case of subluxated capsular bag-IOL complex. Here, an endoforceps (e.g. Scharioth IOL fixation forceps set 1286.SFD, DORC Int., The Netherlands) could be used to stabilize the implant. In case of a modified capsular tension ring, the needle is placed through the hole in the fixation eyelet. Now, the needle is stitched through the ciliary sulcus, sclera and conjunctiva ab interno in the area of the scleral pocket (Fig. 26.4). Alternatively, a 27G needle could be placed ab externo through conjunctiva and sclera in the area of scleral pocket, and the tip of the suture needle is placed into the lumen of this 27G needle to guide it. Then, needles are cut off the sutures (Fig. 26.5), and with the help of a push–pull hook or an endoforceps, the suture is caught in the scleral pockets and withdrawn towards the cornea (Fig. 26.6).

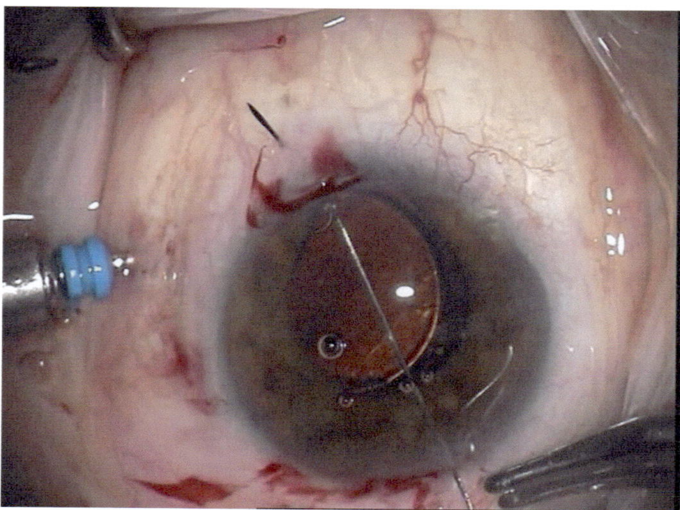

Fig. 26.3 First needle of a double armed polypropylene suture is placed transscleral in the area of the scleral pocket

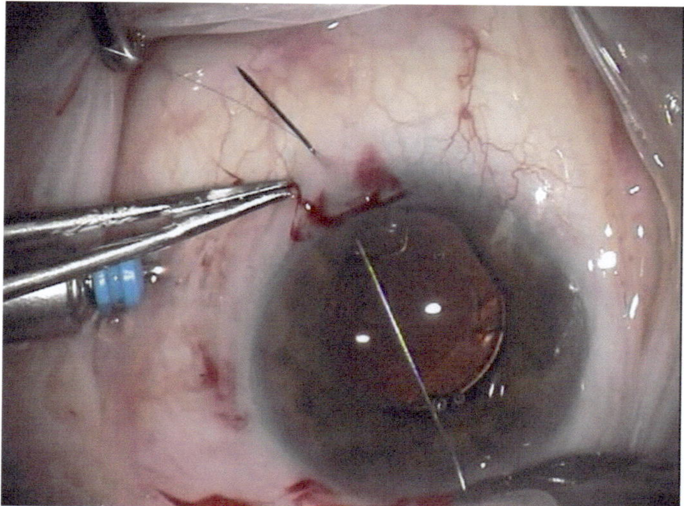

Fig. 26.4 Sneedle of double armed polypropylene suture is placed transscleral in the area of the scleral pocket a bit away from the first one, note first suture part is already externalized

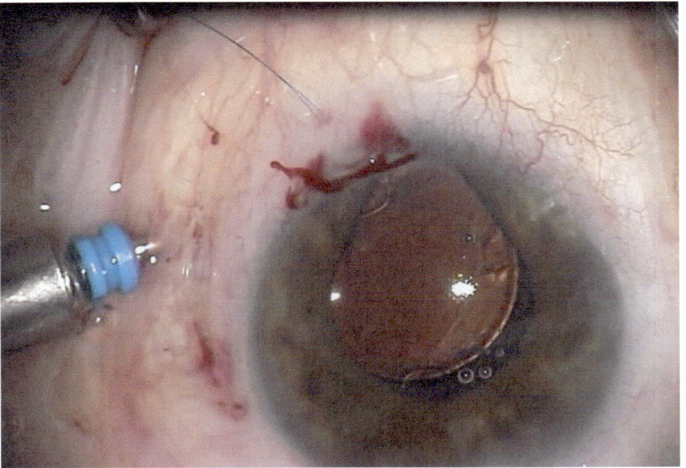

Fig. 26.5 After removing the needles at the first scleral pocket

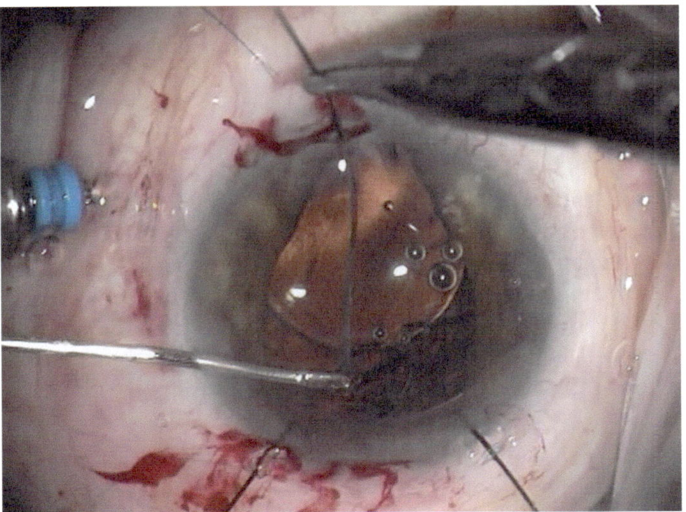

Fig. 26.6 The same procedure is repeated with the second scleral pocket

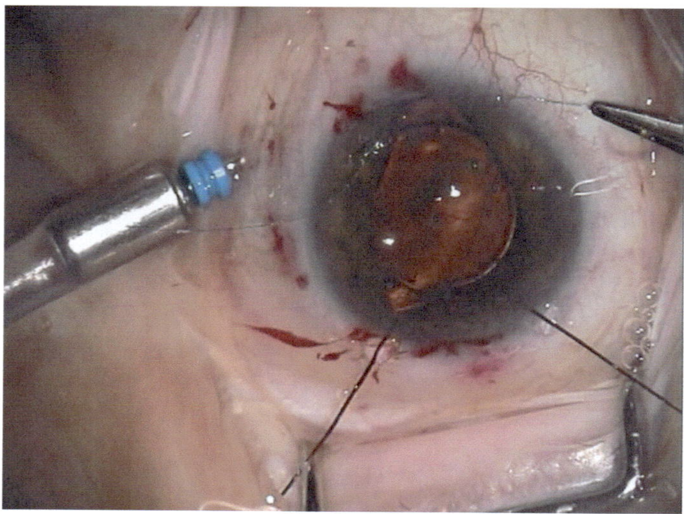

Fig. 26.7 Polypropylene suture is tightened, while suture loop is pulling inside the implant and centring the IOL

6. Tying and knotting the suture
7. Burring the suture ends in scleral pocket
8. Remove infusion and/or OVD.

Using the two ends of a suture, a three throws knot is made and gently tightened (Fig. 26.7). The tension is carefully adjusted on both sites to ensure that the IOL is well centred. Once the IOL is centred, another knot is added to fixate the suture. The suture ends are cut and then repositioned into the scleral pockets (Fig. 26.8). Anterior chamber maintainer and/or OVD is removed from the anterior chamber. Incisions are hydrated and checked for leakage. They can be sutured if needed. Fig. 26.8 Ends of the polypropylene suture are placed into the scleral pocket

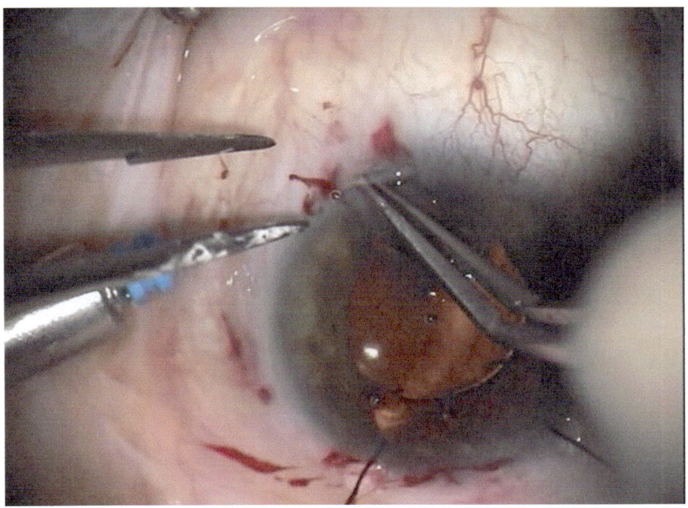

Fig. 26.8 Ends of the polypropylene suture are placed into the scleral pocket

Fixation of IOL with Iris Suture

27

Contents

Abstract

An IOL can be fixated to the iris with a suture. This can be done with an IOL-in-the bag and without lens capsule. This special technique is demonstrated step-by-step in this chapter.

Keywords

Iris suture · IOL fixation

Author: V. O. Ponomarev

In surgical practices of the Ekaterinburg Eye Microsurgery Center, the technology of suturing various models of IOLs, as well as IOL-capsule complexes to the iris through suture fixation, is actively used. The first developers and subsequent implementers of this technology are Dr. Med. Ivanov D., Shilovskikh O. and Fechin O, who started to actively use the method in anterior segment surgery from the beginning of the 1990s. Today, at the Ekaterinburg Eye Microsurgery Center, more than 250 IOL suturing operations to the iris are performed annually in various modifications, including as part of combined vitreoretinal surgery. (Videos available).

Internal indications for the use of the technology:

- Dislocation of IOL and/or IOL-capsular bag complex into the vitreal cavity for any reason;

– Secondary IOL implantation in the absence or disruption of capsular support;
– Combination of the need for IOL and/or the IOL-capsule complex with the need for mydriasis suturing, pupilloplasty or anterior chamber angle reconstruction;

Internal contraindications to the use of the technology:

– Aniridia;
– Iris rubeosis (when more than 1/3 of the iris is involved);
– Uveitis.

Complications:

– Iris root detachment;
– Bleeding from iris vessels;
– Pupil deformity (requires thermo corneoplasty);
– Dislocation of the IOL after inadequate suturing.

There is no fundamental need to distinguish between pure IOL implantation or implantation of the IOL-capsular bag complex, but there are a number of peculiarities, which we will discuss below.

Suturing an IOL to the iris typically involves fixation of the IOL to the iris by two sutures running through the haptic elements of the IOL and the iris body. This design allows the IOL to be stably positioned in the frontal plane, providing high anatomic and functional results (Fig. 27.1).

Instruments and equipment:

(1) Surgical "spatula", "hook", "hatchet" for IOL positioning (Fig. 27.2)
(2) IOL gripping forceps—surgeon's choice (Fig. 27.3)
(3) A needle holder with a long, curved needle, usually polypropylene 9.0–10.0 for suturing (Fig. 27.4).

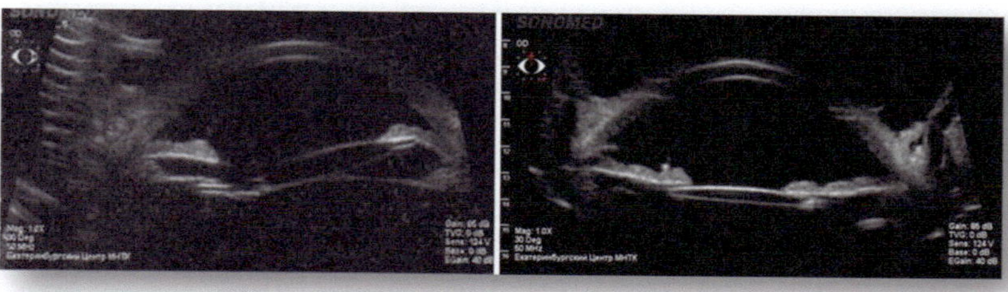

Fig. 27.1 Example of ultrasound biomicroscopy of a dislocated IOL—photo on the left, and on the next day after suturing to the iris—photo on the right (Photo courtesy: Nikitin V. Ekaterinburg Eye Microsurgery Center)

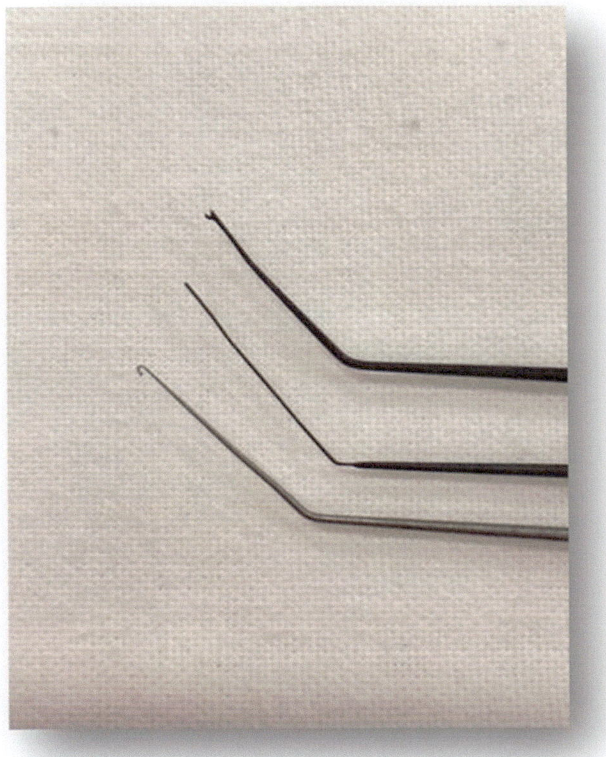

Fig. 27.2 From top to bottom: surgical "hatchet", "spatula", "hook" for IOL positioning

IOL selection

As far as IOL selection is concerned, almost any three-piece IOL can be iris-sutured. All modern three-piece IOLs have posterior angulation, which keeps the optic away from the iris after sutures are placed. To minimize chafe on the iris and pigment dispersion, a rounded anterior surface is preferred.

In Russia, more and more surgeons prefer hydrophilic and hydrophobic acrylic IOLs. Some state hospitals still implant silicone and PMMA IOLs (fortunately, less and less frequently). In our clinic, we generally use only acrylic IOLs.

It should be noted that the technology of suturing of a 1-piece IOL to the iris is widely discussed and criticized. The discussion boils down to the fact that the sutured edge of the 1-piece IOL can dislodge pigment from the iris or lead to "hyphema-uveitis-glaucoma syndrome". However, publications on this topic mainly focus on the implantation of 1-piece IOLs in the sulcus. For this reason, the

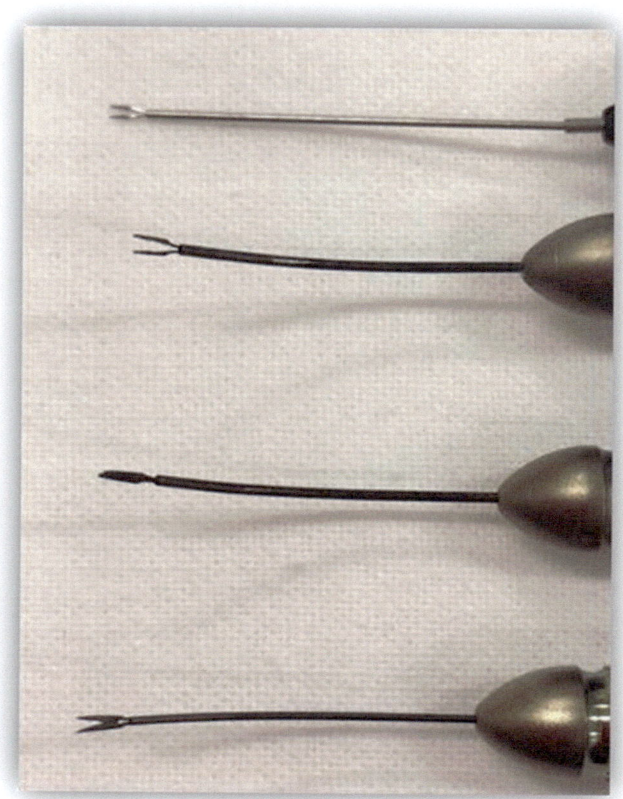

Fig. 27.3 From top to bottom: IOL grip forceps—Grieshaber #13, horizontal intracameral forceps, vertical intracameral forceps, intracameral scissors (can be used for suture cutting

question of such treatment tactics remains under the personal responsibility of the surgeon. Nevertheless, our centre has experience with such surgery, and it is positive.

27.1 Suturing an IOL to the Iris

The surgery step by step:

(1) **IOL implantation into the anterior chamber**
(2) **IOL capture after pinching of haptics behind the iris**
(3) **Paracentesis at 12 and 6 o'clock**

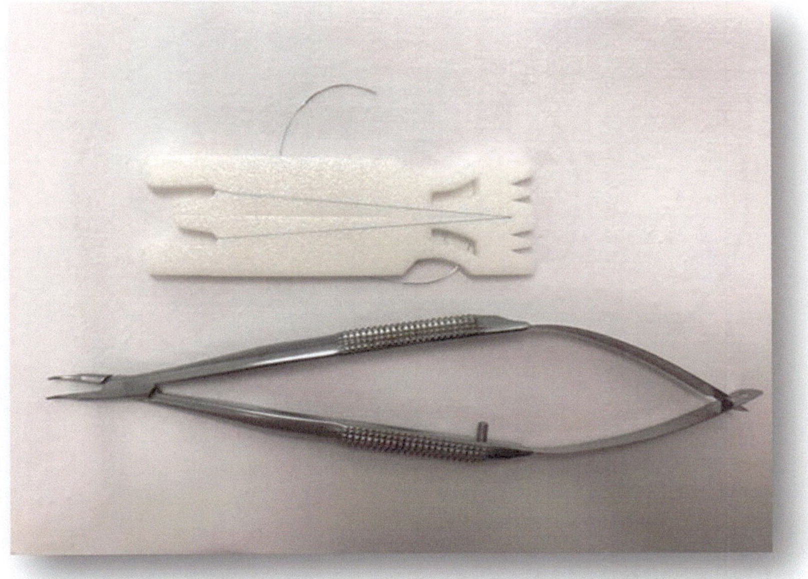

Fig. 27.4 Needle holder with long curved needle, polypropylene 9.0

(4) **Insertion of needle for fixation of both haptics**
(5) **Extraction of both ends of suture through paracentesis at 6 and 12 o'clock and tying the knot**
(6) **Repositioning of optic behind iris.**

The surgery in detail:

(1) **IOL implantation into the anterior chamber**

Beforehand, one can inject myotics into the anterior chamber (this manipulation can help in positioning the IOL), but it is not necessary. Start the procedure with implantation of the IOL into the anterior chamber so that its optical part and at least one haptic element are above the iris (Fig. 27.5).

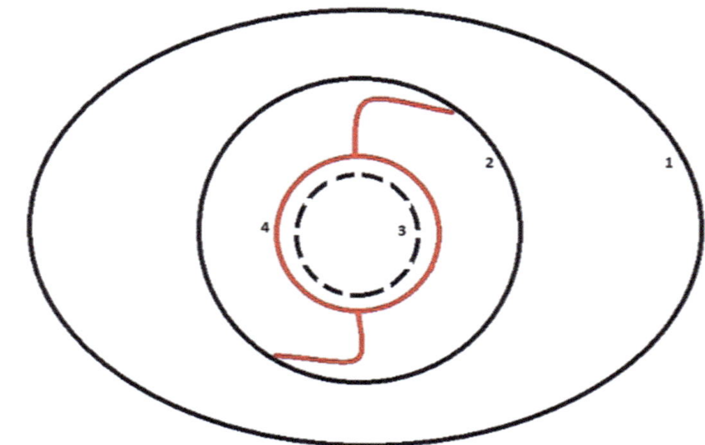

Fig. 27.5 Drawing. Location of the IOL in the anterior chamber above the iris. 1—sclera, 2—iris root, 3—pupillary edge of iris, 4—IOL optics

(2) IOL capture after pinching of haptics behind the iris

Once the IOL is implanted into the anterior chamber, it must be positioned in a place that is comfortable for suturing. The most comfortable position is to pinch the IOL optic over the iris (optic capture), with the haptic elements placed at the 6 and 12 o'clock. To do this, the haptic elements of the IOL need to be tucked behind the iris using a surgical "hook." and "axe.", rotating the IOL optic along its axis (Fig. 27.6). If the pupil is too wide and it is difficult to pinch the IOL (e.g. with a wide pupil), one can use a myotic—it makes the procedure much easier. It is not necessary to dilate the pupil before surgery. A spatula (or any other instrument one deems appropriate) is usually used as an auxiliary instrument during implantation. Alternatively, one can fixate and elevate the IOL with forceps to help visualize the haptic under the iris. All procedures are performed under the control of sufficient viscoelastic.

(3) Paracentesis at 12 and 6 o'clock

After this, two paracenteses at 6 and 12 o'clock are performed. If the paracentesis is at 5 and 11 o'clock or 7 and 13 o'clock, it is not critical. The main thing is that they should be as close as possible to the position of the haptic elements of the IOL.

(4) Insertion of needle for fixation of both haptics

Once the lens is positioned and the paracentesis is done, one can proceed with the iris suture. The process of IOL iris suturing consists of passing through **five consecutive points**, which are shown in Fig. 27.7.

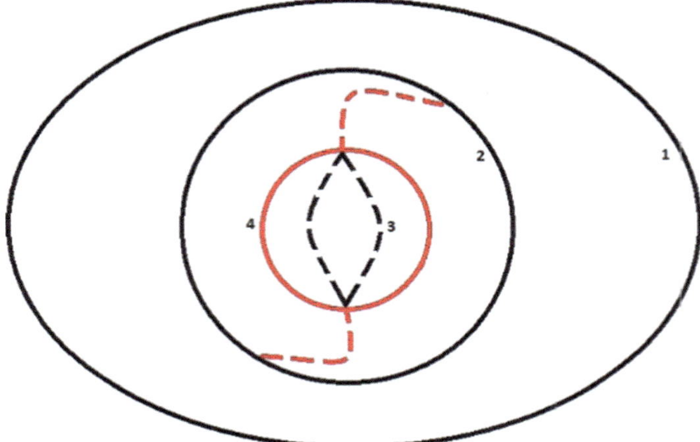

Fig. 27.6 Drawing. IOL optics is located above the iris, IOL haptics is tucked behind the iris (the lens is pinched in the pupillary edge of the iris). 1—sclera, 2—iris root, 3—pupillary edge of iris, 4—IOL optics

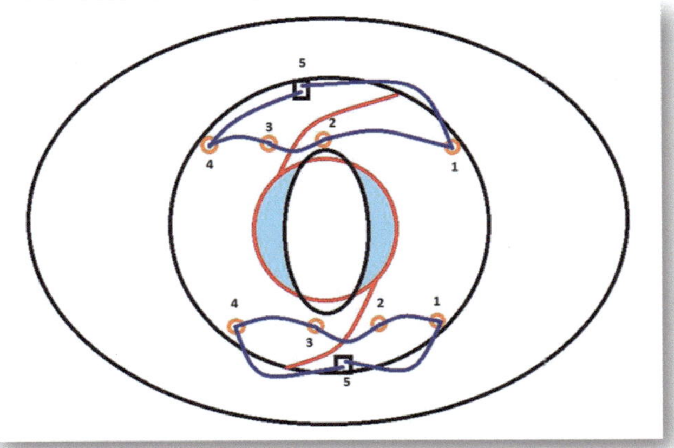

Fig. 27.7 Drawing. IOL with iris capture. 1, 4—points of surgical limbus. 2, 3—points of needle punctures in the iris. 5—points of paracentesis for suture removal

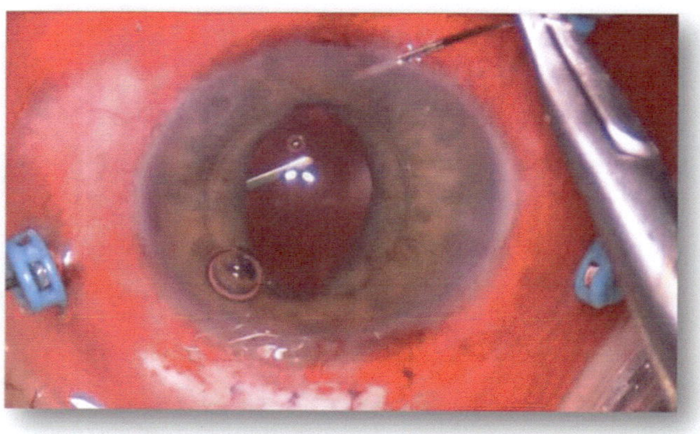

Fig. 27.8 Illustration of the passage of the first point

Point 1. Place of needle insertion into the cornea in the limbus area. This area is the most convenient for needle insertion because the risk of intraocular fluid filtration and bleeding is minimal in this area (Fig. 27.8).

Point 2. Insertion of a needle into the iris with capturing the haptic element. During this point, one must minimize the impact on the iris root to avoid bleeding. The procedure should be done fairly quickly (Fig. 27.9).

Point 3. Removal of the needle from under the iris. The haptic element is captured (Fig. 27.10).

Point 4. Exit of the needle through the limbus (Fig. 27.11).

(5) **Extraction of both ends of suture through paracentesis at 6 and 12 o'clock and tying the knot**

Cutting, extraction and tying of sutures (**Point 5**). After trimming the sutures through the iris with the haptic grasp, they need to be taken out through the paracentesis made earlier. To do this, one free end of the suture is held with forceps, and the other end is led into the paracentesis with a "hook". **Only the ends of the suture that are involved in fixation to the iris are pulled out (points 2 and 3 in Fig. 27.7).** The suture ends are tied with 2–3 knot stitches. Usually, 2 straight, one reverse. When the procedure is finished, the remaining sutures are cut off.

(6) **Repositioning of optic behind iris**

Once the haptics are sutured, the IOL optic can be tucked behind the iris, and the viscoelastic can be safely removed. The IOL will be stable (Figs. 27.12 and 27.13).

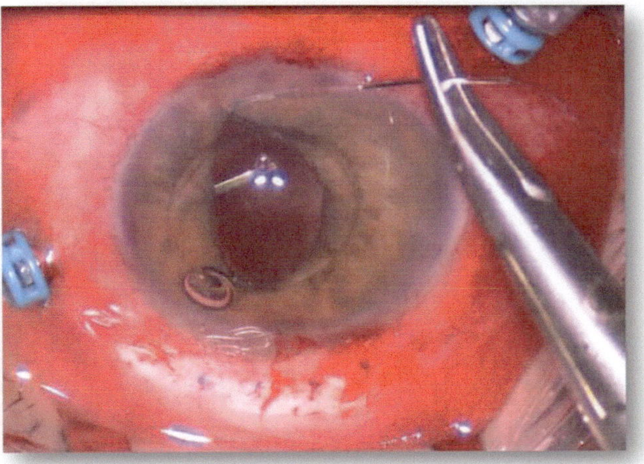

Fig. 27.9 Illustration of the passage of the second point

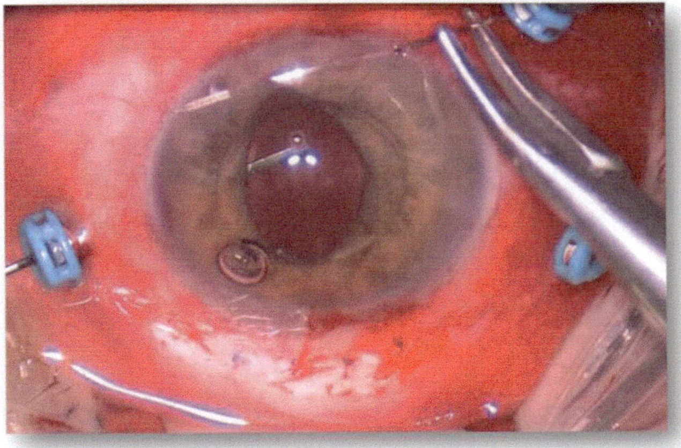

Fig. 27.10 Illustration of the passage of the third point

Helpful tips:

– Monitor the balance of IOP in the posterior and anterior chambers—excessive
  hypotension or hypertension can significantly affect the success of the manipulation. This is usually resolved with additional viscoelastic injection or BSS
  delivery into the anterior (posterior) chambers.

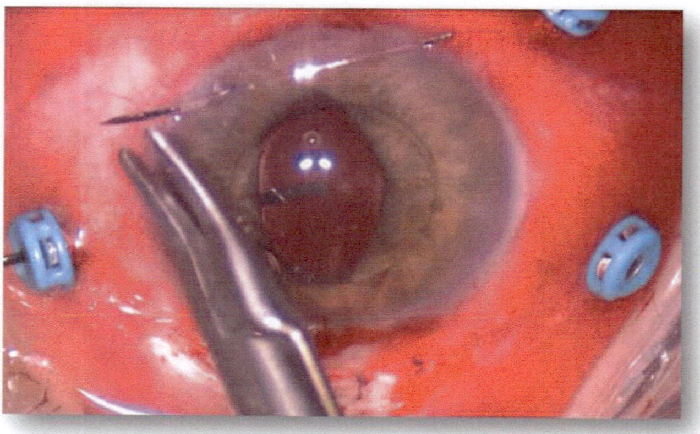

Fig. 27.11 Illustration of the passage of the fourth point

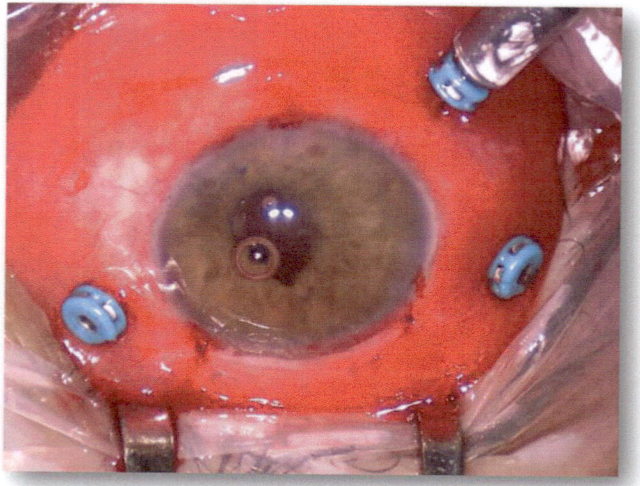

Fig. 27.12 Appearance of the IOL at the final stage of surgery

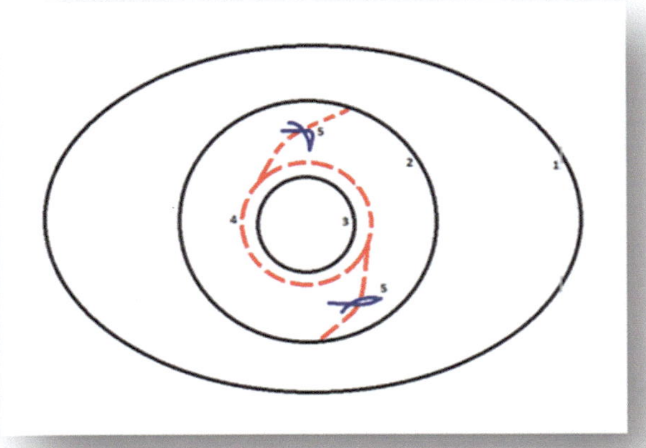

Fig. 27.13 Location of the sutured IOL behind the iris. 1—sclera, 2—iris root, 3—pupillary edge of iris, 4—IOL optics, 5—places of suture fixation of IOL haptics to iris

- After IOL impingement and vitreous prolapse, doing anterior vitrectomy is quite comfortable, and the main thing is to make sure that the structure is stable.
- During IOL suturing, do not put excessive pressure on the iris; this may cause it to tear (see the first point about IOP balance). "Movements should be quick and precise."
- Perhaps the most important point: Tightening the sutures. When suturing an IOL and/or IOL-capsular bag complex on an eye with a preserved vitreous body, the loop width can exceed 1.5 mm, with no risk of subsequent dislocation. However, if the eye is avitreal, try to tighten the suture to a loop width of 0.3–0.5 mm. Do not suture too far from the pupillary margin—this will minimize the risk of future IOL dislocation.

27.2 Suturing an IOL-Capsular Bag Complex to Iris

As described above, there is no fundamental difference in suturing a pure IOL or as part of an IOL-capsule complex, but peculiarities should be mentioned:

- Suturing the IOL/bag complex allows one to put a wider loop on the iris, because the risk of its rotation is much lower than with a "naked" IOL;
- Great care needs to be taken when suturing because, when piercing the complex, a certain amount of force is required; therefore, it should be done "lightning fast";

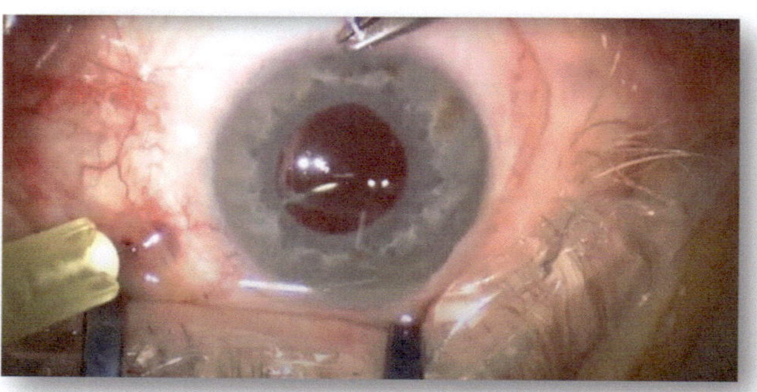

Fig. 27.14 Suturing the IOL-capsular bag complex using a stabilizer needle inserted through the flat part of the ciliary body. In this case, it performs the role of positioning and holding. The second hand is used for direct suturing (Photo courtesy: Ivanov D.)

– When puncturing the complex, one does <u>not</u> need to go through the haptic element within the capsular bag, as the fibrous capsular bag is strong enough to fix only it.

The surgery:

Direct suturing of the complex to the iris by puncturing it through the fibrous capsular sac using the technique described above. Take care that the complex is firmly fixed with the supporting hand (or "one hand") while using forceps (or stabilizer needle). Visualize the projection of lens capsule behind the iris. With the other hand, insert the needle directly through the fibrotic lens capsule located behind the iris. Subsequent extraction of suture ends through paracentesis, and tying is performed according to the above described technique (Fig. 27.14).

27.3 Intra- and Postoperative Complications

The number of intra- and postoperative complications is minimal if the technique of IOL fixation (IOL-capsular bag complexes) is followed.

Amount of IOL-suture cases in 2019: 259; amount of IOL-suture cases in 2020 (due to COVID-19, we were closed for 3 months): 157; amount of IOL-suture cases until mai 2021: 132.

Postoperative complications:

The number of repeated repositions (after dislocations) during these periods was—7, iritis—0, macular oedema—2.

Intraoperative complications:

1. **Iris root detachment**. Usually occurs if the surgeon had a gross violation of surgical technique. For example, dislocation of a needle. In this case, complication #2 can be a consequence of #1.
2. **Bleeding from iris vessels**. Most often encountered when there is too much pressure on the iris root due to displacement of the needle direction. This can be avoided by precise movements and minimal iris displacement.
3. **Ovalization (pupil deformity)**. When doing IOL dislocation (IOL-capsular bag complex), there are three goals:

   (A) positioning the IOL (IOL-capsular bag complex) in the frontal plane behind the iris;
   (B) the edge of the IOL optic should not extend into the pupillary edge of the iris (the lens should be positioned centrally);
   (C) preservation of constriction and dilatation function of the pupil.

Attention should be paid to the width and placement of the sutures to ensure that all goals are met (it is the IOL that is particularly sensitive to these rules):

If the IOL (IOL-capsular bag complex) is sutured too close to the pupillary edge and the knots are overtightened, a deformity (ovalization of the pupil) is guaranteed and most likely impaired pupil function with the risk of the optic hitting the pupillary edge.

If the suture is too wide, the IOL (less so for the complex) can be dislocated the next day (or in the near future).

If one suture the IOL (almost irrelevant to the complex) too close to the iris root, the risk of ovalization of the pupil will be minimal, but the risk of IOL dislocation (or getting the optic margin into the pupil) is much higher. This phenomenon is related to the design of the IOL—the farther the suture is from the optical edge of the IOL, the greater the potential for its dislocation due to suture movement along the vertical component of the haptic element (Fig. 27.15).

Naturally, support from the vitreous body or avitrium dictates the need for tighter suture tension in avitrium.

Taking these factors into account, we recommend suturing approximately in the middle of the distance between the iris root and its pupillary edge (or close to it). The stitch width in the intact vitreous eye can be about 1.5 mm, and in the avitreal eye, it should be reduced to 0.3–0.5 mm.

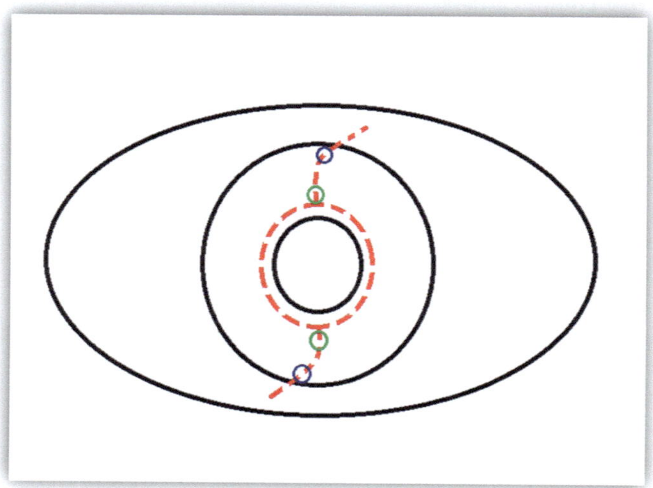

Fig. 27.15 Undesirable places of stitch. If the stitch is too close to the iris root (blue circle), the lens can be dislocated by gravity. If the suture is too close to the pupil edge (green circle)—risk of pupil deformation. The golden mean is the key to success. A wide suture loop located near the iris root guarantees secondary dislocation

If ovalization cannot be avoided, but otherwise, the surgeon is satisfied with the expected anatomical and functional result, he can delicately use a thermocoagulator under viscoelastic control to improve the appearance of the pupillary iris margin.

Advanced Complication Management of Posterior Segment Using a Phacoemulsification Machine

All videos of this part be found in a playlist of my YouTube channel:
https://www.youtube.com/playlist?list=PL0dKYclPD7yMJRuQAIt9Dr7pOtuI0Seex

Part VII: Insertion of trocar cannulas
Part VII: Surgery of a dropped nucleus for dummies with phaco machine
Part VII: Dropped nucleus with Infinity machine and phacoemulsification handpiece
Part VII: Management of a dropped nucleus
Part VII: Extraction of dropped nucleus with ICCE and retropupillar Artisan IOL
Part VII: Combined phaco + PPV
Part VII: Extraction of dropped nucleus with fragmatome and sulcus IOL
Part VII: Posterior dislocated IOL retrieval and scleral fixation

Introduction and Possible Indications for Trocar Surgery of Posterior Segment

28

Contents

Abstract

This chapter shows a check list for trocar surgery of posterior segment and reports about possible indications for trocar surgery of posterior segment. All surgeries can be performed with a phacoemulsification machine.

Keywords

Trocar surgery · Trocar · Check list for posterior segment · Posterior segment · Trocar cannula · Pars plana · Indications

Trocar surgery of posterior segment with a phacoemulsification machine is possible for emergency cases such as dropped nucleus. This surgery has been performed successfully with the Catarex 3 (Oertli), Centurion (Alcon) and Infinity (Alcon).

28.1 Checklist for Trocar Surgery of Posterior Segment

You want to operate a dropped nucleus or a posterior dislocated IOL. Are you confident with the following surgical steps you learned from trocar surgery of the anterior segment? See the following checklist:

Trocar surgery techniques for *anterior* segment in a stepwise manner

1. Insertion and removal of 1 trocar on the temporal side
2. Anterior vitrectomy through trocar cannula
3. Master SICS
4. Elevation of anterior dislocated nucleus
5. Elevation of anterior dislocated IOL
6. Secondary IOL implantation
7. Insertion of two trocars on the temporal side; one trocar for irrigation line
8. Anterior vitrectomy from pars plana with infusion line.

If you are acquainted to perform trocar surgery with two trocars, then you can proceed with the next steps.

Trocar surgery techniques for *posterior* segment in a stepwise manner

1. Insertion of three trocars
2. Usage of Biom and light fibre
3. Core vitrectomy
4. Elevation of dropped nucleus
5. Elevation of dropped IOL.

Start with insertion of three trocars, insertion of a light fibre and visualization of the retina (steps 1–2). If you can obtain a sharp picture of the retina, the next step will be the core vitrectomy (step 3). If you are acquainted with this step, you can continue with the final steps which are elevation of a dropped nucleus and IOL (steps 4 and 5).

28.2 Possible Indications for Trocar Surgery of Posterior Segment

A dropped nucleus (Fig. 28.1) and a dropped IOL (Fig. 28.2) can be operated with a phacoemulsification machine. The modern phacoemulsification machines have novel anterior vitreous cutters with 23 Gauge. Before 20 Gauge was the standard for phacoemulsification machines. 23G trocars can be purchased from many companies (Alcon, Dorc, FCI, Mani). The companies Dorc (Netherlands), FCI (France) and Mani (Japan) offer sets with three trocars and one infusion line. Three

Fig. 28.1 Dropped nucleus

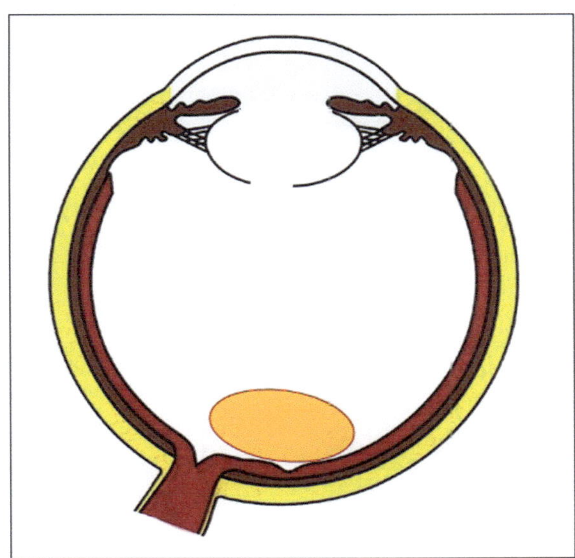

Fig. 28.2 Posterior dislocated IOL

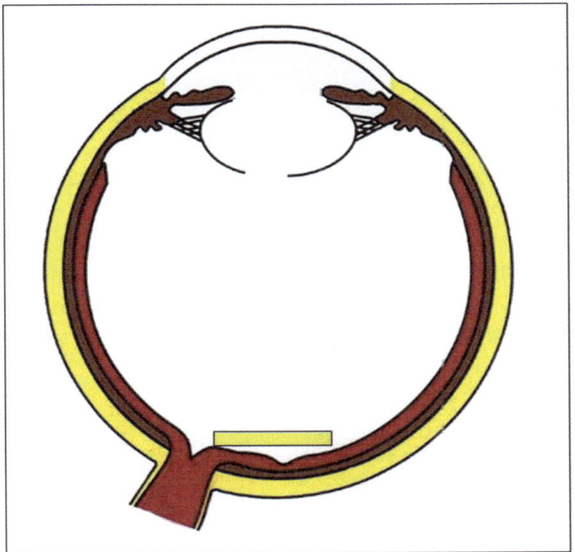

trocars are inserted at pars plana, the infusion line is inserted in one trocar, and the two other trocars are used for illumination and for the vitreous cutter (Figs. 28.3 and 28.4). The surgery of a vitrectomy is explained in detail in the final chapter of this book.

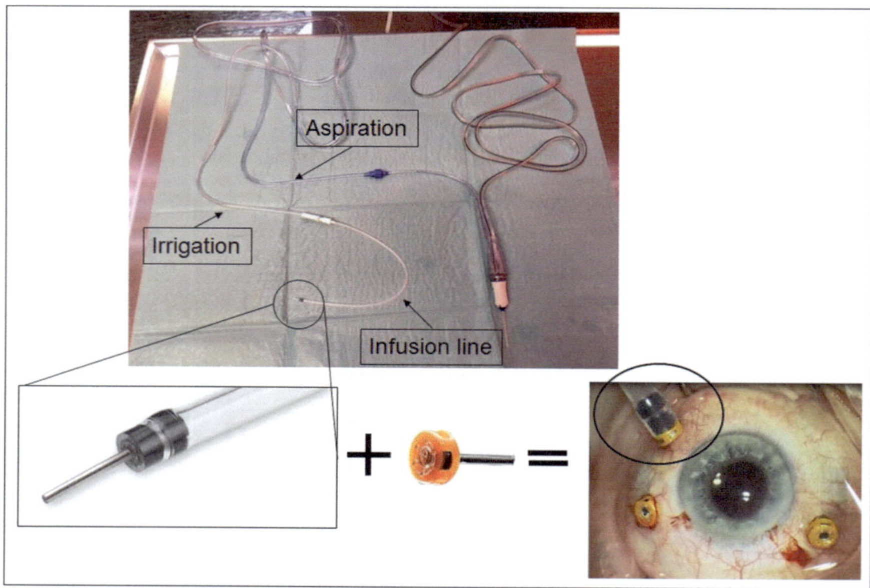

Fig. 28.3 Three 23G trocars are inserted. The irrigation from the cataract machine is connected to an infusion line (DORC, FCI, Mani) and inserted into the inferotemporal trocar

28.3   Anatomy of Pars Plana Vitrectomy

It is important to know the location designations of the eye during pars plana vitrectomy (Fig. 28.5). The lens is located anterior, and the macula is located posterior. The trocar cannula is inserted behind the limbus. The pars plana is located between ciliary body and the peripheral retina (ora serrata).

28.4   Surgical Set-Up

A vitrectomy with a cataract machine is possible. We perform combined vitrectomies and macular peeling for epiretinal membrane with an Infinity machine and a Centurion machine from Alcon (Fig. 28.6). Even combined phaco + vitrectomies are possible. We use the 23G vitreous cutters which are used for anterior vitrectomy. In addition, you need a viewing system and an illumination to visualize the retina. The viewing system is a BIOM (Oculus, Germany or RUV800, Leica, Germany) or a contact lens (Volk, USA). The illumination is a light fibre which is connected to an external light source (Photon, Synergetics). (Video available).

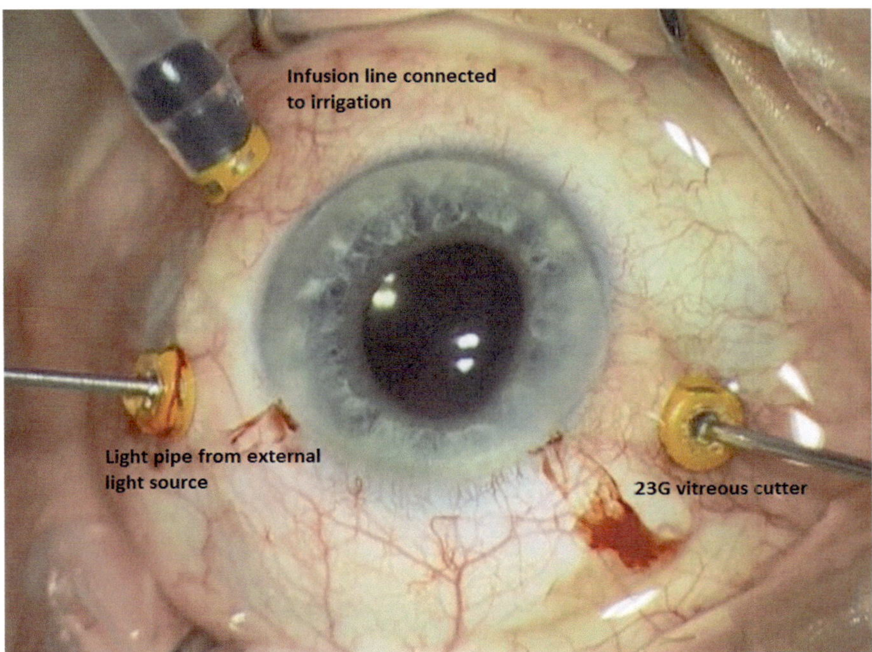

Fig. 28.4 Other two trocars are for the vitreous cutter and the light pipe. The vitreous cutter is a conventional anterior vitreous cutter and not a posterior segment vitreous cutter. The light pipe and the external light source must be purchased separately

Fig. 28.5 Location designations in vitrectomy

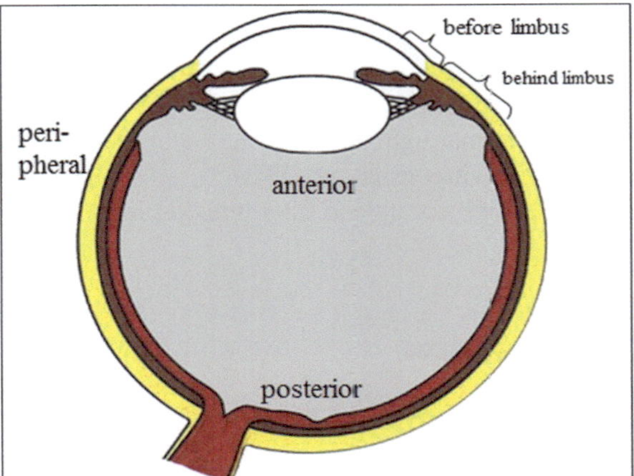

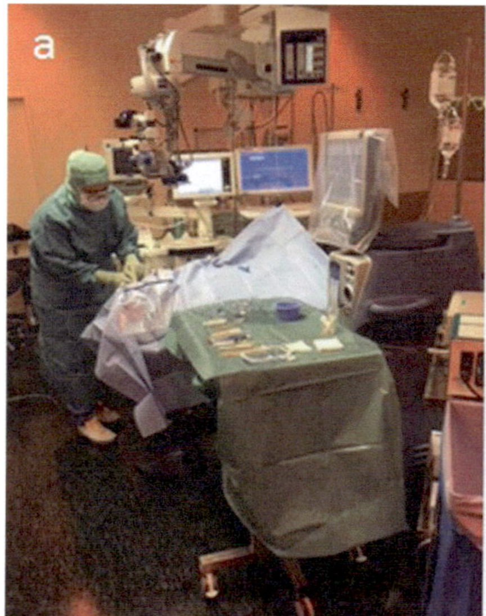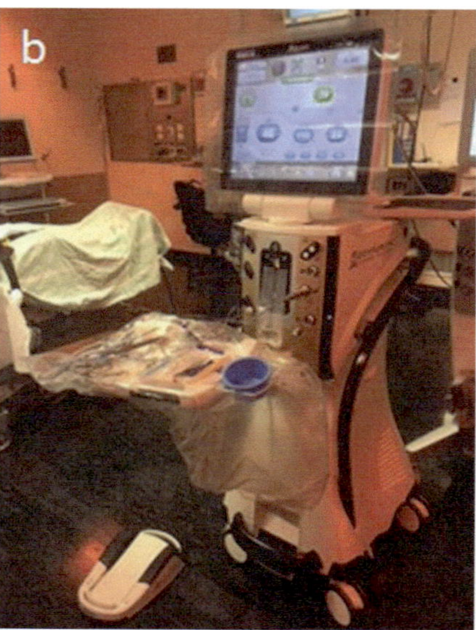

Fig. 28.6 **a** Vitrectomy with an Infinity machine (Alcon) and 23G cutter (2500 **cpm**). **b** Vitrectomy with a Centurion machine (Alcon) and 23G cutter (4000 cpm)

28.5   Equipment for Trocar Surgery of Posterior Segment

For posterior segment surgery, the following devices and instruments are required:

1. Phacoemulsification machine
2. Viewing system
3. One 23G light fibre
4. One external light source
5. Anterior vitreous cutter (23G)
6. Three 23G trocars and 23G infusion line.

28.5.1   Devices

Phacoemulsification machines

The most modern phacoemulsification machines can be employed for vitrectomy (Fig. 28.6). It is only important that the anterior vitreous cutter is available in 23 Gauge. <u>Remark</u>: The Centurion machine can be used for vitrectomy but <u>not</u> for removal of dropped nucleus with phacoemulsification handpiece.

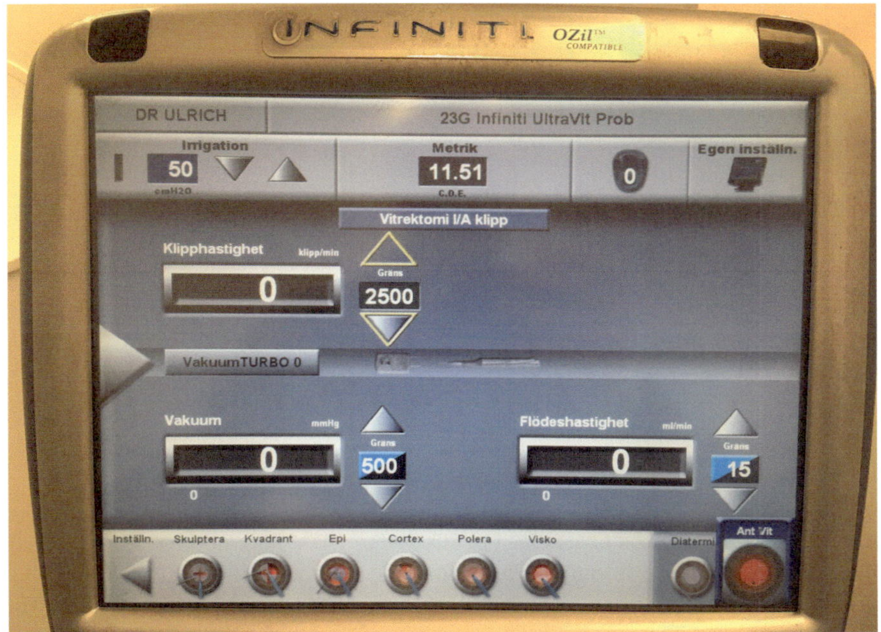

Fig. 28.7 Phaco settings for posterior vitrectomy with three trocars. Note Continuous irrigation. We use an irrigation pressure of approximately 45–50 cmH$_2$O. The vitrectomy setting is I/A Cut

Settings for posterior segment

For settings we use continuous irrigation (Fig. 28.7). The irrigation pressure is different from machine to machine. It is approximately 35–40 mmHg for Centurion and 45–55 for Infinity. Look for a spontaneous retinal venous pulsation at the optic disc. For vitrectomy we use the setting I/A Cut.

Viewing system (Binocular Indirect Ophthalmo Microscope (BIOM system))

The optical quality of the surgical microscopes is excellent in all current models of the major manufacturers. More important is the viewing system. To obtain a sufficient view of the posterior segment, you need either a plano-concave contact lens which is directly placed onto the cornea, or a highly refractive lens (60D, 90D, 120D) which is placed in front of the lens of the surgical microscope comparable to indirect ophthalmoscopes. This results in an inverted image. By flicking a reversal system (so-called inverter) into the parallel beam path of the operating microscope, an upright image is created.

The best viewing systems for high volume VR surgery are Resight from Zeiss, Germany and BIOM from Oculus, Germany. Both viewing systems require, however, an inverter. If you operate small volume VR surgery, then the Eibos (Möller-Wedel, Germany) or RUV800 (Leica, Germany) viewing system is a good

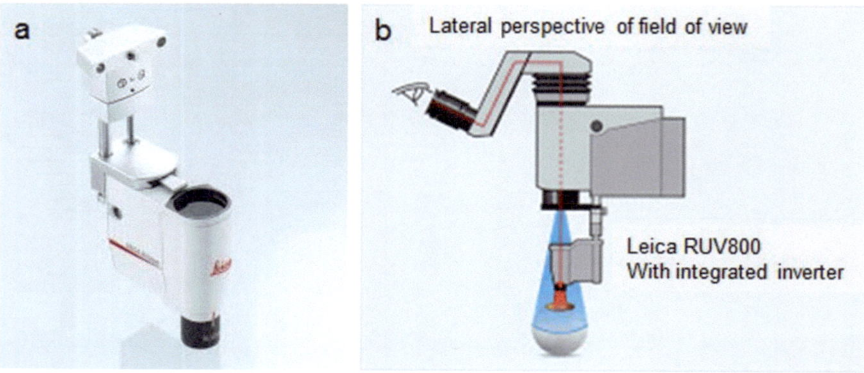

Fig. 28.8 RUV800 from Leica

option (Fig. 28.8). This viewing system is very easy to use, it requires no inverter, and the view to fundus is excellent. For Eibos and RUV 800, no inverter is needed. The RUV800 system can only be used for Leica microscopes (Fig. 28.9).

Oculus (Germany) offers a one-way BIOM (Fig. 28.9) which is easy to use. The Oculus BIOM can be used with all microscopes. If you use a Zeiss microscope, you have an option of attaching an inverterscope which is an eye piece having a built-in inverter which can be activated by a knob. The viewing system BIOM from Oculus provides a mirror image. Therefore, an *inverter* is installed in the microscope, which turns the mirror image of the BIOM. This must be turned on or off every time you switch between anterior segment or posterior segment view (by help of a knob or by a foot switch).

The company Oculus (Germany) has recently introduced a high-resolution lens which can be used as a 120D lens and at the same time as 60D peeling lens (Fig. 28.10).

Contact lenses

Contact lens for retinal viewing can be for periphery (wide angle) and central use (Chalam 2004; "Volk surgical lens" OR "Ocular surgical lens"). Both have direct and indirect types. Only indirect contact lens will require an inverter as their focal plane is close to the cornea and much away from the microscope objective lens. Regarding direct contact lenses for periphery work, we can use Lander Lens 20, 30 or 50° Tolentino prism (Ocular instruments). All these are also direct type, so no inverter needed (based on Landers design).

Indirect wide angle lens like HRX, MiniQuad XL from Volk also requires an inverter and used for a wide angle viewing. You can get similar design contact lens from Ocular instruments also. Remember: *Direct contact lens requires no inverter, and indirect contact lens do need the inverter.*

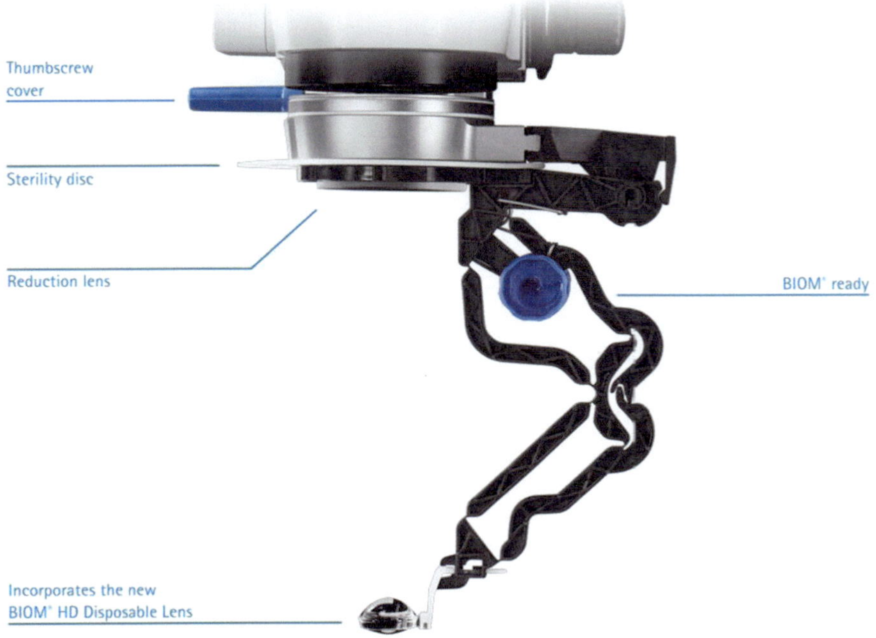

Fig. 28.9 One-way BIOM from Oculus (Germany). Integrated is an inverter, which may be operated manually or by foot pedal. At the front of the BIOM, the interchangeable front lenses are attached. https://www.oculussurgical.com/us/products/oculus-biom-ready/highlights/

Fig. 28.10 Novel 120D and 60D lens from Oculus, Germany. The lens can be used for the BIOM and for the Resight viewing system

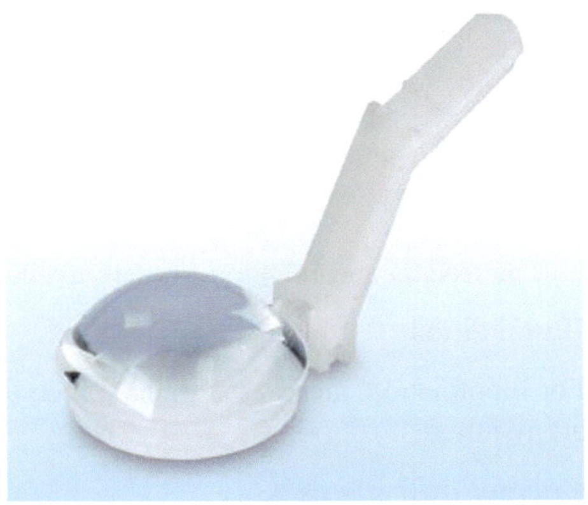

Manufacturer: AVI, Grieshaber (Alcon), DORC, FCI Ophthalmics, Ocular instruments. Madhu Industries (Fig. 28.11). Aurolab does not manufacture contact lenses.

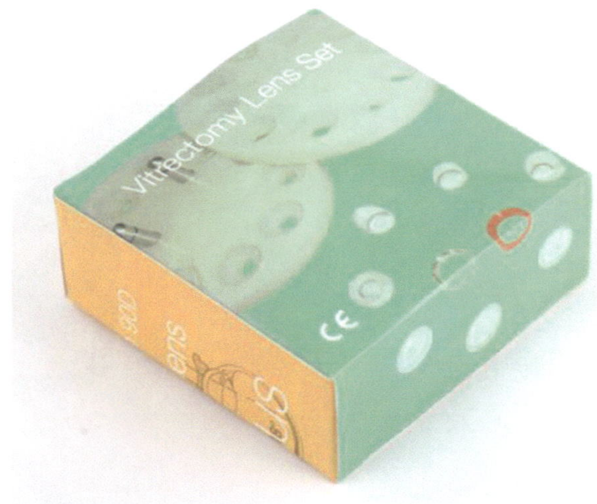

Fig. 28.11 Irrigating contact lens for viewing retina from Madhu Industries, Delhi (www.madhuinstruments.com)

Conclusion

The RUV800 and Eibos viewing systems are robust and easy to use. They can only be used for Leica and Möller Wedel microscopes. A good alternative for all microscopes is the one-way viewing system BIOM from Oculus (Germany). This one-way BIOM has an excellent lens for peripheral view and for central fundus view.

A contact lens is a good and cheap alternative to a viewing system.

28.5.2 Instruments

The following instruments are required:

1. Three 23-gauge trocars (Figs. 28.12, 28.13, 28.14 and 28.15)
2. 23-gauge infusion line (Fig. 28.16)

The trocars and infusion line are available as a kit:

Illumination

For illumination, an external light source (Fig. 28.17) and a light fibre (Fig. 28.18) are required.

External light source

Conclusion: I am convinced that anterior and posterior segment surgery will fuse in the future. The modern cataract machines have a very powerful vitrectomy function today and employ 23G anterior vitreous cutters. In case of a dropped nucleus, the cataract surgeon can convert with the same machine to a vitrectomy and remove the nuclear fragments.

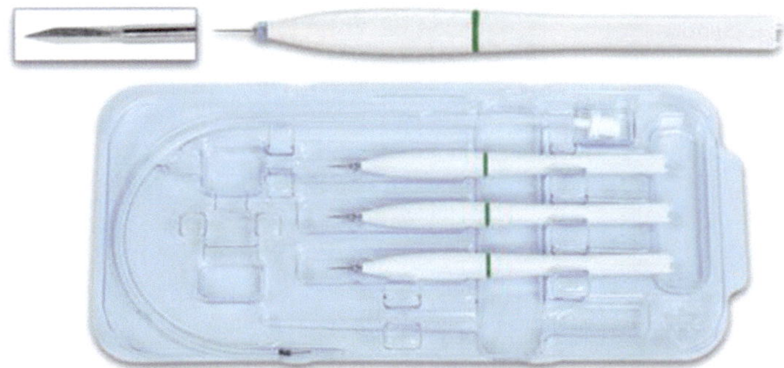

Fig. 28.12 23G One step cannula system from DORC No: 1272.ED206. This package includes three trocars and one infusion line

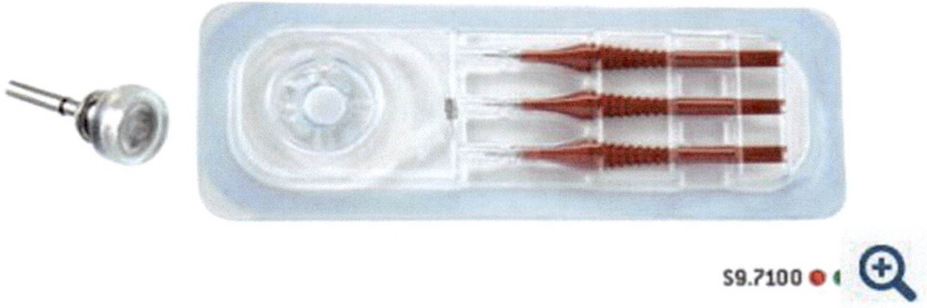

Fig. 28.13 This package includes three 23G trocars and one infusion line. (FCI, France No. S9.7100.23)

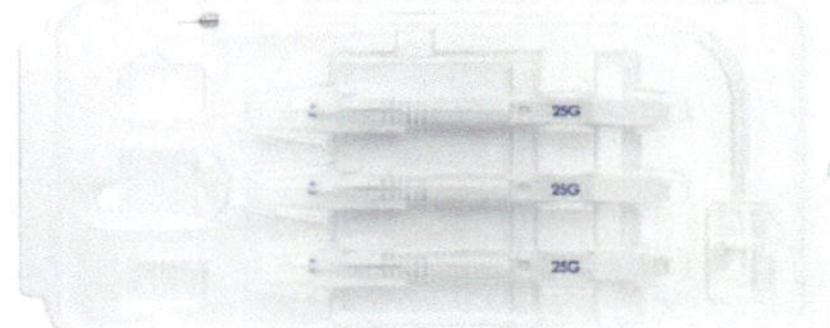

Product Name	Packaging	Order #
Trocar Kit 25G S	3 Kits / Box	MTK25S
Trocar Kit 23G S	3 Kits / Box	MTK23S

• Sterile 1 kit consists of 3 pcs. trocar with the valved cannula and 1 pc. infusion cannula.

Fig. 28.14 This package includes three 23G trocars and one infusion line. (Mani, Japan MTK23S)

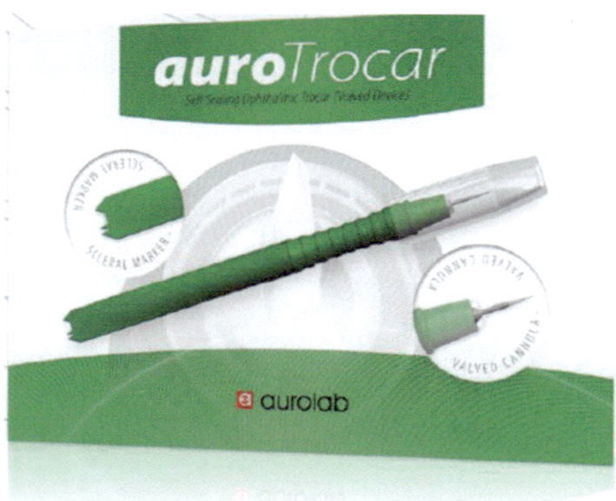

Fig. 28.15 This package includes three 23G trocars and one infusion line (Aurolab, India)

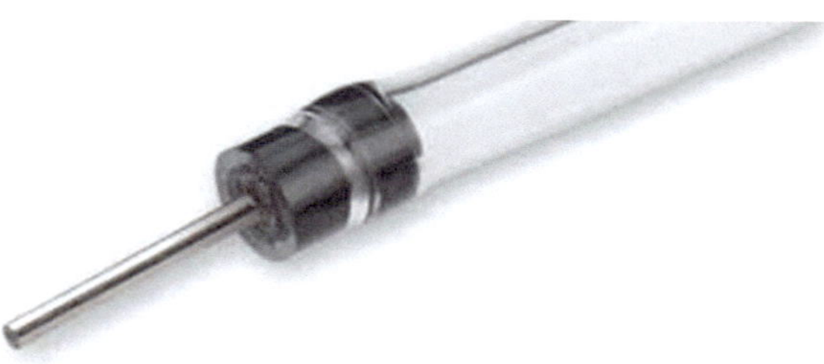

Fig. 28.16 Infusion line (23G, DORC) No: 1279.VFI. The infusion line can be purchased separately from DORC and Mani

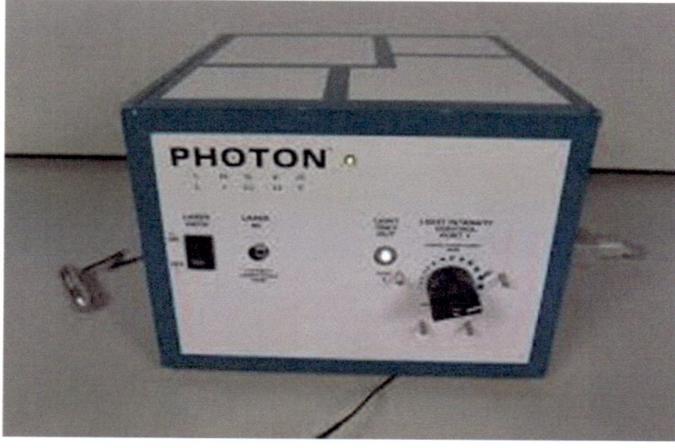

Fig. 28.17 External light source (Photon from Synergetics, USA) provides light for the light pipe

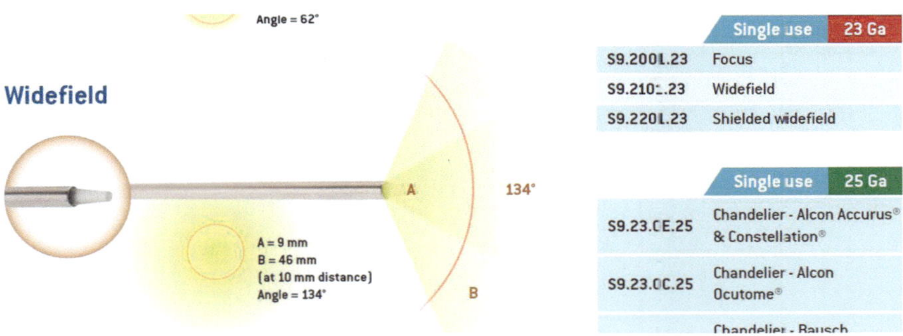

Fig. 28.18 Light pipe Synergetics (belongs to Bausch & Lomb) No. 56.21.23

References

Chalam KV, Shah VA. Optics of wide-angle panoramic viewing system-assisted vitreous surgery. Surv Ophthalmol. 2004;49:437–445.
If you type "Volk surgical lens" OR "Ocular surgical lens" in, you get videos showing how great the field is.

Intraocular Pressure During Vitrectomy—Clinical Assessment and Surgical Action

29

Abstract

This chapter explains the importance of intraocular pressure during vitrectomy—the signs and what action has to be taken, if the IOP is too high or too low.

Keywords

IOP · Intraocular pressure during vitrectomy

The tonus of the globe is an essential element of anterior and especially of posterior segment surgery. As a surgeon, you must be able to assess the tonus of the globe and take adequate actions.

Assessment: The intraocular pressure can be assessed in the easiest way with the index finger. During posterior segment surgery, you check the globe pressure regularly with your index finger. There are also clinical signs for high and low IOP. If the IOP is too high, then the cornea becomes edematous because the endothelium cannot pump out the excess intracorneal fluid. Further signs are an iris prolapses through the corneal incision and a flat anterior chamber. In the posterior segment, a high IOP can only be visualized with a non-pulsatile optic disc. A low IOP presents with a globe losing its shape, and scleral folds occur. In addition, a choroidal detachment develops. In the anterior segment, there are hardly signs for a low IOP except for folds in the cornea or a gaping scleral tunnel.

Another important factor is the presence of aphakia or not. If aphakia is present, then intraocular fluid can flow freely from posterior to anterior segment and vice versa. *Remark*: A PCR is more or less comparable to aphakia.

In contrast, if a natural lens or in-the-bag IOL is present, then aqueous flows only slowly from posterior to anterior segment and vice versa. For example: In case of aphakia or PCR, an anterior chamber maintainer has the same effect as a pars plana trocar infusion because no barrier between anterior and posterior segment is present. If, however, a natural lens or an in-the-bag IOL is present, then an anterior chamber maintainer cannot maintain the IOP in the posterior segment. If you perform in this situation a vitrectomy then an underpressure in the posterior segment will develop. This underpressure may result in a (sub)choroidal haemorrhage.

Surgical procedure: What to do if the IOP is too high? The simplest surgical procedure is a paracentesis. If a paracentesis is not possible because of a flat anterior chamber, then you can relieve pressure from the posterior segment (via pars plana). This can be achieved with a needle cannula or a vitreous cutter. If the IOP is too low, you can increase the IOP by injecting fluid into the anterior chamber or into the posterior chamber (like an intravitreal injection). Assess the effect of your action with the index finger.

Surgical Management of a Dropping and Dropped Nucleus

30

Contents

Abstract

This chapter describes the management of a dropped nucleus. Two surgical methods are described: The extraction of a dropped soft nucleus with a vitreous cutter and the removal of a dropped hard nucleus with a phacoemulsification handpiece.

Keywords

Trocar surgery · Trocar · Pars plana · Dropping nucleus · Dropped nucleus

The surgical management of a dropped nucleus is usually in the hands of VR surgeons because a vitrectomy machine is required. But the new generation of phacoemulsification machines has a powerful vitreous cutter with good fluidics. A dropped nucleus surgery can be performed with these machines. There are three techniques for removal of the nucleus. (1) vitreous cutter, (2) elevation with PFCL and removal with SICS and (3) phacoemulsification. A vitreous cutter can be used if the nucleus is soft. If the nucleus is hard, I recommend an elevation of the nucleus into the anterior chamber with PFCL and the extraction with SICS technique. The intravitreal emulsification of the nucleus with a phacoemulsification handpiece is

© The Author(s), under exclusive license to Springer Nature Switzerland AG 2022
U. Spandau and G. B. Scharioth, *Complications During and After Cataract Surgery*,
https://doi.org/10.1007/978-3-030-93531-3_30

difficult because good fluidics are required, and this is not achieved by all cataract machines. This technique may be easier with the most recent generation of phacoemulsification machines with active IOP control.

30.1 Recovery of a Dropping Nucleus from Pars Plana

You must master this technique to become a complete cataract surgeon: To save a dropping nucleus and elevate it into the anterior chamber. A dropping nucleus can only be saved from pars plana and not from the anterior chamber because you need to place the viscoelastic cannula behind the nucleus (Fig. 30.1). You have to work fast; otherwise, the nucleus will be lost. If you suspect a dropping nucleus in an early stage of the surgery (e.g. large zonular lysis) then perform the sclerotomy or insert a trocar in advance in order to be prepared and not to lose time when the nucleus drops. (Videos available).

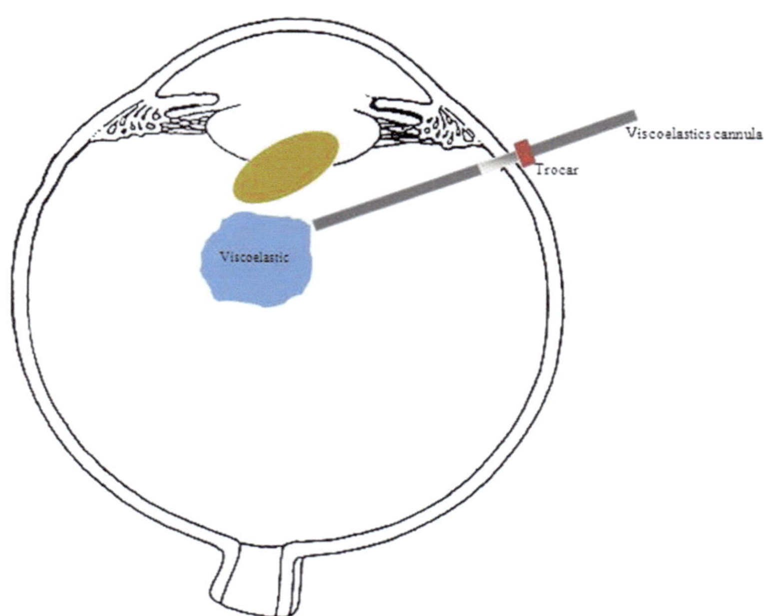

Fig. 30.1 Nucleus elevation from pars plana. In case of a posterior capsular defect and luxation of the nucleus insert a trocar and inject viscoelastics (Viscoat®) posterior to the nucleus. Elevate then the nucleus with the viscoelastic cannula into the anterior chamber

<u>Instrumentation</u>

(1) Paracentesis knife, e.g. 15° knife

OR

(2) 23G trocar

Stab the paracentesis knife 4 mm posterior the limbus into the middle of the eyeball (perpendicular); through the conjunctiva and the sclera. This manoeuvre is exactly the same as an intravitreal injection. Insert the viscoelastic cannula through the sclerotomy, place it behind the posterior capsule, and inject viscoelastic behind the nucleus. Then, elevate the nucleus with the viscoelastic cannula into the anterior chamber (Fig. 30.1).

Alternatively to a sclerotomy, you can insert a trocar (Fig. 30.1). The insertion of a trocar is fast, and the trocar has a distance marker for the sclerotomy. The viscoelastic cannula fits easily through the trocar.

The next steps are removal of the nucleus, anterior vitrectomy and secondary IOL implantation. For further details, see also chapter "Posterior capsule rupture".

Tips & tricks

<u>The fastest method for retrieving of dropping nucleus</u>: Attach a 27G needle cannula to the viscoelastic syringe (such as in Fig. 30.1), pierce the needle through the sclera (3.5 mm behind the limbus), and inject viscoelastic behind the nucleus.

30.2 Operative Planning and Strategies for Surgical Management of Dropped Nucleus

Removal of dropped nucleus: A soft nucleus and cortex can be removed with a vitreous cutter. A hard nucleus can only be removed with a fragmatome. A fragmatome is a phacoemulsification handpiece without sleeve. It is used without trocar cannula. The fragmatome is inserted through a 20G sclerotomy without trocar cannula. A fragmatome *cannot* be used with a cataract machine. You can use instead a phacoemulsification handpiece without sleeve. The phaco needle is shorter than a fragmatome needle.

Remark: All videos of this chapter be found in a playlist of my youtube channel:

https://www.youtube.com/playlist?list=PL0dKYclPD7yMJRuQAIt9Dr7pOtuI0
Seex

Necessity of surgery: If nuclear fragments drop, we always operate in order to prevent intraocular inflammation and hypertension. In case of dropped soft cortical fragments, it is possible to wait and delay surgery as long as the eye remains quiet.

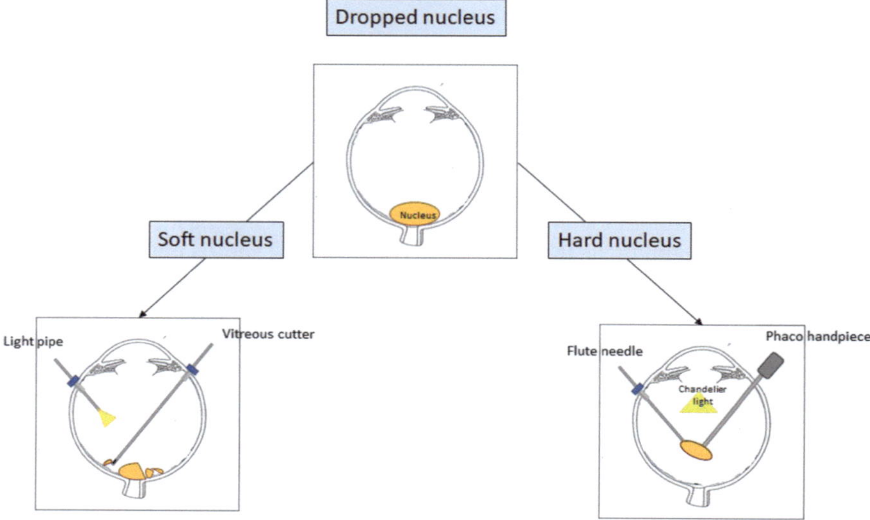

Fig. 30.2 Treatment algorithm for removal of soft or hard dropped nucleus

Timing of surgery: The surgery is not an emergency. Normally a dropped nucleus occurs under topical anaesthesia. To proceed with vitrectomy under drop anaesthesia will inflict much unnecessary pain to the patient. It is therefore advisable to stop surgery when a dropped nucleus occurs and to schedule a planned surgery within 1 week. During this time, the eye must be treated for inflammation and ocular hypertension so that the cornea is clear for the surgery.

Tips & tricks

The most patients who underwent a complicated cataract surgery do not complain about the complication but about the painful procedure. Why? The cataract surgery was performed with topical anaesthesia, and when the complication occurred, the surgery was continued with the same anaesthesia. Our recommendation: If you experience a complication, decide if you continue or stop the surgery. If you decide to continue, then add a subtenon or retrobulbar anaesthesia. I recommend the injection of 3 cc Carbocaine (Mepivacaine) into the caruncle. You will have a happy patient and an easy surgery.

The most difficult part of this surgery is the removal of the nucleus. There are two methods (Fig. 30.2).

(1) Epinucleus and soft nuclear fragments can be removed with the vitreous cutter. But hard and big nuclear fragments *cannot* be removed with the vitreous cutter. In this case, the following method must be applied. We recommend the use of a light pipe and a vitreous cutter.

(2) A hard nucleus can be removed with a phacoemulsification handpiece. We recommend the use of a chandelier light to have two free hands. The first hand holds the phacoemulsification handpiece and the second hand a flute needle.

Surgical planning: Two things should be assessed preoperatively:

(1) How much of the nucleus is luxated? Is it a soft or hard nucleus? Or did only cortical fragments drop? In case of a soft nucleus, I recommend removing it with a vitreous cutter. In case of a hard fragment or nucleus, I recommend a phacoemulsification handpiece.
(2) Assess preoperatively whether the anterior capsule is intact. If the anterior capsule is intact, implant a three-piece IOL in the sulcus. If it is not intact, you can implant a scleral fixated or even easier an iris-fixated IOL.

30.3   Extraction of a Posteriorly Dislocated Soft Nucleus with Vitreous Cutter

The limitation of a dropped nucleus removal with the phacoemulsification machine is that a fragmatome cannot be used. Do you know which tissue you can remove with a vitreous cutter? This is an important knowledge for this case. With the vitreous cutter, you can remove cortex, epinucleus, a soft nucleus and iris tissue. You cannot remove a hard nucleus or a thick capsular fibrosis. To remove a hard nucleus, it is advisable to perform phaco at the pupillary plane or a SICS.

Remark: All videos of this part be found in a playlist of my youtube channel:

https://www.youtube.com/playlist?list=PL0dKYclPD7yMJRuQAIt9Dr7pOtuI0Seex

<u>Instruments</u>

1. 23G trocars and infusion line
2. Illumination: Chandelier light fibre or hand-held light fibre
3. Viewing system
4. Anterior vitreous cutter

Individual steps

1. 23G 3-port system with chandelier light fibre
2. Anterior vitrectomy via pars plana
3. Removal of residual cortex from the lens capsule via paracentesis
4. Core vitrectomy, if necessary PVD
5. Removal of nuclear fragments with vitreous cutter
6. Vitrectomy of peripheral vitreous
7. Implantation of an intraocular lens
8. Removal of trocar cannulas

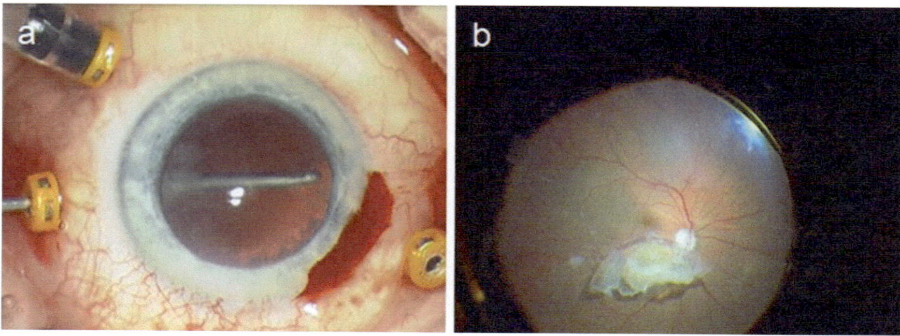

Fig. 30.3 **a** Anterior vitrectomy from pars plana in an eye with PCR. **b** A soft dropped nucleus

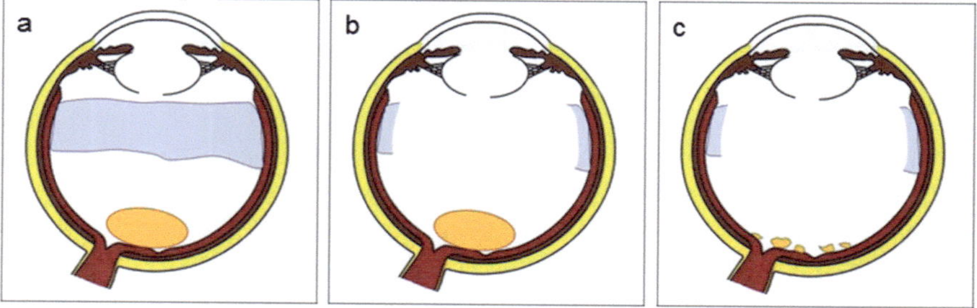

Fig. 30.4 **a** The posterior vitreous is *detached*. **b** After removal of the central vitreous. **c** The nuclear fragments have no contact with the vitreous

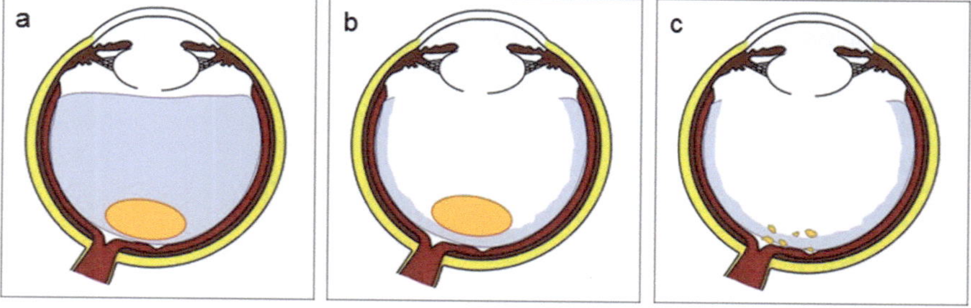

Fig. 30.5 **a** The posterior vitreous is *attached*. **b** After removal of the central vitreous. The posterior vitreous is still attached and present. **c** Some nuclear fragments are located above the vitreous and easy to remove. But some nuclear fragments are localized behind the vitreous which are difficult to remove because the vitreous is in the way

Fig. 30.6 Monomanual surgery with light pipe and anterior vitreous cutter

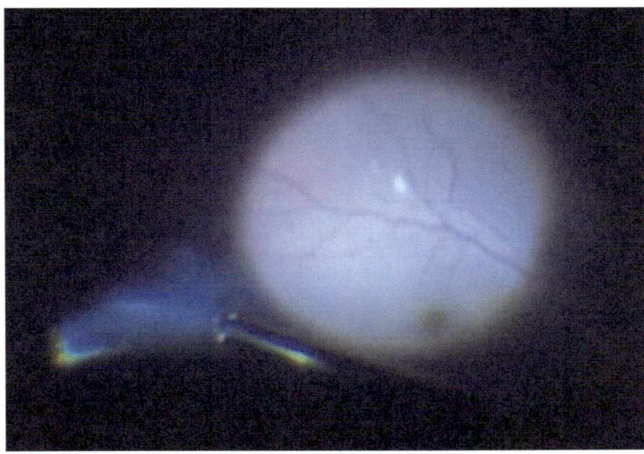

The surgery step by step: (Figs. 30.3, 30.4, 30.5 and 30.6)

1. 3-port system with chandelier light fibre

After insertion of three trocars, we insert a chandelier light fibre, because we work bimanually in step 6.

2. Anterior vitrectomy via pars plana

3. Removal of residual cortex from the lens capsule via paracentesis

4. Core vitrectomy, if necessary PVD

The anterior vitreous is removed with the vitreous cutter via pars plana (Fig. 30.3). Make circular movements with the vitreous cutter. The vitreous cutter port points towards the posterior pole in order to avoid a damage of the lens capsule. Aspirate then the residual cortex with the vitreous cutter via a paracentesis. If vitreous clogs the port of the vitreous cutter during aspiration, then cut vitreous first. Alternatively, you can use two I/A handpieces. It is important that you switch the vitreous cutter to aspiration and not to cutting; otherwise you risk destroying the anterior capsule.

If the lens capsule is free from cortex, continue with a core vitrectomy from pars plana. There are two possible scenarios regarding the vitreous. The posterior vitreous may be *detached* (PVD) (see Fig. 30.4) or the posterior vitreous may be *attached* (no PVD) (see Fig. 30.5). If a PVD is present, then you remove the anterior and central vitreous (Fig. 30.4b). The nucleus is located on the retina and has no contact with the vitreous (Fig. 30.4c). If a PVD is absent, then you remove the anterior and central vitreous but not the posterior vitreous (Fig. 30.5b). The nucleus is, therefore, in contact with the vitreous (Fig. 30.5b). After removal of the large nucleus small nuclear fragments remain. They may be located above the vitreous or behind the vitreous (Fig. 30.5c). Those fragments which are located behind the vitreous are difficult to extract because the vitreous is in the way. In this case, a posterior vitreous detachment must be performed.

6. Removal of nuclear fragments with vitreous cutter

Soft lens material can be removed easily with the vitreous cutter. Many small nuclear fragments are present. Every fragment has to be removed (Fig. 30.6). The left hand holds the light pipe, and the right hand holds the vitreous cutter. Use the setting "I/A CUT". Aspirate the fragment carefully, lift it up and the cut it.

7. Vitrectomy of peripheral vitreous

The vitreous cutter breaks the nucleus in many small pieces which are dispersed all over the posterior segment. These fragments must be removed meticulously, because every nucleus fragment which remains may cause a postoperative sterile uveitis. The most lens fragments are located in the vitreous base at 6 o'clock. In order to visualize and remove them you need to self-indent the vitreous with the scleral depressor. For this procedure, use a chandelier light.

Tips & tricks

The trimming of the vitreous base is an important step because a residual nuclear fragment will cause a postoperative sterile uveitis. Check the periphery 360 degrees and particularly at 6 o'clock. Conclusion: Do not be satisfied after removal of the big fragments but after complete removal of all small fragments.

8. Implantation of the IOL

9. Removal of trocar cannulas

If the anterior capsule is intact, the lens can be implanted into the sulcus with optic capture inside the anterior capsulorhexis. If not, fixate a 3-piece IOL to the sclera or implant an iris-fixated IOL (Artisan®, Verisyse®).

Tips & tricks

1-piece IOL versus 3-piece IOL: Do not implant a 1-piece IOL into the sulcus because the haptics cause a focal depigmentation of the iris resulting in a secondary pigment glaucoma (iris chaffing). This does not happen with a 3-piece IOL. The reason for this is that a 1-piece IOL has thick and sharp haptics whereas 3-piece haptics are round and thin.

Postoperative treatment for conventional vitrectomy: Combined Dexamethasone-Gentamicin drops 5× daily for 2 weeks and 3× daily for third week. Atropine drops ×1 daily for 2 weeks.

30.4 Extraction of a Posteriorly Dislocated Hard Nucleus with Intravitreal Phacoemulsification

The extraction of a dropped nucleus with an intravitreal phacoemulsification is not widely established yet. Ruiz Moreno and colleagues use a vitrectomy machine for dropped nucleus surgery, but for intravitreal phacoemulsification, they use a regular phacoemulsification handpiece (and not a fragmatome) as a routine (Ruiz-Moreno et al. 2006). They say that the phacoemulsification handpiece is better than fragmatome because it is peristaltic and keeps lens fragments attached to the phacotip with less chattering. Ruiz Moreno uses a standard phaco needle with 50% phaco power and vacuum of only 100 mm Hg. They conclude that intravitreal phacoemulsification is the technique of choice for dislocated nuclei (Ruiz-Moreno et al. 2006; Soliman Mahdy et al. 2010; Schaal and Barr 2009). In this chapter, we will demonstrate a complete dropped nucleus surgery only with a cataract machine (Infinity, Alcon). We will use an anterior vitreous cutter and a phacoemulsification handpiece.

Remark: The Centurion machine (Alcon) can be used for vitrectomy but not for removal of dropped nucleus with phacoemulsification handpiece.

The following video demonstrates the extraction of a dropped nucleus with Catarex machine and phacoemulsification handpiece:

https://www.youtube.com/watch?v=Qusvb8l7UJY&feature=youtu.be

Instruments

Fragmatome/ phacoemulsification handpiece: A fragmatome and a phacoemulsification handpiece are identical except for different needles. The fragmatome needle is longer than the phaco needle. You can use a normal phacoemulsification handpiece with a normal phaco needle but without sleeve (Fig. 30.7). Remove the irrigation tube from the phaco handpiece. Only the aspiration tubing is connected to the phaco handpiece. The irrigation is placed via an irrigation line into a trocar cannula at pars plana. The phaco handpiece requires a 20G sclerotomy without trocar cannula. I recommend three trocar cannulas (one for irrigation line, one for light fibre and one for vitreous scutter) and one 20G sclerotomy without trocar

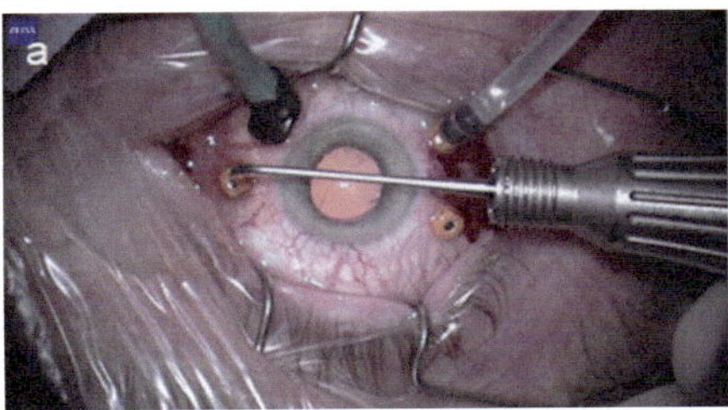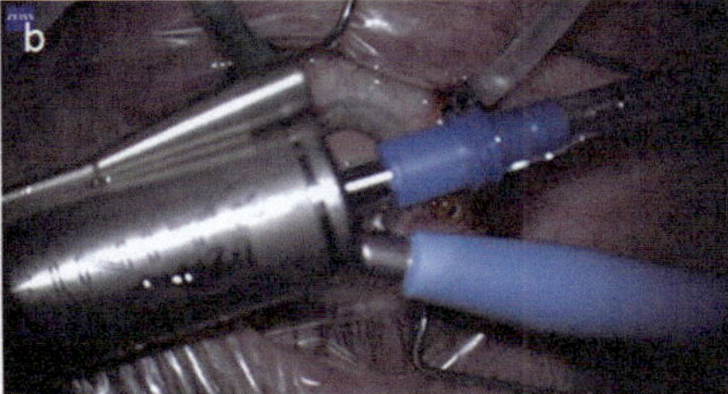

Fig. 30.7 **a** Remove the sleeve from the phaco needle. A regular needle is used. **b** Remove the irrigation tubing, and attach the aspiration tubing

cannula. The latter is located between the two temporal cannulas and is for the intravitreal phacoemulsification handpiece. For settings, I recommend low aspiration or the sculpting mode.

A fragmatome or intravitreal phacoemulsification handpiece is difficult to use. On the one hand, the removal of a nucleus is more difficult inside the vitreous cavity than within the lens capsule. Lens fragments tend to jump away from the needle tip, but this behaviour is more prominent in a fragmatome than a phacoemulsification handpiece. High levels of suction inside the vitreous cavity must be avoided. Aspiration of the vitreous or retinal damage may occur (retinal detachment or choroidal damage).

The dropped nucleus is removed with the vitreous cutter and the phacoemulsification handpiece. Do you know which tissue you can remove with a vitreous cutter and the phacoemulsification handpiece? This is an important knowledge for this case. With the vitreous cutter, you can remove cortex, epinucleus and a soft nucleus. You cannot remove a dense nucleus or a thick capsular fibrosis. With the phacoemulsification handpiece, you can remove a dense nucleus and a thick capsular fibrosis. A rock-hard nucleus is difficult to remove by a phacoemulsification handpiece. To remove a rock-hard nucleus, it is advisable to perform a removal with the SICS technique.

Remark: Use always Irrigation and Aspiration from the phaco machine. Do *not* use a separate bottle. A separate bottle results in dangerous IOP fluctuations. The aspiration tubing is attached to the anterior vitreous cutter and the phacoemulsification handpiece, and the irrigation tubing is attached to an infusion line which is inserted in a trocar cannula at pars plana.

Chandelier light: I perform dropped nucleus surgery always with a chandelier light. Why? I want to work with two free hands. I elevate the nucleus with a Charles flute needle, hold it in the middle of the eye and then I cut it with the vitreous cutter. If you choose to work without chandelier light, then you have the light fibre in one hand and the phacoemulsification handpiece in the other hand. The vitreous cutter aspirates the nuclear fragments directly from the retina and doing this you may injure the retina and the choroid. Alternatively, you can elevate the nucleus with a PFCL bubble in order to protect the posterior pole.

<u>The surgery</u>

<u>Instruments</u>

1. 23G-port trocar system
2. 120D lens
3. Anterior vitreous cutter.

Individual steps

1. 23G 3-port system with chandelier light fibre
2. Anterior vitrectomy via pars plana

3. Removal of residual cortex from the lens capsule via paracentesis
4. Vitrectomy, if necessary PVD
5. 20G sclerotomy at 9 o'clock
6. Emulsification of the nucleus with phacoemulsification handpiece and flute needle
7. Closure of 20G sclerotomy
8. Peripheral vitrectomy
9. Implantation of an intraocular lens
10. Removal of trocar cannulas.

The surgery step by step: (Figs. 30.8, 30.9 and 30.10)

1. 3-port system with chandelier light fibre

After insertion of three trocars, we insert a chandelier light fibre, because we work bimanually in steps 7 and 9.

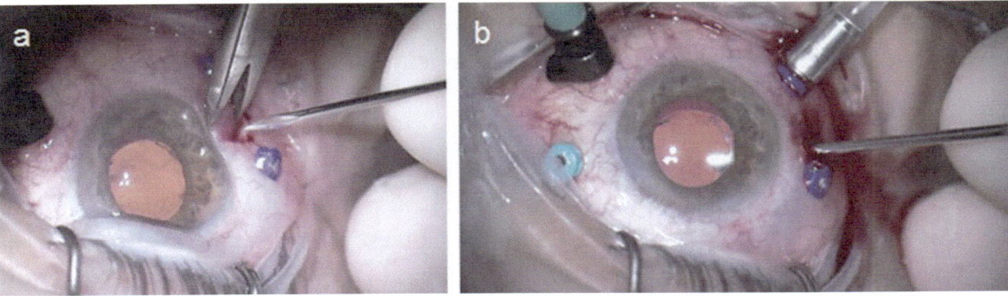

Fig. 30.8 The sclerotomy for the phacoemulsification handpiece is placed at 9 o'clock for right hand dominant surgeons. Open the conjunctiva and perform a perpendicular sclerotomy

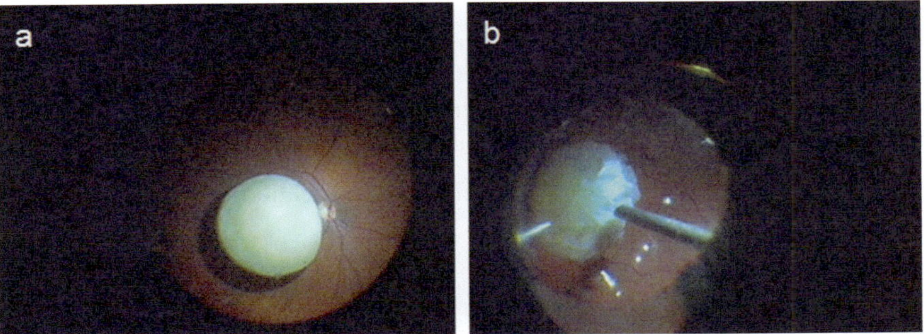

Fig. 30.9 **a** A luxated white nucleus secondary to trauma for 20 years ago. **b** Emulsification of a nucleus with phacoemulsification handpiece. A PFCL (heavy water) bubble was injected to protect the posterior pole

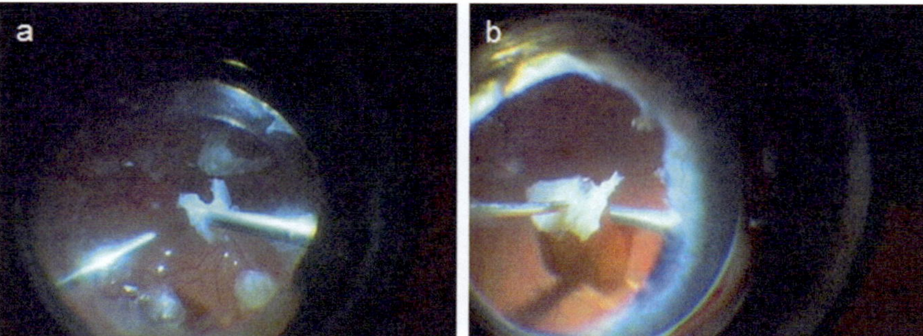

Fig. 30.10 **a** Many small nuclear fragments. Every fragment has to be removed. **b** The left hand fixates the fragment with a backflush instrument, and the right hand removes it with the phacoemulsification handpiece. The phacoemulsification handpiece is a dangerous instrument which can cause severe retinal and choroidal damage

2. Anterior vitrectomy via pars plana

3. Removal of residual cortex from the lens capsule via paracentesis

4. Vitrectomy, if necessary PVD

The anterior vitreous is cut with the vitreous cutter via pars plana. Make circular movements with the vitreous cutter. The vitreous cutter port points backwards towards the posterior pole in order to avoid a damage of the lens capsule. Aspirate then the residual cortex with the vitreous cutter via a paracentesis. Alternatively, you can use two I/A handpieces. It is important that you switch the vitreous cutter to aspiration and not to cutting. Otherwise, you risk destroying the anterior capsule. If the lens capsule is free from the cortex, continue with a core vitrectomy from pars plana.

5. 20G sclerotomy at 9 o'clock

Then, open the conjunctiva at 9 o'clock in the area of the sclerotomy, and perform a non-lamellar (perpendicular) 20G sclerotomy with the V-lance (Fig. 30.8). This sclerotomy is used for the phacoemulsification handpiece and closed as soon as the nucleus is removed, in order to avoid leakage from the sclerotomy.

6. Emulsification of the nucleus with phacoemulsification handpiece and flute needle

The settings for phacoemulsification are: Low aspiration (approximately 100 mmHg) or sculpting mode. Soft lens material can be removed first with the vitreous cutter. For hard lens fragments, you can use the flute needle in your left hand and the phacoemulsification handpiece in the right hand. Aspirate the lens fragments with the flute needle, move the needle to the central vitreous cavity, and emulsify them there safely with the phacoemulsification handpiece (Figs. 30.9 and

30.10). This procedure is performed repeatedly until all the lens fragments are removed.

If you perform this procedure without flute needle (only with the phacoemulsification handpiece), there is a risk that during the frequent aspiration of the lens fragments with the phacoemulsification handpiece you may injure the retina (retinal break) or the choroid (choroidal haemorrhage). In addition, the frequent aspiration of the lens fragments clogs the vitreous cutter. If the suction is not working properly, the risk is increased to induce damage to the retina or choroid.

Tips & tricks

<u>Dropped nucleus</u>: The difficulty of this step is that the nucleus is located on the posterior pole so that a damage of the retina is easily induced. Two advices: (1) Work bimanual so that one hand can fixate the nucleus and the other hand can remove it. (2) Elevate the nucleus with a flute needle.

7. Closure of 20G sclerotomy

The 20G sclerotomy is closed with a Vicryl 6-0 interrupted stitch or a Vicryl 8-0 cross stitch.

8. Peripheral vitrectomy

The phacoemulsification handpiece breaks the nucleus in many small pieces which are dispersed all over the posterior segment. These fragments must be removed meticulously, because every nucleus fragment which remains may cause a postoperative sterile uveitis. The most lens fragments are located in the vitreous base at 6 o'clock. In order to visualize and remove them, you need to indent the vitreous with the scleral depressor. Use for this procedure a chandelier light.

Tips & tricks

The trimming of the vitreous base is an important step because a <u>residual nuclear fragment</u> will cause a postoperative sterile uveitis. Conclusion: Do not be satisfied after removal of the large nucleus but after complete removal of all small fragments.

9. Implantation of the IOL

10. Removal of trocar cannulas

If more than two third of the anterior capsule are intact, the lens can be implanted into the sulcus ("haptic out, optic in"). If not, fixate a 3-piece IOL to the sclera or implant an iris-fixated IOL (Verisyse®).

Tips & tricks

<u>1-piece IOL versus 3-piece IOL</u>: Do not implant a 1-piece IOL into the sulcus because the haptics cause a focal depigmentation of the iris resulting in a secondary pigment glaucoma. This does not happen with a 3-piece IOL. The reason for this is that a 1-piece haptic has sharp edges and a 3-piece haptic is round.

References

Ruiz-Moreno JM, Barile S, Montero JA. Phacoemulsification in the vitreous cavity for retained nuclear lens fragments. Eur J Ophthalmol. 2006;16(1):40–5.

Schaal S, Barr CC. Management of retained lens fragments after cataract surgery with and without pars plana vitrectomy. J Cataract Refract Surg. 2009;35(5):863–7. https://doi.org/10.1016/j.jcrs.2008.12.030.

Soliman Mahdy M, Eid MZ, Shalaby KA, Hegazy HM. Intravitreal phacoemulsification with pars plana vitrectomy for management of posteriorly dislocated nucleus or lens fragments. Eur J Ophthalmol. 2010;20(1):115–9.

All videos of this part be found in a playlist of my YouTube channel:
https://www.youtube.com/playlist?list=PL0dKYclPD7yMJRuQAIt9Dr7pOtuI0
Seex

Corneal Perforation

31

Abstract

This chapter described step-by-step the surgical management of a corneal perforation.

Keywords

Corneal perforation · Surgery

Case report no. 1: Corneal perforation and large iris defect

Video: No video available

Figures 31.1, 31.2, 31.3, 31.4, 31.5, 31.6, 31.7, 31.8

29 y/o male patient who perforated his cornea with a screwdriver during work. Visual acuity was light perception. In a first surgery, only the cornea was sutured. The visual acuity was HM, and a vitreous haemorrhage was present. The patient was followed up every week, and in the fourth week, a retinal detachment was detected with B-scan. A second operation with phacoemulsification and vitrectomy + silicone oil was performed. The visual acuity was 0.1, and a silicone oil removal + IOL reposition was performed one month later. During the postoperative follow-up, the patient complained of severe photophobia, and visual acuity was 0.1–0.2. Eight months later an iris prosthesis with 11 mm diameter was implanted into the sulcus without sutures. In a follow-up after 6 months, the patient has no complaints. In a follow-up after 12 months, the patient complains of ocular irritation, and the IOL is partially dislocated. Visual acuity is 0.1–0.2.

In hindsight: I would not do anything else. Due to the retinal detachment I had to perform a combined phaco/vitrectomy. If the retina did not detach, I would only operate the traumatic cataract and perform a vitrectomy one month later. The

Fig. 31.1 Case report 1: a handyman injured his eye with a screwdriver

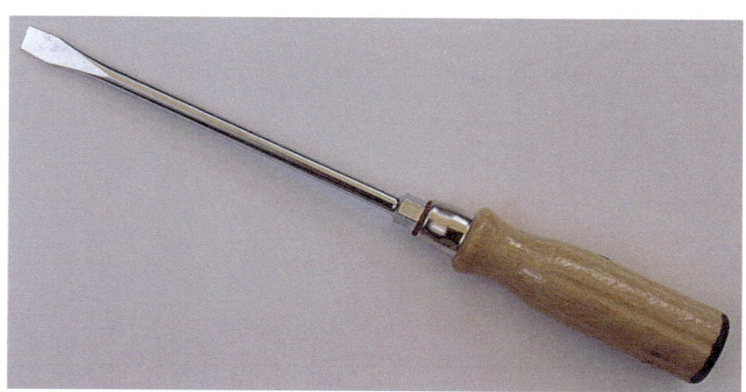

Fig. 31.2 Case report 1: the superior cornea is perforated

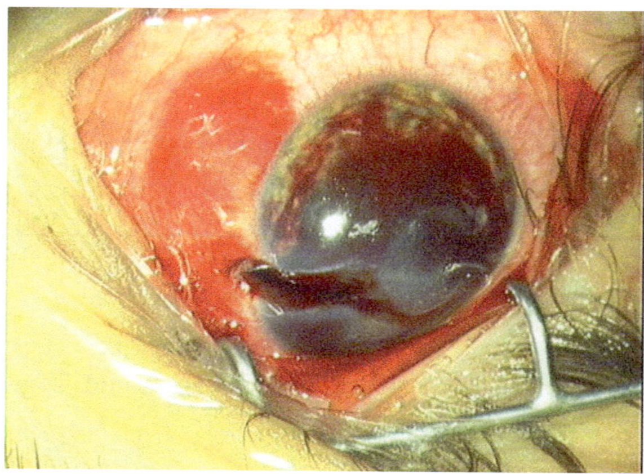

Fig. 31.3 Case report 1: 4 weeks follow-up. A continuous suture of the central cornea was performed. At the limbus, a single suture is used. Continuous sutures are easier to perform and watertight

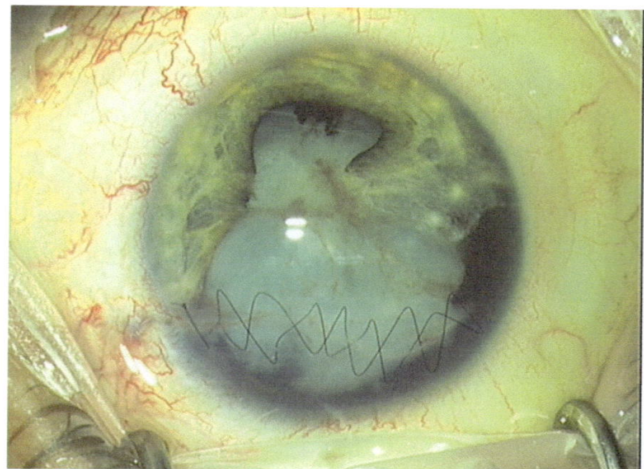

Fig. 31.4 Case report 1: a drawing for corneal sutures. In the centre: continuous suture. At the limbus: single suture

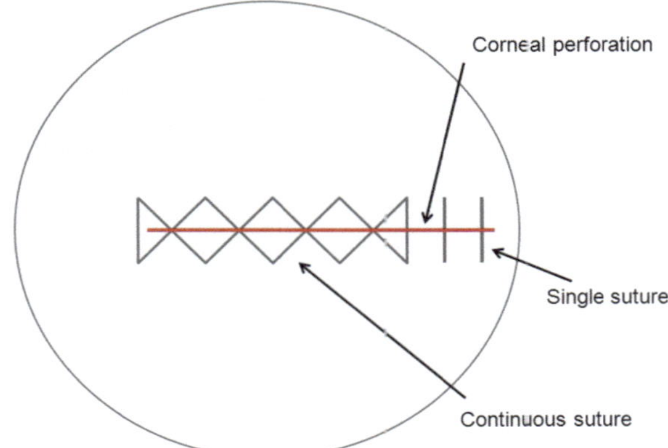

Fig. 31.5 Case report 1: second surgery. 1 month after first surgery: Staining with trypane blue

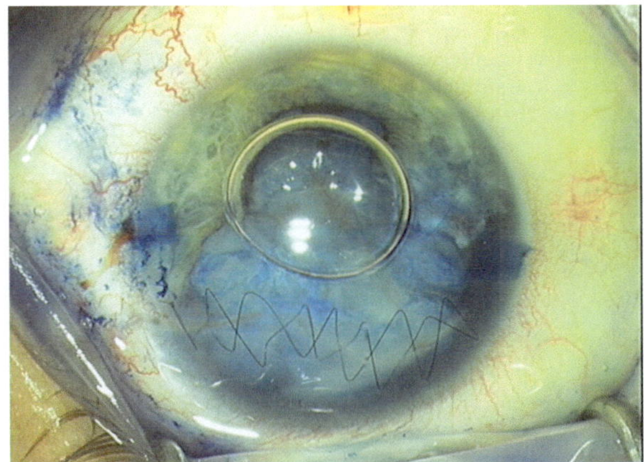

Fig. 31.6 Case report 1: removal of the soft nucleus with I/A

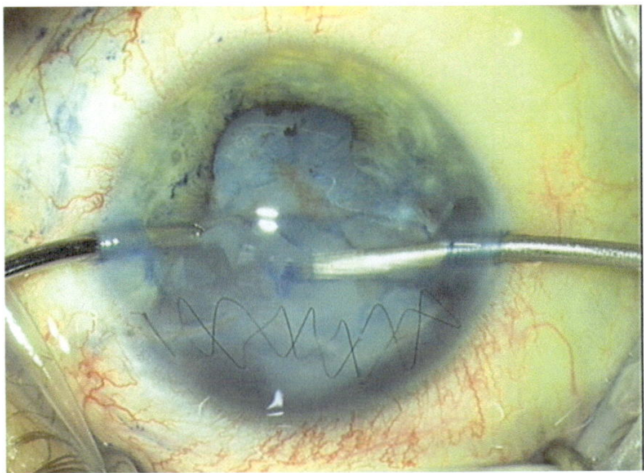

Fig. 31.7 Case report 1: implantation of a 1-piece IOL. Note the large iris defect

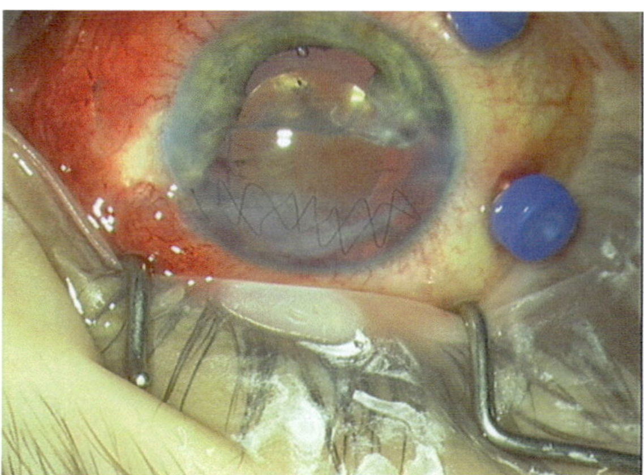

Fig. 31.8 Case report 1: third surgery: implantation of a customized artificial iris prosthesis (Human Optics)

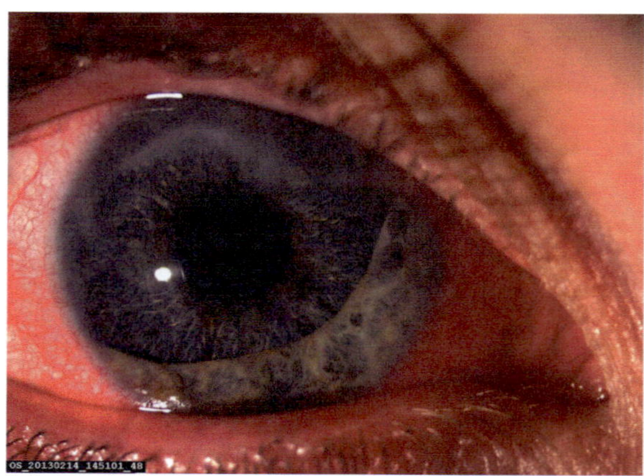

advantage of this stepwise approach is that it is easier to achieve a stable IOL position and you avoid posterior synechiae. The ocular irritation may be caused by the iris prosthesis. I prefer today a 10 mm prosthesis size for sulcus implantation, and I use a trephine (Ophtec®, NL).

Case report no. 2: Corneal perforation in a child

Video: No video available

Figures 31.9, 31.10, 31.11, 31.12, 31.13

A 5 y/o female patient with her friends was jumping on a trampoline and throwing spruce cones at each other. One spruce cone hit her eye and caused a corneal perforation.

She was first operated with suturing of the corneal wound with Nylon 10–0. A continuous suture was performed in the centre of the cornea and interrupted

Fig. 31.9 Case report 2: corneal perforation of a 5 y/o girl with a spruce cone

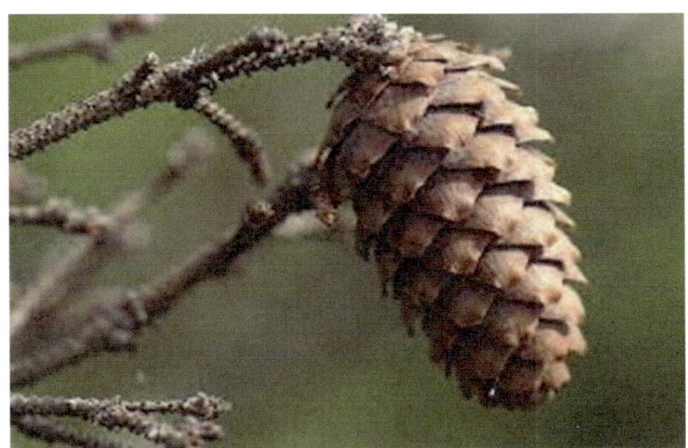

Fig. 31.10 Case report 2: 1 month after first surgery with continuous corneal suture. Note that the corneal wound is fibrotic

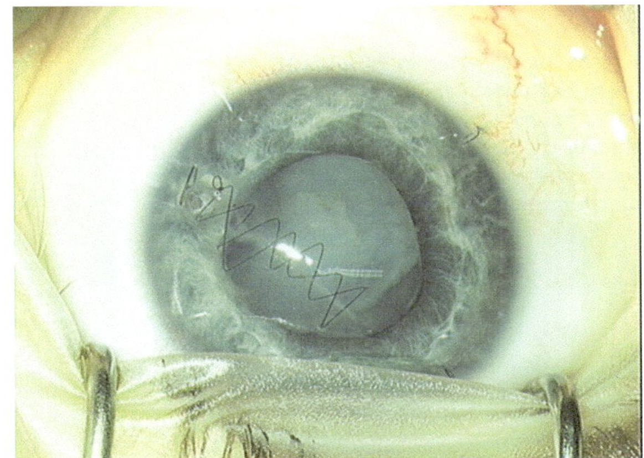

Fig. 31.11 Case report 2: staining of anterior capsule with trypane blue. The anterior capsule is partially defect. Try to make the rhexis as round as possible

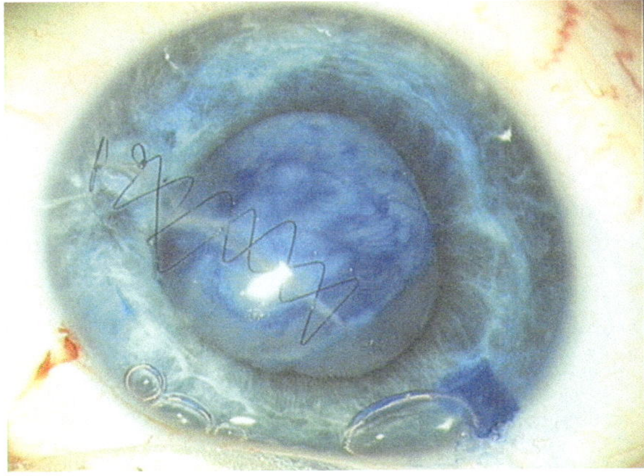

Fig. 31.12 Case report 2: the posterior capsule is intact

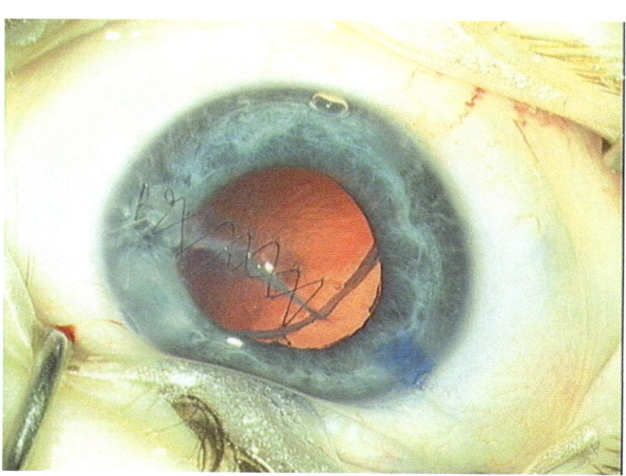

Fig. 31.13 Case report 2: in-the-bag implantation and an air bubble to stabilize the anterior chamber. The corneal suture was removed one month later

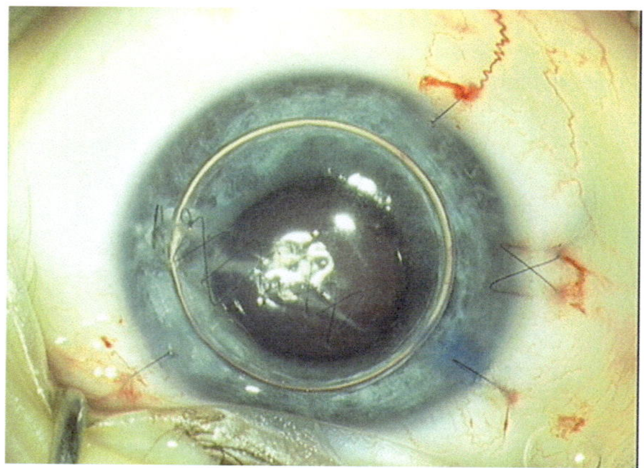

stitches at the limbus. One month later a phacoemulsification + IOL was performed. The visual acuity in the last follow-up after 2 years was 0.9.

<u>In hindsight</u>: This case went very well. I think that a traumatic cataract is easier to operate after 1 month because the inflammation has subsided, and the lens capsule is partially fibrotic.

<u>Remark</u>: I never experience increased intraocular inflammation and pressure after perforation of a lens capsule. This relates, however, to young patients.

Traumatic Cataract

32

Abstract

This chapter describes step-by-step the surgical management of a traumatic cataract.

Keyword

Traumatic cataract · Surgery

The surgery of an old traumatic cataract is not as difficult as the eye looks like. The main difficulty is the rhexis because the anterior lens capsule tissue is very fibrotic. To perform the rhexis, you need special scissors (Figs. 32.1 and 32.2). These scissors enable to cut the anterior lens capsule from the side incisions. Often more than two side incisions are necessary to perform a circular rhexis (Figs. 32.3, 32.4, 32.5, 32.6, 32.7, 32.8, 32.9, 32.10, 32.11, 32.12, 32.13 and 32.14) (Video available).

If the posterior capsule is also fibrotic, then a posterior capsular rhexis needs also to be performed. This can be done in the easiest way at a later time point with a vitreous cutter from pars plana.

Instruments:

1. Phaco set
2. Special capsule scissors
3. Regular capsulorhexis forceps.

Individual steps:

(1) Capsulorhexis
(2) Phacoemulsification
(3) I/A
(4) IOL implantation.

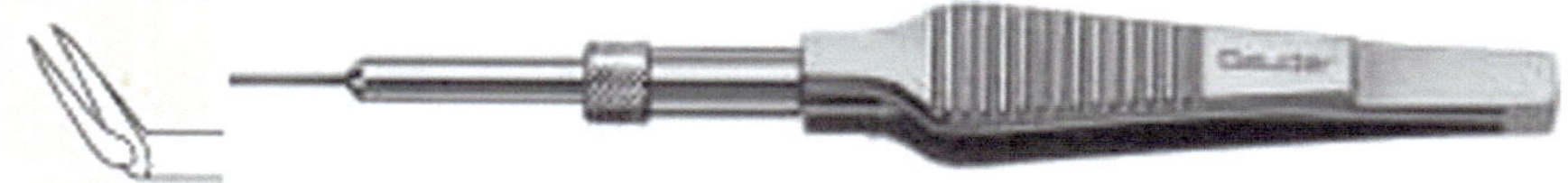

Fig. 32.1 Capsule scissors after Kampik (a, b). The instrument fits through a paracentesis. 22G. Indication: Cutting of capsule or iris. Geuder 38215

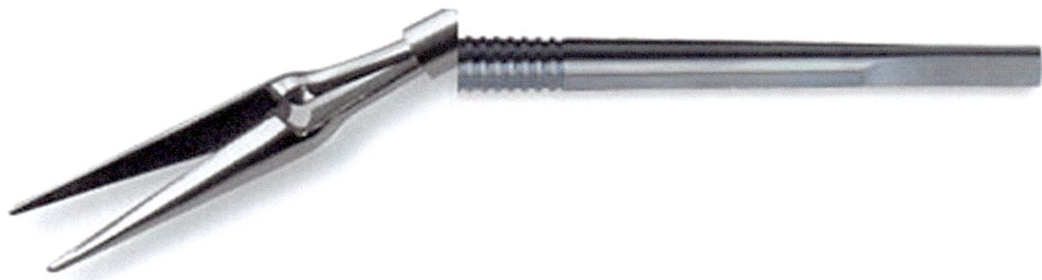

Fig. 32.2 Intravitreal scissors (a, b). 23G. Indication: General cutting of tissue. DORC 1286.J06

Fig. 32.3 Traumatic cataract after blunt trauma with a paint ball

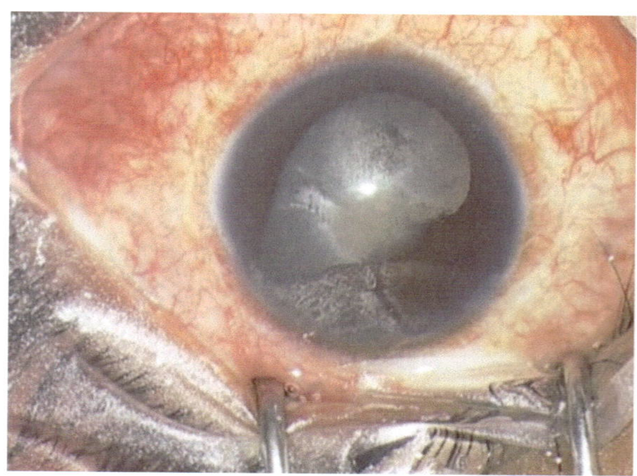

The surgery step by step:

(1) Capsulorhexis

Use Healon GV if possible, to inflate the anterior chamber. Enlarge the pupil if necessary (Figs. 32.6 and 32.7). Stain the anterior capsule with Vision Blue. Pinch a hole in the middle of the lens capsule with the cystotome. Perform a capsulorhexis with the capsulorhexis forceps. If you cannot continue with the rhexis due to a

Fig. 32.4 Cutting a membrane with 23G intravitreal straight scissors. A side incision at 11 o'clock is used

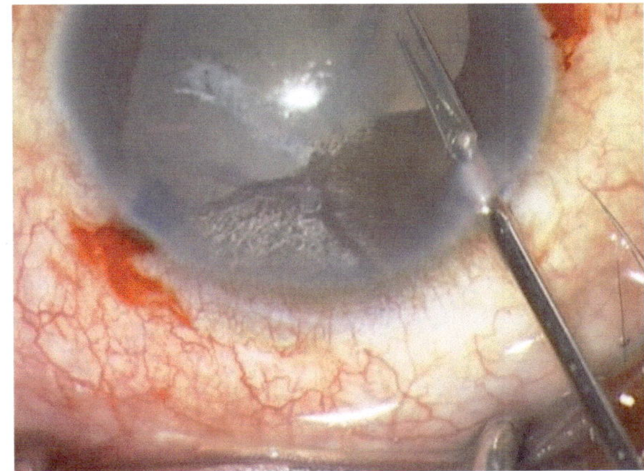

Fig. 32.5 Observe that a different side incision is used (8 o'clock). Cutting another membrane with 23G intravitreal scissors

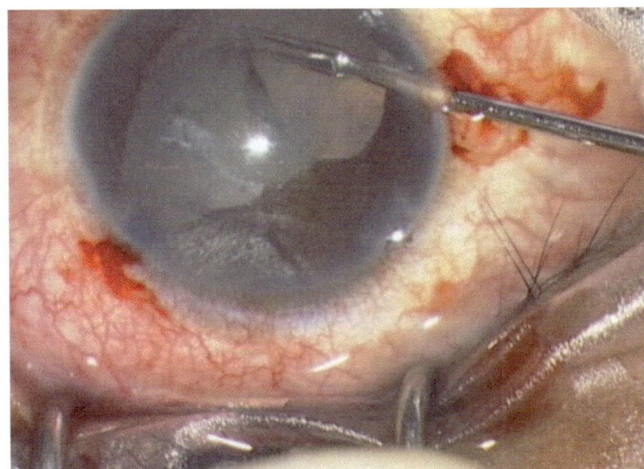

Fig. 32.6 Traumatic cataract after blunt trauma with a fist

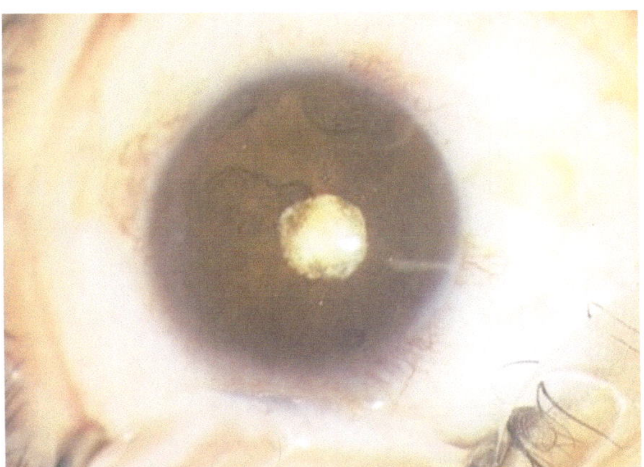

Fig. 32.7 Enlarging the small pupil with two push–pull instruments

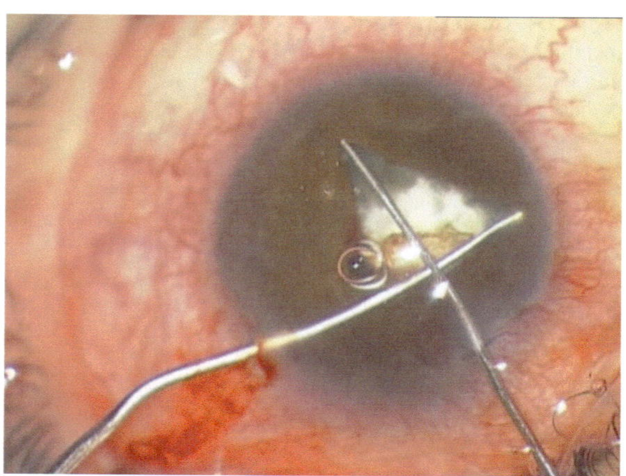

Fig. 32.8 Cutting a fibrotic part of the lens capsule with intravitreal straight scissors

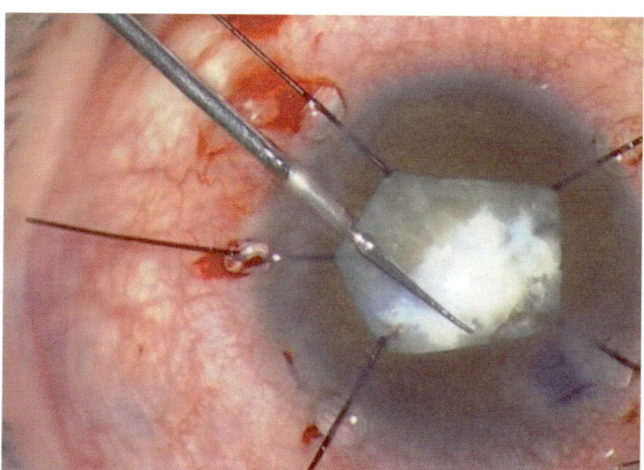

Fig. 32.9 Observe the cut in the white part of the fibrosis

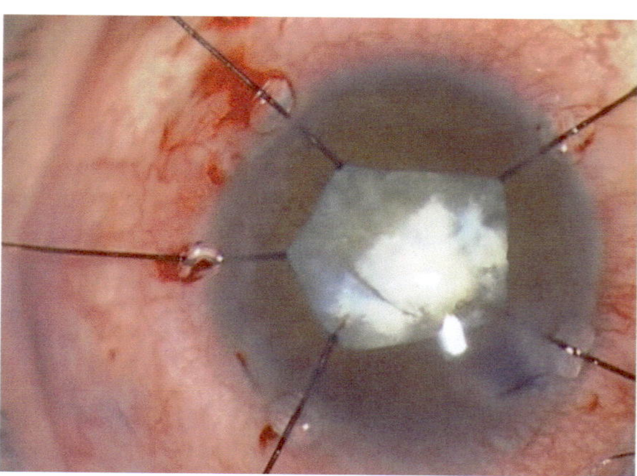

Fig. 32.10 Difficult rhexis due to much fibrosis

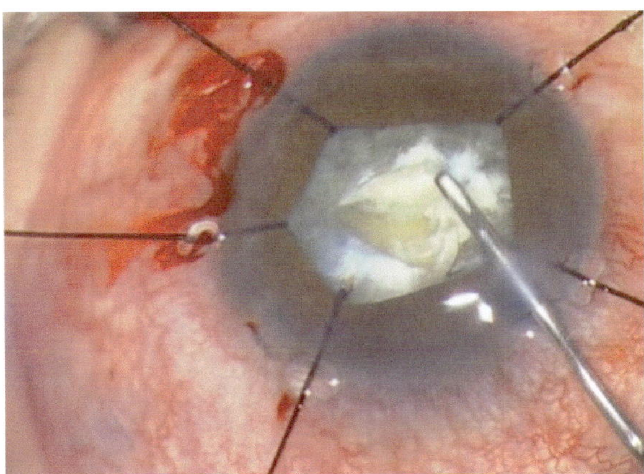

Fig. 32.11 Cutting the fibrosis with intravitreal straight scissors

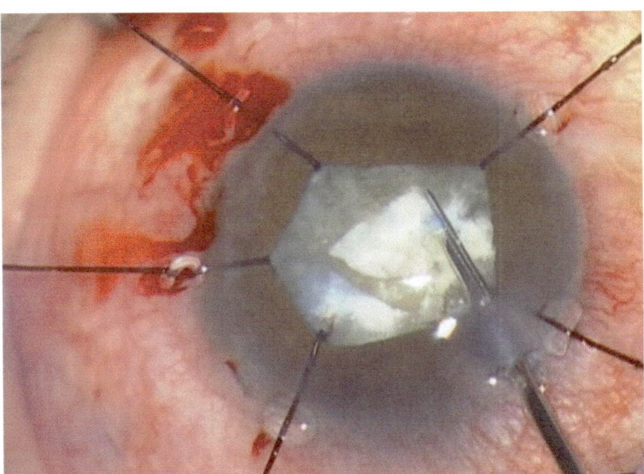

Fig. 32.12 Removing the fibrosis with a capsulorhexis forceps

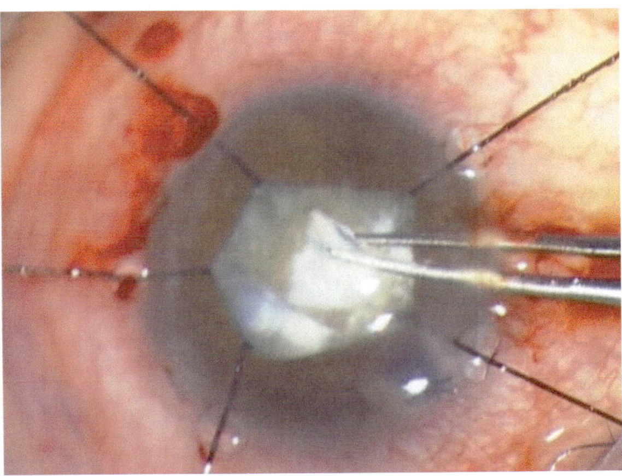

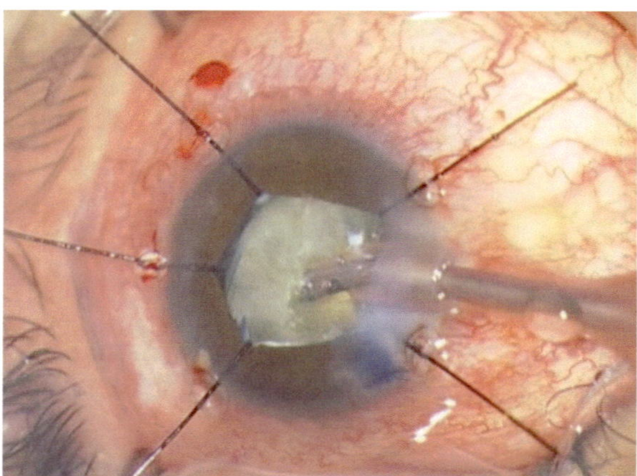

Fig. 32.13 Phacoemulsification of a dense nucleus. In some trauma cases, the nucleus is reduced to a fibrotic remnant

Fig. 32.14 Implantation of a one-piece IOL into the capsular bag

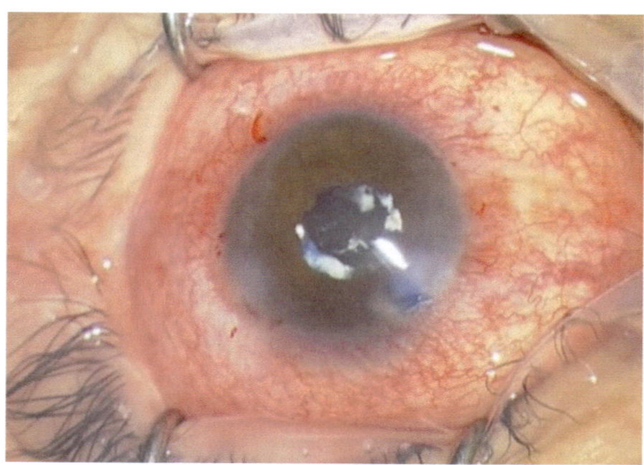

fibrosis, then cut the fibrosis with the special capsule scissors (Figs. 32.8, 32.9 and 32.11). Then, continue with the rhexis using the capsulorhexis forceps or cystotome (Fig. 32.10). Fibrotic parts of the lens capsule have to be removed with the capsulorhexis forceps (Fig. 32.12).

(2) Phacoemulsification
(3) I/A
(4) IOL implantation

Continue with phacoemulsification or with I/A if the nucleus is soft (Fig. 32.13). Implant a 1-piece IOL or even better a 3-piece IOL in the capsular bag (Fig. 32.14).

Remark: The lens capsule in this specific case was fibrotic. It was not possible to remove the fibrosis without risking damage to the posterior capsule. The fibrosis was also too thick for removal with YAG-capsulotomy. One month later, I created therefore a posterior capsular opening with a vitreous cutter from pars plana.

Traumatic Mydriasis

33

Abstract

This chapter explains in detail the surgical management of a traumatic mydriasis.

Keyword

Traumatic mydriasis · Surgery

A traumatic mydriasis can be managed surgically with an iris suture. There are several techniques. I will present an easy-to-learn suture technique using two forceps from Geuder (Germany) and a special suture with a very short needle from Onatec (Germany) (Video available).

Instruments:

(1) Hattenbach iris instruments (Geuder) Figs. 33.1 and 33.2
(2) Onatec suture (Geuder) Fig. 33.3.

A 66 y/o male patient was hit by a hockey stick in his right eye (Fig. 33.4). In the local eye clinic, a dislocation of the natural lens was observed. The eye pressure with peaks to 40 mmHg level was treated with acetazolamid tablets. The patient was admitted to us for surgical management. The preoperative visual acuity was CF. In the first surgery, the dislocated nucleus was removed, and a vitrectomy performed. In a second surgery, three months after the injury, an iridoplasty with implantation of an iris-claw IOL was performed. For iridoplasty, instruments from Geuder, Germany, were used (Figs. 33.5, 33.6, 33.7 and 33.8). The postoperative VA was 0.8.

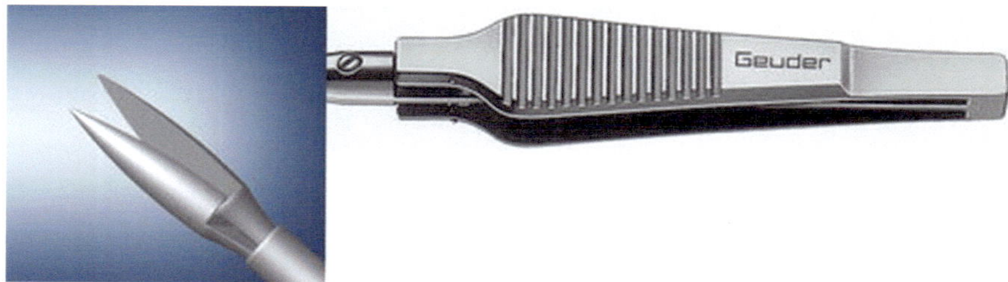

Fig. 33.1 These iris instruments from Hattenbach (Geuder, Germany) enable a technically easy suturing of the iris. These are the scissors

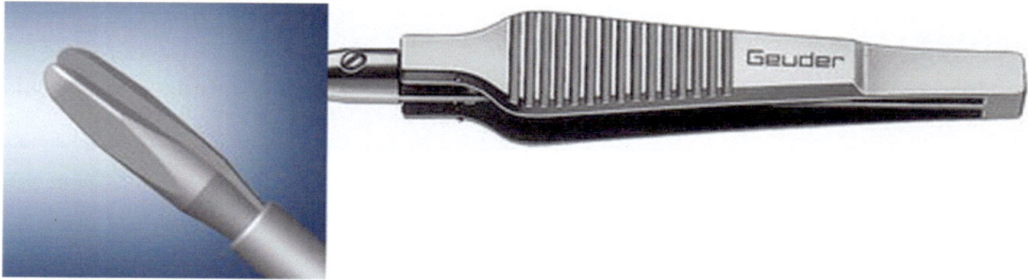

Fig. 33.2 Needle holder

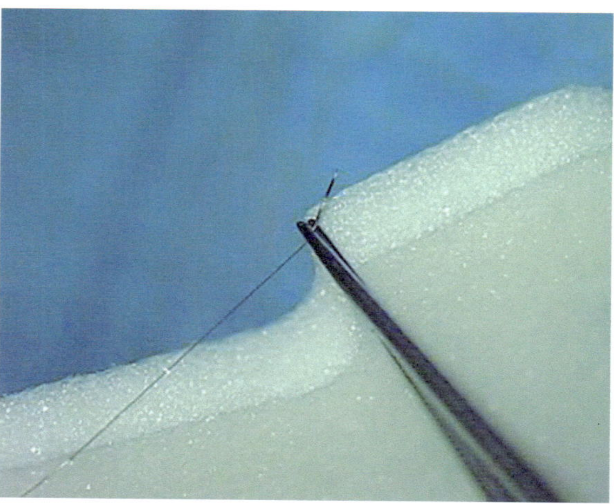

Fig. 33.3 For suturing, the company provides a special suture (Onatec) with a very short needle

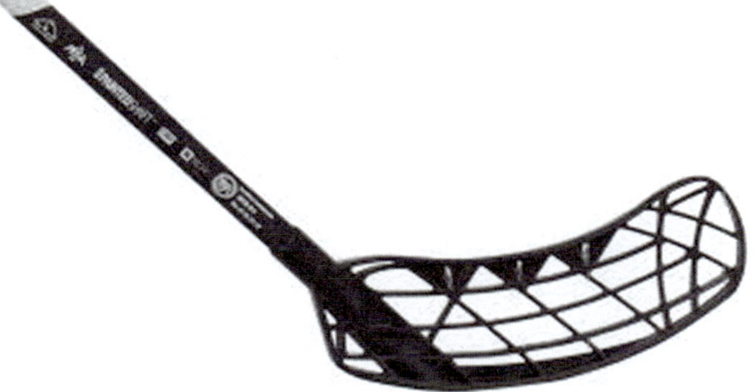

Fig. 33.4 Blunt ocular trauma from an indoor hockey stick

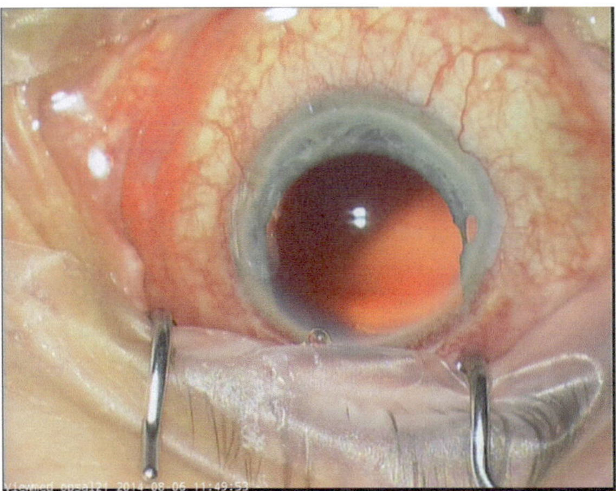

Fig. 33.5 Maximal traumatic mydriasis and aphakia

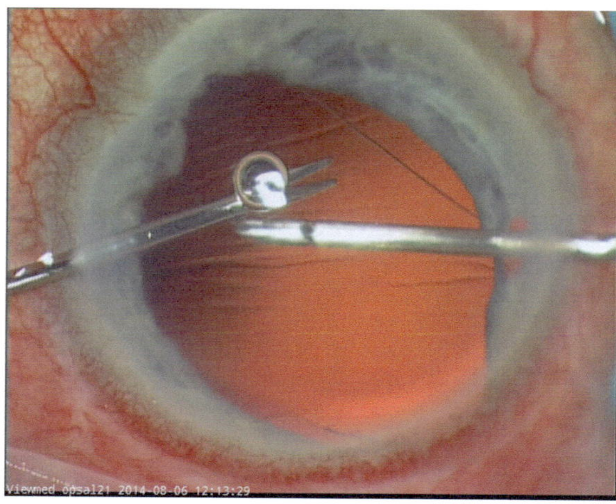

Fig. 33.6 I am using the Hattenbach iris instruments and an Onatec suture with a tiny needle (both Geuder, Germany)

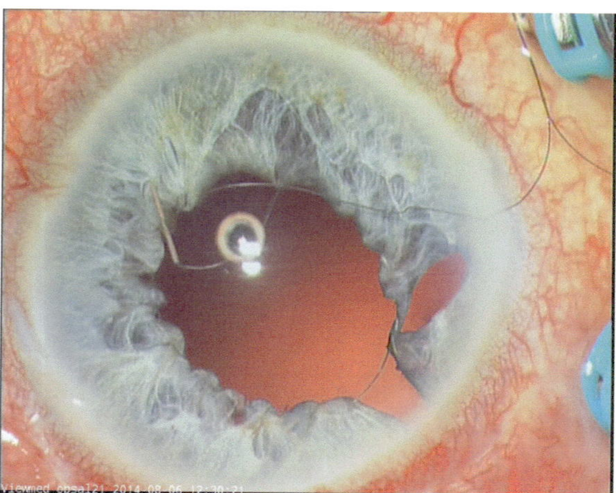

Fig. 33.7 Perform then a pursestring suture. The instruments are easy to handle. Note the small Onatec needle

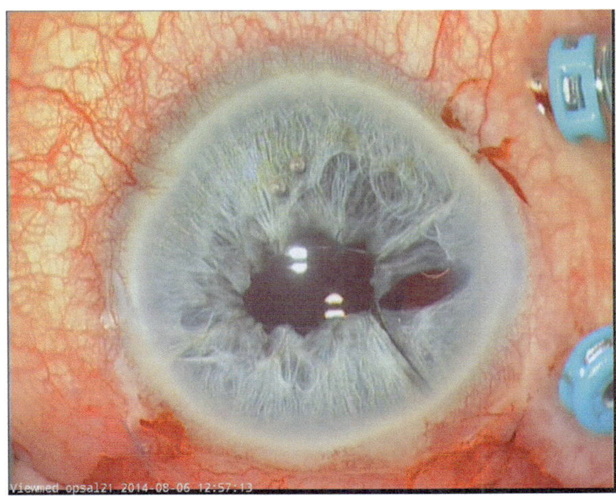

Fig. 33.8 Before closing the pursestring, an iris-claw IOL is implanted. Then, the suture is tied

<u>In hindsight</u>: An iridoplasty with the instruments from Geuder is technically quite easy but time consuming. It is for me the method of choice in such pathologies. The advantage of an iridoplasty compared to a foldable iris prosthesis is the lack of possible ocular irritation.

Iridodialysis 34

Contents

Abstract

This chapter explains step-by-step the surgical management of an iridodialysis.

Keyword

Iridodialysis · Surgery

An iridiodialysis can be sutured with a 10–0 polypropylen suture. The crucial part is the insertion of the needle into the paracentesis without catching corneal tissue. I use therefore a trocar cannula to avoid this possible complication.

A 50 y/o male patient was hit by a plastic ball during a game of indoor hockey (Fig. 34.1). He was admitted to us for surgical management. An iridodialysis was present, and the lens was dislocated. Visual acuity was measured with 0.05. The eye was amblyopic and had a VA of maximal 0.3. The patient worked as a dentist and was very affected in his daily work. The eye was operated with secondary implantation of a 3-piece IOL with Scharioth technique and in a second surgery with iridoplasty (Figs. 34.2, 34.3 and 34.4). Visual acuity in the final follow-up was 0.1–0.2.

Video: No video available

Material:

10–0 polypropylen with long curved needle.

   331
U. Spandau and G. B. Scharioth, *Complications During and After Cataract Surgery*,
https://doi.org/10.1007/978-3-030-93531-3_34

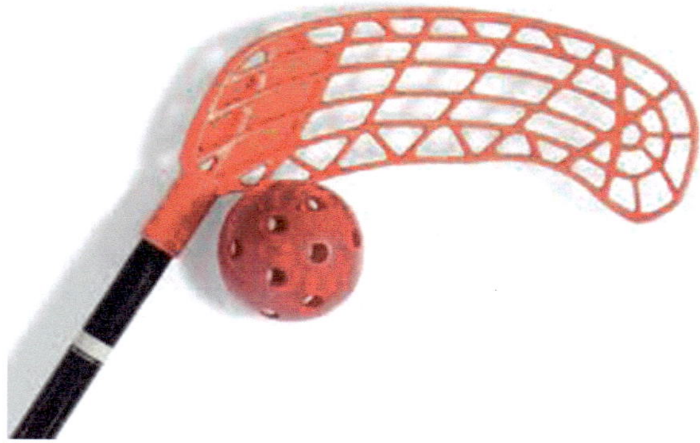

Fig. 34.1 A blunt ocular trauma secondary to an indoor hockey ball

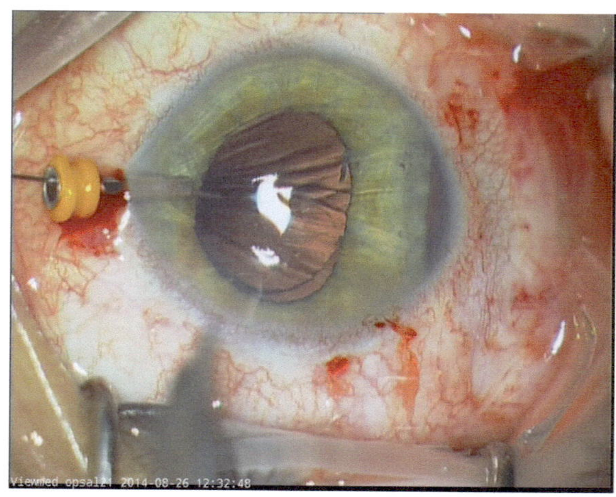

Fig. 34.2 Insert a trocar without valve on the opposite side of the iridodialysis

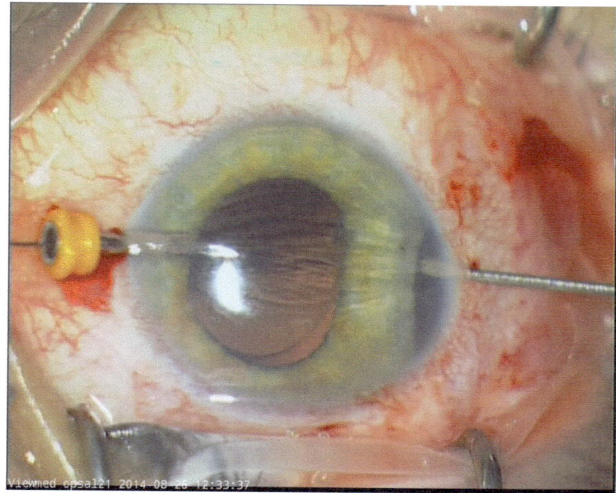

Fig. 34.3 Insert a straight needle of a polypropylen 10–0 suture through the trocar, and then, insert a 27G cannula from the other side

Fig. 34.4 Then, pierce the iris with the needle, and catch the needle with the 27G cannula from the other side. Then, repeat the manoeuvre with the second straight polypropylen needle, cut both needles, and make a knot on the side of the iridodialysis

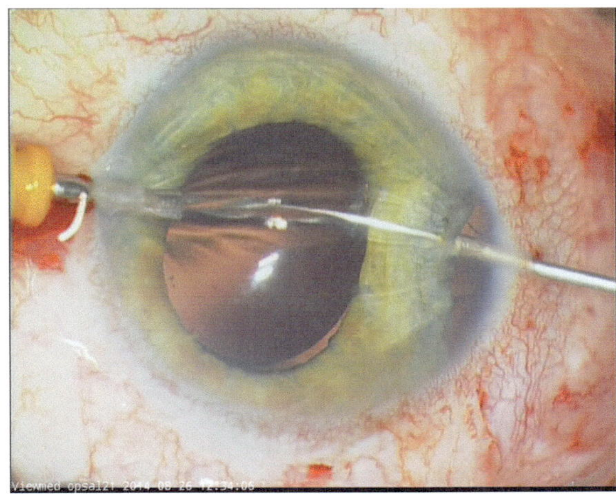

34.1 Iris Defect

An iris defect can be repaired with diathermy. Attach both iris edges with an intravitreal forceps, and cauterize the edges. Alternatively, you can suture the iris defect. Use a long curved needle and 10–0 polypropylen suture. The curved needle is easier to use than the straight needle (Figs. 34.5 and 34.6).

Fig. 34.5 A main incision is performed at 12 o'clock. Then, the curved needle is inserted through the limbus at 10 o'clock, then through the first edge of iris defect, then through the second edge and finally through the limbus at 2 o'clock. The needle is removed, and the sutures retrieved through the main incision at 12 o'clock

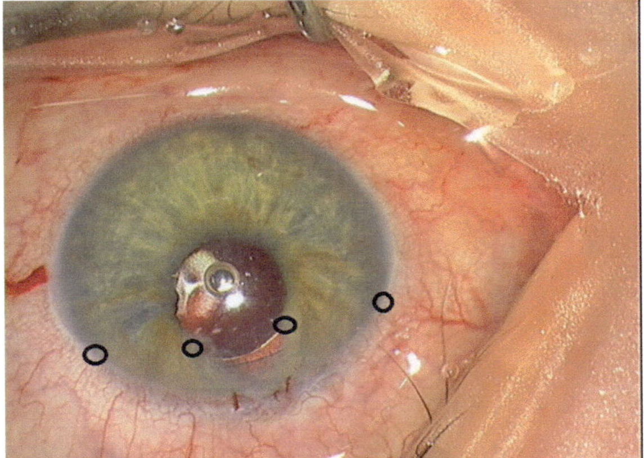

Fig. 34.6 Then, tie the suture. It helps to push the knot with a push–pull instrument to the pupillary edge

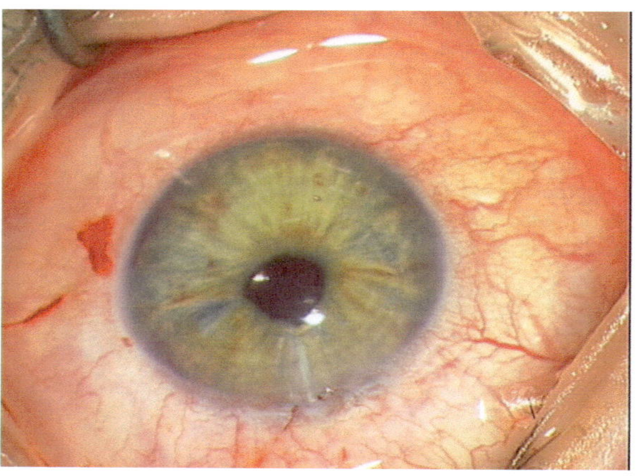

Surgical Management of a Traumatic Aniridia and Aphakia with Iris and IOL Prosthesis

35

Contents

Abstract

This chapter explains step-by-step the surgical management of a traumatic aniridia and aphakia. The implantation of a special IOL/iris prosthesis is demonstrated.

Keywords

IOL/iris prosthesis · Aphakia · Aniridia

Eyes with mydriasis, aniridia and aphakia secondary to trauma can be provided with combined iris and IOL prosthesis. The company Human Optics produces a foldable iris prosthesis (without IOL), which is handpainted (Fig. 35.1). The companies Morcher and Ophtec offer iris and IOL prosthesis, whereas Morcher offers handpainted iris prosthesis and Opthec a range of four colours (Fig. 35.2). Both prosthesis from Morcher and Ophtec are PMMA and not foldable. The Morcher and Opthec iris and IOL prosthesis require a 9.0 mm broad main incision.

The iris prosthesis from Human Optics can be implanted with an IOL injector into the sulcus. For aniridia and aphakia, the iris prosthesis from Human Optics can be combined with a 3-piece IOL: The iris prosthesis is fixated into the haptics of a 3-piece IOL (MA60AC, Alcon). I call this a combo iris–IOL prosthesis. It is implanted through a 2.4 mm main incision with an IOL injector (Alcon). (Video available).

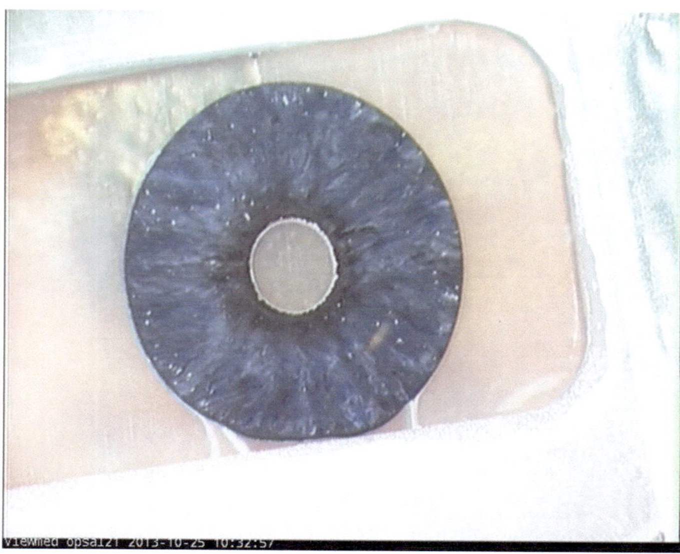

Fig. 35.1 A handpainted and foldable iris (without IOL) prosthesis from Human Optics, Germany. The diameter is 12 mm. The prize is approximately 2000 Euros

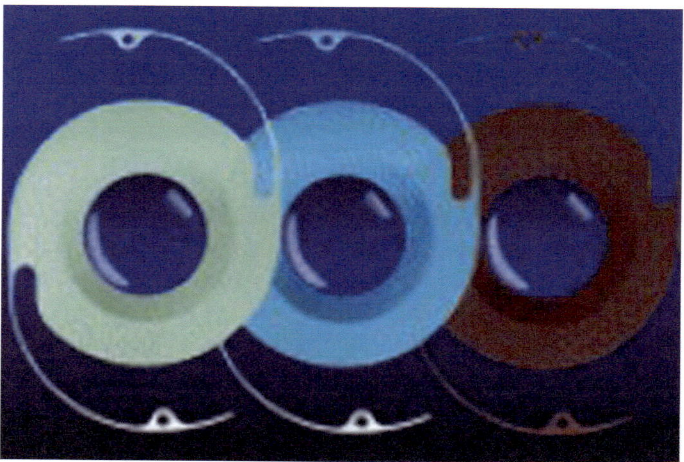

Fig. 35.2 An IOL–iris prosthesis from Opthec, Netherlands. The diameter is 9 mm. A large incision is therefore required. The colour of the prosthesis turns out brighter when inserted in the eye. We use only the brown iris. The prize is approximately 450 Euros

There are several important features which determine the surgical planning:

(1) (Partial) aniridia
(2) Traumatic mydriasis
(3) Aphakia
(4) Intact lens capsule.

Remark: An old traumatic mydriasis cannot be operated with iridoplasty because the iris tissue is fibrotic and bleeds very much. Try to mobilize the iris tissue with a forceps. If this is possible, then perform an iridoplasty with the Hattenbach instruments. In the first case, implant an iris prosthesis.

Our surgical management is as follows:

(1) (Partial) Aniridia => Foldable iris prosthesis (Human Optics®)
(2) Aniridia and phakia = > Combo iris–IOL prosthesis and in-the-bag implantation
(3) Aniridia and aphakia => Combo iris–IOL prosthesis and scleral fixation
(4) Old traumatic mydriasis => Foldable iris prosthesis (Human Optics®)
(5) Recent traumatic mydriasis => Iridoplasty with iris instruments (Geuder®, Germany)
(6) Recent traumatic mydriasis and aphakia => Iridoplasty and iris-claw IOL OR first scleral-fixated IOL and then iridoplasty
(7) Recent traumatic mydriasis and intact lens capsule = > Iridoplasty and phaco + IOL.

Implantation site:

The Ophtec IOL can be implanted in the bag and be scleral fixated with 9–0 polypropylene suture (Figs. 35.3, 35.4, 35.5, 35.6, 35.7, 35.8, 35.9 and 35.10). A scleral incision of 9 mm is required.

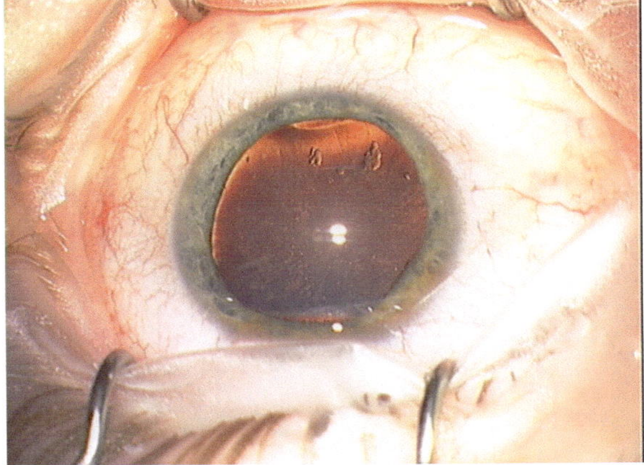

Fig. 35.3 Blunt ocular trauma secondary to an indoor hockey ball

Fig. 35.4 Traumatic mydriasis

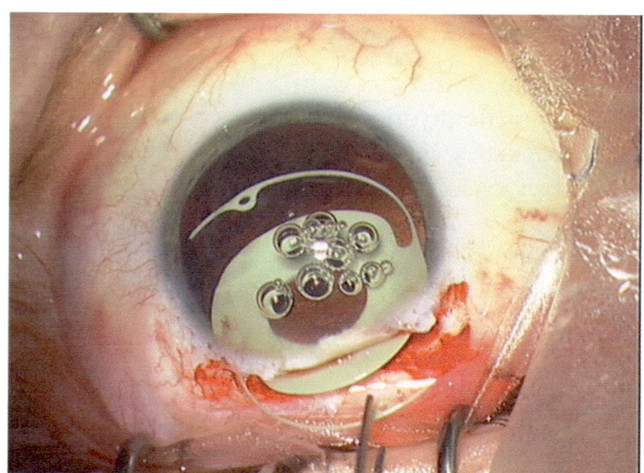

Fig. 35.5 Implantation of an iris–IOL prosthesis (Ophthec) inside the capsular bag

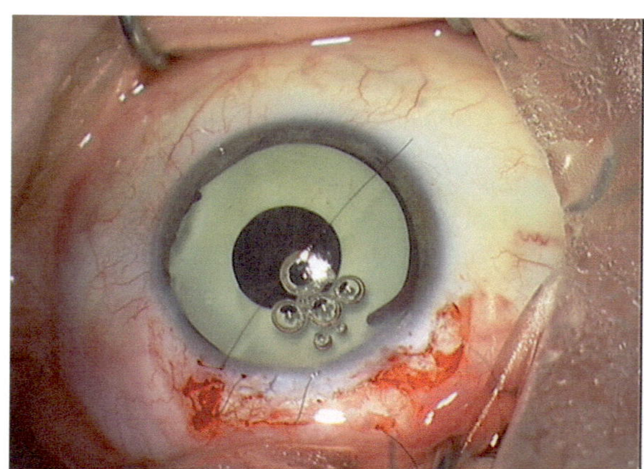

Fig. 35.6 The main incision is 9 mm large. Asurgical alternative is an iridoplasty and implantation of a regular IOL

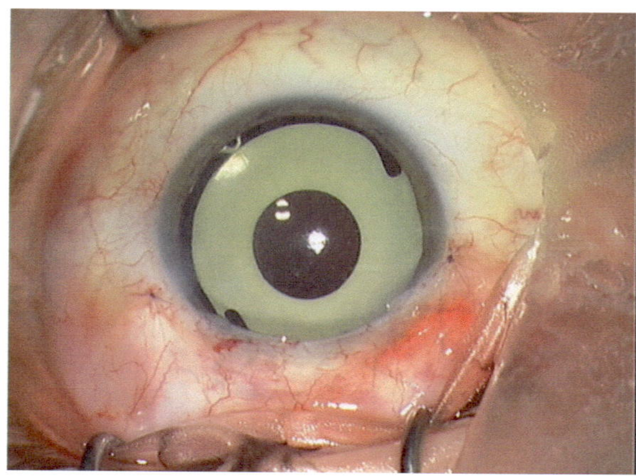

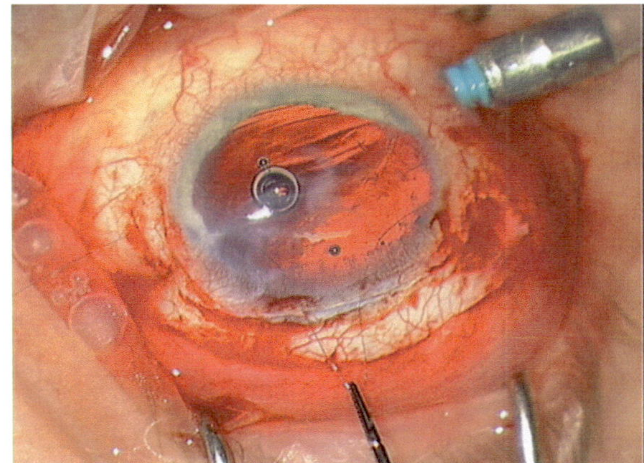

Fig. 35.7 Aphakia and a large iris defect. An Opthec iris–IOL prosthesis is implanted with scleral fixation

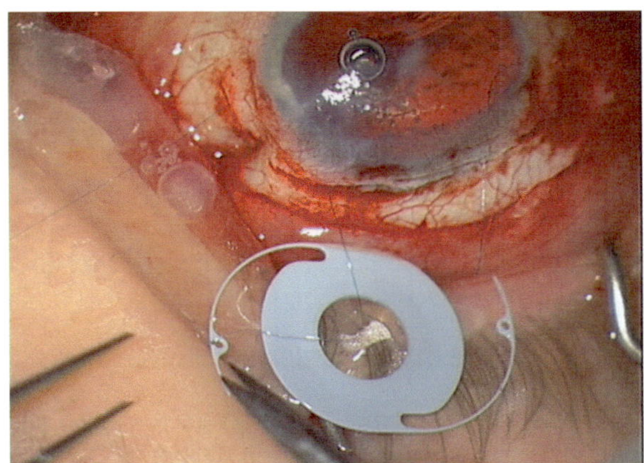

Fig. 35.8 The suture can be fixated very easily in the haptic hole

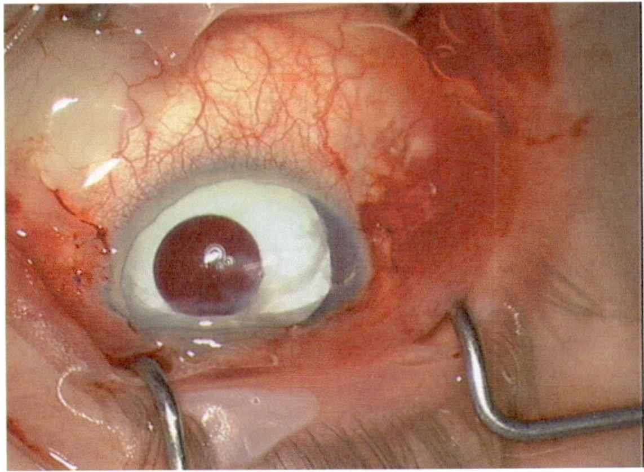

Fig. 35.9 The prosthesis sits very stable

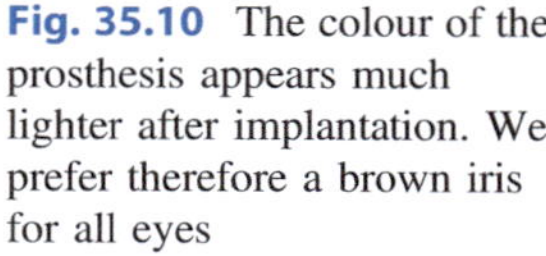

Fig. 35.10 The colour of the prosthesis appears much lighter after implantation. We prefer therefore a brown iris for all eyes

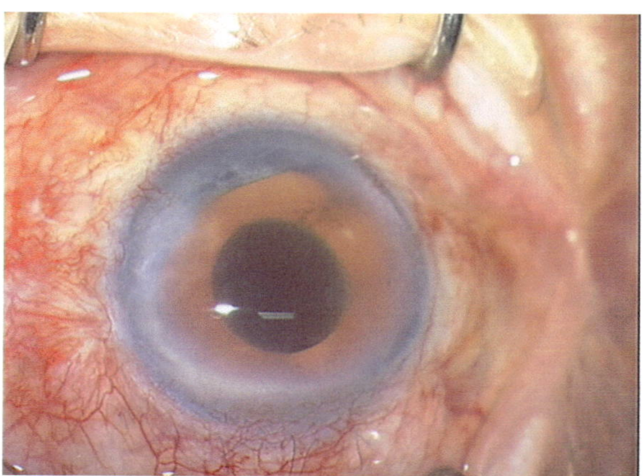

35.1 Fixation of a 3-Piece IOL in a Foldable Iris Prosthesis (Human Optics®) and Implantation of Combo IOL–Iris Prosthesis Through a 2.4 mm Incision

The artificial iris (Human Optics) can be implanted into the sulcus. The combo IOL–iris prosthesis can be implanted in the lens capsule and be scleral fixated with 9–0 polypropylene suture. An alternative is a Scharioth intrascleral fixation with the 3-piece IOL. (Video available).

Prosthesis size for Human optic iris prosthesis:

   Sulcus implantation: 10.0–11.0 mm.
   In-the-bag implantation: 9.0–10.0 mm.

A male 29-y/o patient was wounded in his face after the explosion of a gas cylinder of a gas truck (Fig. 35.11). The patient was surgically assessed at the local hospital. CT scan was done and showed no brain damage, no skull fracture and no foreign bodies in the orbit. It showed a deformed globe right and signs of perforation on the left. It also showed pronounced damage to the soft tissue of the face. He had healthy eyes before the injury, and the sight was 1.0 in both eyes.

The patient was admitted to us for acute surgery. The preoperative assessment showed a bilateral perforated cornea (left more advanced than right). But the retina on the right eye was more affected than on the left eye. Visual acuity was light perception in both eyes. Both eyes were first operated with suturing of the corneal perforation.

In the last follow-up, the left eye has an opacified cornea and a slight nuclear sclerosis. Visual acuity was 0,4.

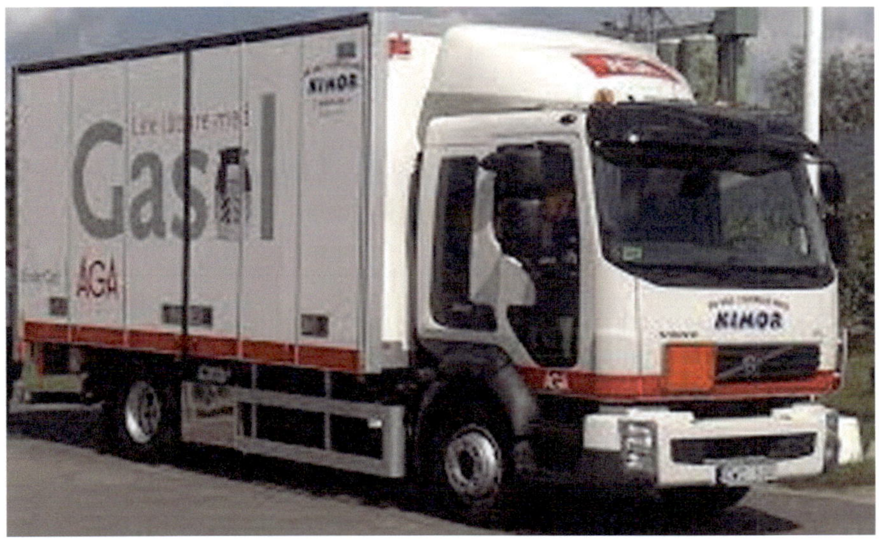

Fig. 35.11 A bilateral corneal perforation secondary to an exploding gas truck resulting in bilateral corneal perforation, aphakia, iris defect and PVR detachment

The retina in the right eye detached after 1 week and was operated with a vitrectomy and 1 month later with fixation of an iridodialysis. Three months after the retinal detachment the silicone oil was removed. One month later an implantation of a combo iris and IOL prosthesis due to aphakia and traumatic mydriasis was performed. The visual acuity in the last follow-up was 0,4 in the left eye.

Instruments

1. 10 mm corneal trephine (Opthec)
2. 23G or 25G endgripping forceps
3. IOL injector.

Material

Iris prosthesis (Human Optics).
MA60AC IOL (Alcon).

Individual steps

1. **Preparation of an iris–IOL prosthesis**
2. **Insertion of iris–IOL prosthesis into a cartridge**
3. **Implantation of iris–IOL prosthesis**
4. **Fixation of iris prosthesis.**

The surgery step by step: Figs. 35.12, 35.13, 35.14, 35.15, 35.16, 35.17 and 35.18

1. Preparation of an iris–IOL prosthesis

The size of the iris prosthesis depends on an implantation in the sulcus or in the capsular bag. In case of a capsular bag implantation, we use a 9.0 mm corneal trephine. In case of a sulcus implantation, we use a 10.0 mm corneal trephine (Fig. 35.13). Place the 3-piece IOL on the backside of the foldable iris, and place two incisions at each haptic with a 15 deg knife (Alcon). Tunnel the 25G end-gripping forceps through the two incisions, grab an end of a haptic, and pull the haptic through the incisions (Figs. 35.14 and 35.15). Repeat the manoeuvre with the other haptic.

2. Insertion of iris–IOL prosthesis into a cartridge

3. Implantation of iris–IOL prosthesis

Fold or roll the combo prosthesis, and insert it into an IOL cartridge (Alcon) and finally into an injector. Continue with a 2,4 mm main incision, and implant then the combo iris–prosthesis into the anterior chamber (Fig. 35.16).

4. Fixation of iris prosthesis

Rotate the combo iris–IOL prosthesis into the lens capsule. If a lens capsule is not present, a scleral fixation has to be performed: (1) Intrascleral Scharioth method or (2) scleral fixation with sutures (Figs. 35.17 and 35.18).

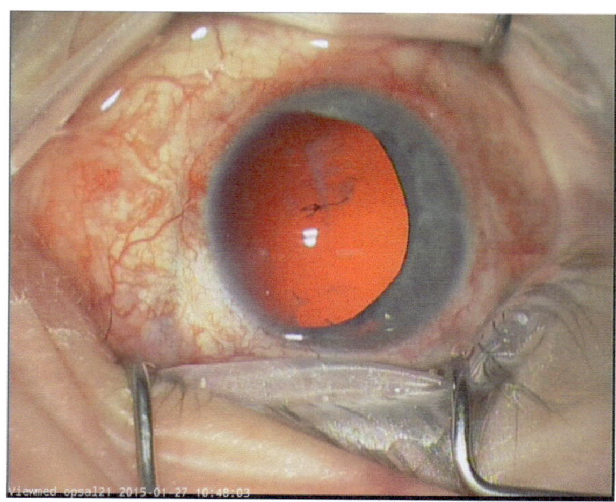

Fig. 35.12 Now: Aphakia and iris defect

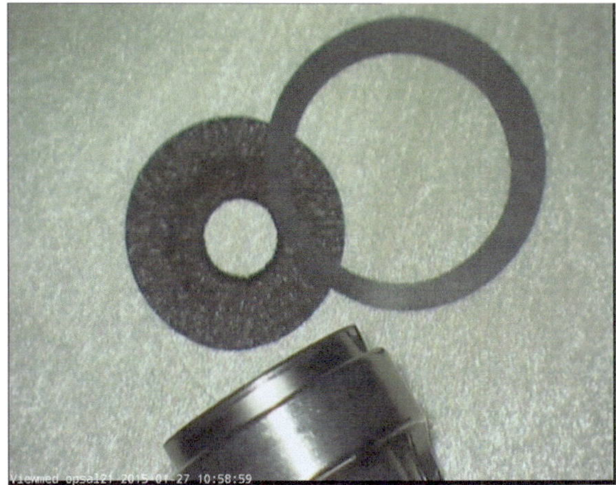

Fig. 35.13 Cutting the foldable iris with a 10 mm trephine (Ophtec)

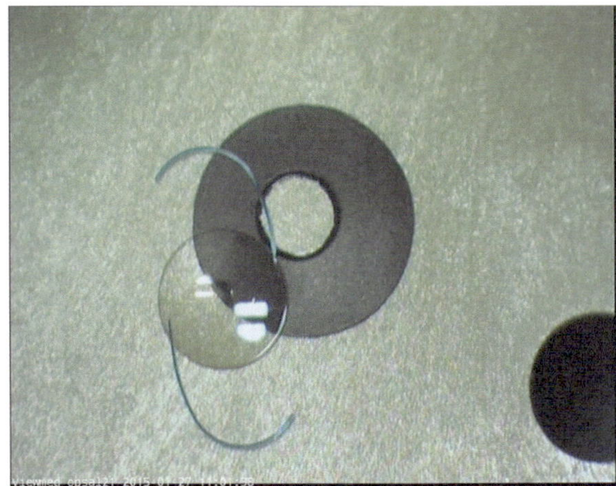

Fig. 35.14 A MA60AC IOL and the iris prosthesis

Pits and Pearls no. 21

I think that the implantation of a foldable iris prosthesis and a combo iris–IOL prosthesis with an IOL injector is the method of choice because it is easy and because the main incision is only 2,4 mm wide.

Pits and Pearls no. 22

The ultimate surgery would be to fasten the IOL–iris prosthesis with the Scharioth or Yamane method.

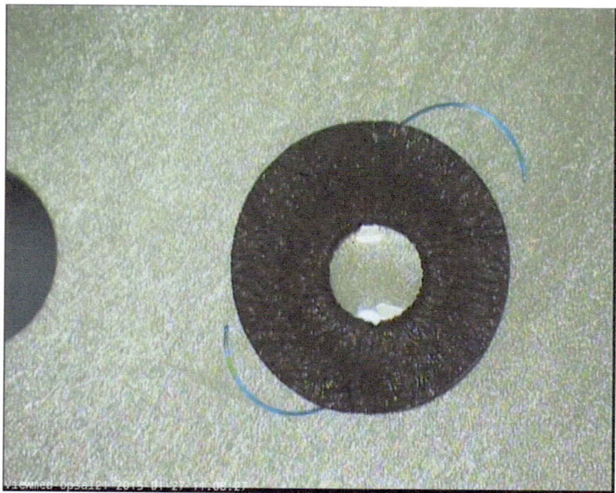

Fig. 35.15 The haptics of the IOL are inserted into the iris

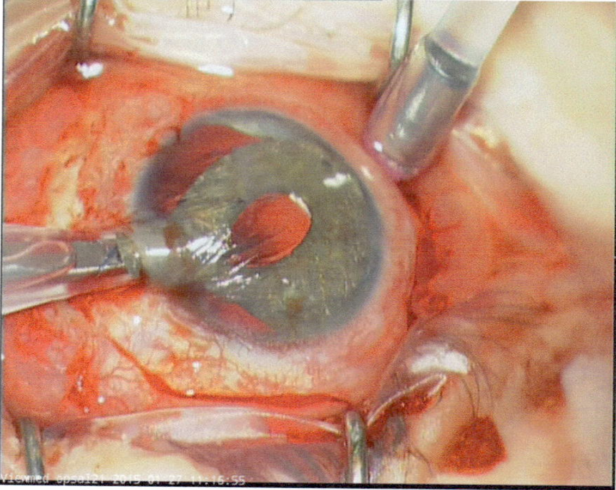

Fig. 35.16 The combo iris–IOL prosthesis is inserted with an IOL injector (Alcon)

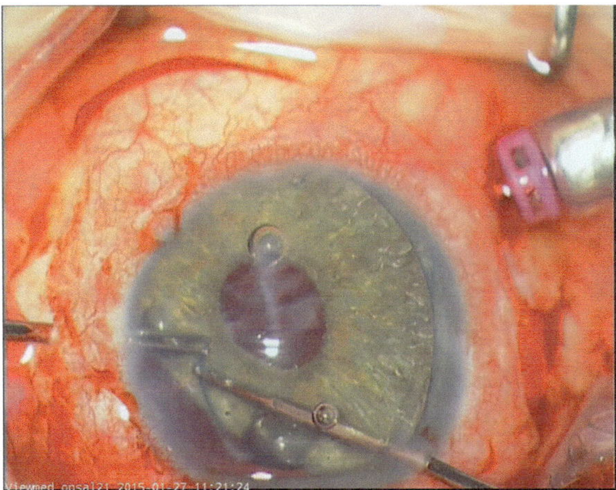

Fig. 35.17 The haptic is grasped inside the anterior chamber and externalised through the sclerotomy

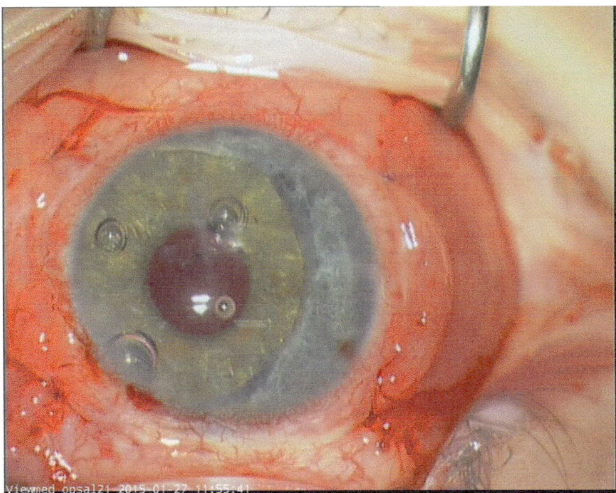

Fig. 35.18 The iris–IOL prosthesis is fixated with scleral sutures. An alternative is a sutureless intrascleral implantation (Scharioth technique)

Corneal, Lens and Retinal Perforation with a Nail

36

Abstract

The surgical management of a corneal, lenticular and retinal perforation is described step-by-step.

Keywords

Corneal perforation · Lenticular perforation · Retinal perforation · Perforation with nail · Surgery

A 24 y/o old male patient was handling a nail pistol during work (Fig. 36.1). At one moment, he was trying to shoot a nail through a wooden material from backward with the nail gun aiming towards his face. The nail shot through the material and penetrated the cornea into his eye. Visual acuity was light perception (Video available).

In the first surgery, the nail was extracted, the corneal wound sutured with a continuous suture and intravitreal antibiotics injected as an endophthalmitis prophylaxis (Figs. 36.2, 36.3, 36.4, 36.5 and 36.6). After 1 week, the patient was discharged, and there was no sign of an endophthalmitis. The eye was followed up weekly with B-scan, and the retina remained attached. After 4 weeks, a second surgery with planned phaco + IOL was performed (Figs. 36.7, 36.8, 36.9, 36.10, 36.11 and 36.12). An eye lash was extracted from the nucleus. Due to a large posterior capsular rupture, an anterior vitrectomy was performed, and I decided to continue then with vitrectomy (Figs. 36.13, 36.14, 36.15 and 36.16). A retinal defect was present at the posterior pole, maybe from the eye lash, maybe from the intravitreal injections. The retinal defect was treated with laser. The nail penetrated the retina at 12 o'clock posterior to the ora serrata. The retina was attached, and the perforation site was treated with cryopexy. Surgery was completed with an air tamponade. The corneal sutures could be removed after 3 months when a fibrotic corneal scar was present. The postoperative visual acuity is 0,6.

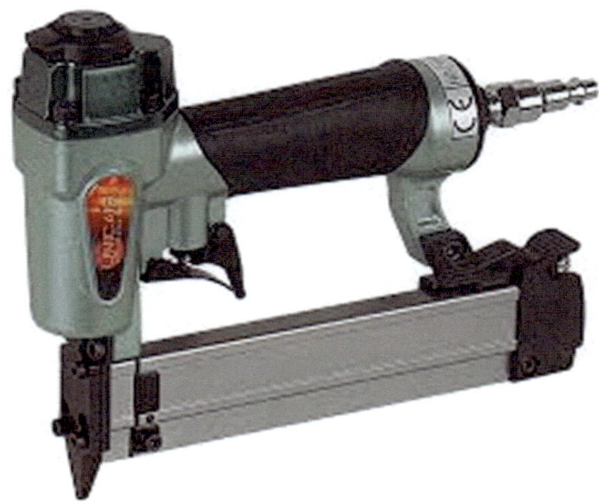

Fig. 36.1 Ocular perforation secondary to a nail from a nail pistol

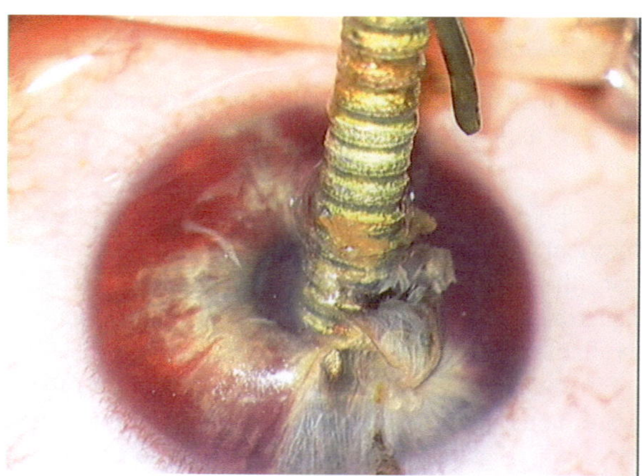

Fig. 36.2 The nail perforated the cornea and hit the retina at 12 o'clock

Remark: I would not perform a combined phaco/vitrectomy. As a result of this, the IOL has a superior iris capture. The vitrectomy with air tamponade caused posterior synechiae which could be prevented with a stepwise approach.

Materials and Companies

Materials (in alphabetical order):

15° knife: Indication: Paracentesis. Alcon. 8,065,921,501.
Acetylcholin, (Miochol®, Novartis). Indication: Pupil constriction.
Backflush instrument: 23G disposable Eckardt backflush. DORC 1281.A5D06.
Calipers, Castroviejo Geuder No.: 19135.

Fig. 36.3 Iris retractors were inserted

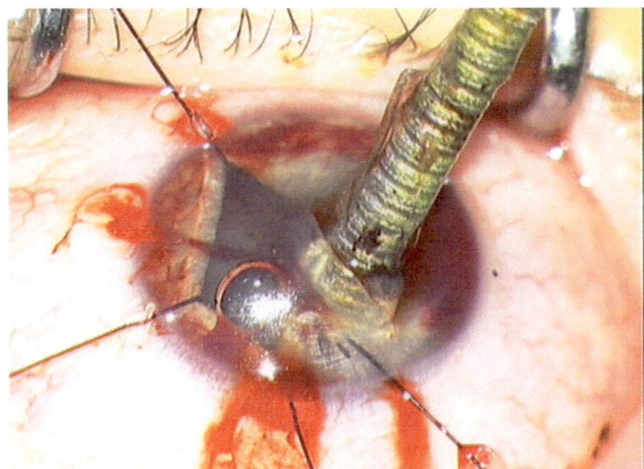

Fig. 36.4 The nail was extracted. Note the barbed hook which makes extraction difficult

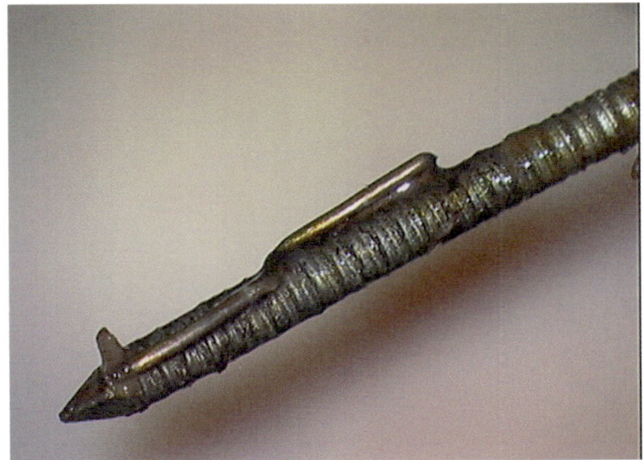

Fig. 36.5 The iris hooks were removed

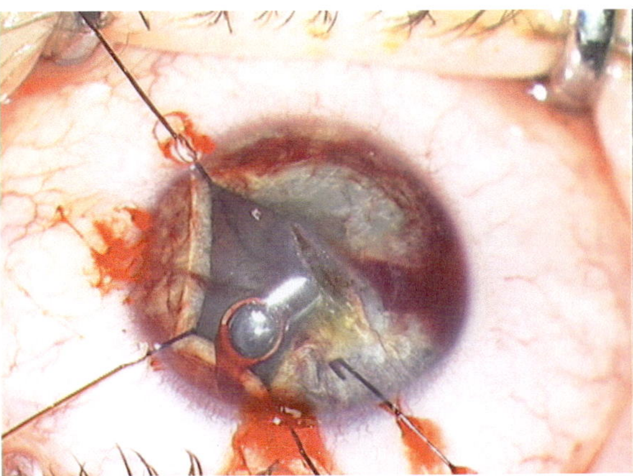

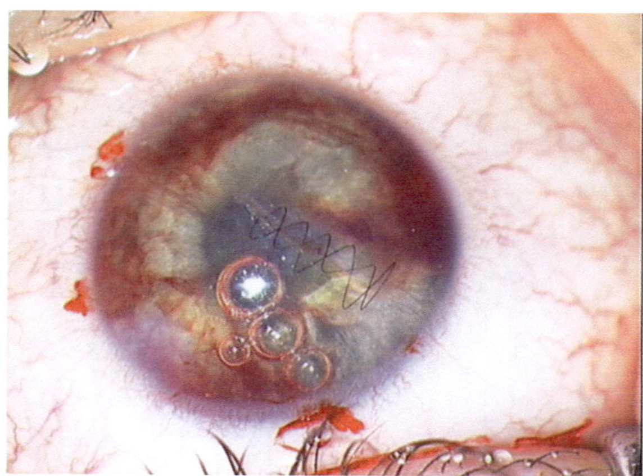

Fig. 36.6 The corneal wound was sutured with a continuous Ethilon 10-0 suture. In addition, intravitreal antibiotics were injected

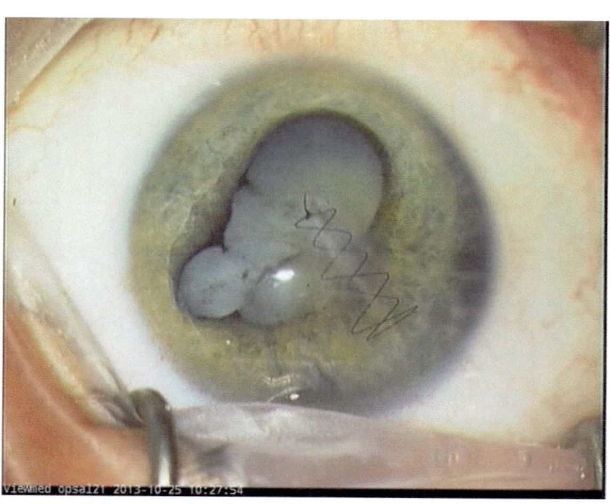

Fig. 36.7 1 Month later. Stable anterior chamber and posterior synechiae

Capsular tension ring with injector: CROMA, DORC, Morcher, Arcadophta.
Capsule scissors after Kampik. The instrument fits through a paracentesis. Indication: Cutting of capsule or iris. Geuder 38,215.
Capsulorhexis forceps. Geuder No.: 31299 or 31,308.
Chandelier light of Synergetics: 25G Awh Chandelier 56.20.25; of ALCON: Constellation Chandelier Chandelier Accurus 8,065,751,574 or 8,065,751,577; DORC of: 27-gauge twin light of Eckardt 3269.MBD27;
Chopper: 1) Combined instrument with push–pull and chopper. Chopper by Neuhann, Geuder 32,162; 2) Chopper by Agarwal. Indication: Chopping of a hard nucleus. Geuder 32,282.
Crescent bevel-up blade. Indication: Dissection of a frown-incision. Crescent-angled bevel up. Alcon. 8,065,990,002.

Fig. 36.8 Insertion of iris hooks

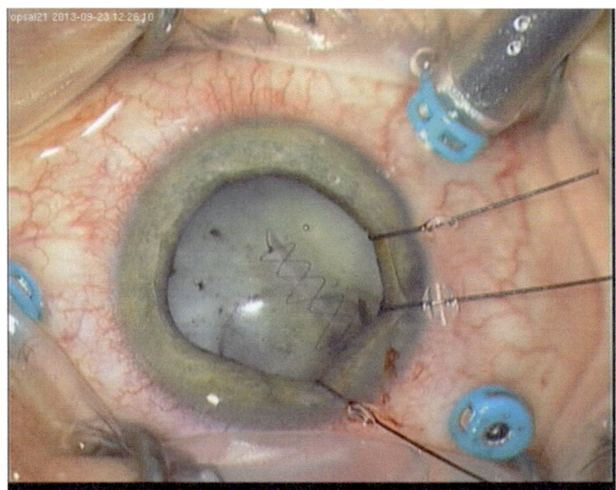

Fig. 36.9 Anterior rhexis with forceps and with 23G straight scissors (DORC)

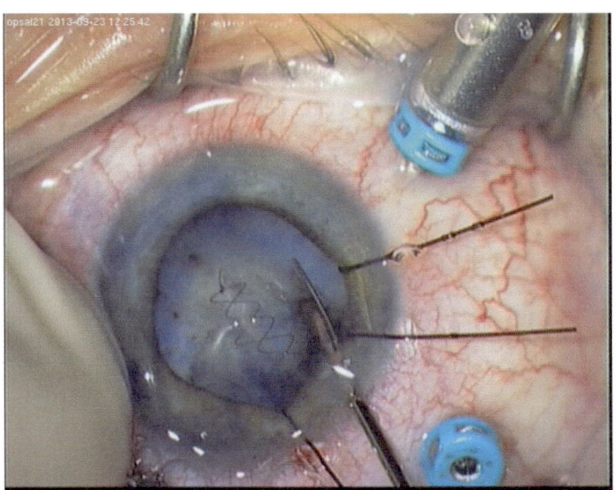

Double-barreled cannula 23G for injecting PFCL: DORC. Eftiar Dual Bore Cannula.

EFD.06.

Fragmatome: Alcon (Accurus fragmentation Handpiece), DORC Fragmatome 3002.M and 20G or 23G Phaco Fragmentation cannula DORC 3005.F106.

Fragment Forceps. Fragment forceps Gaskin. Geuder, No: 31624; Fragment forceps Kelman-McPherson, G-31623, Gaskin fragment forceps to Kansas. B & L. E-2030.

Intravitreal scissors. 23G. Indication: Cutting of tissue in anterior or posterior chamber. DORC 1286.J06.

Intravitreal serrated jaws forceps. 23G. Indication: Grasping of tissue in anterior or posterior chamber. DORC: 1286.C06.

Fig. 36.10 An unknown IOFB was found inside the nucleus

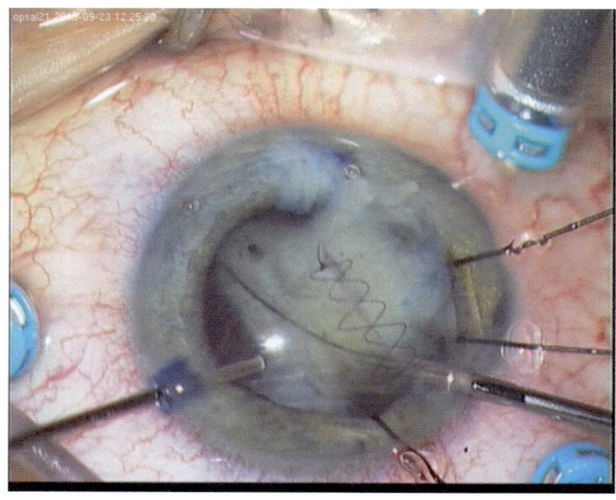

Fig. 36.11 An eye lash could be extracted

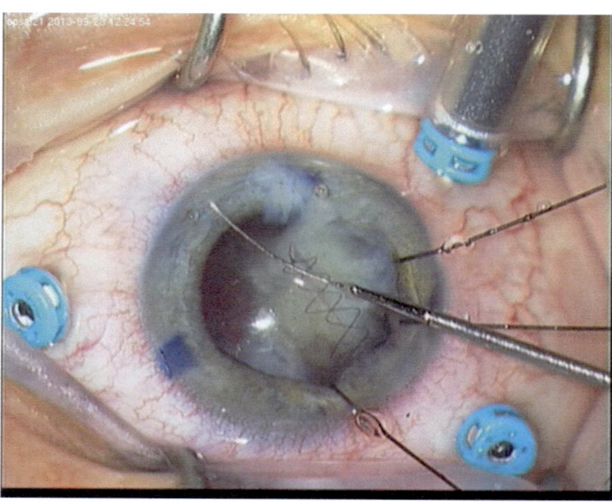

Iris prosthesis, foldable: Human Optics.

Iris prosthesis, non-foldable: Morcher, Opthec.

Iris retractors: Alcon / Grieshaber: Flexible Iris Retractors REF 611.75.

Kuglen hook: Katalyst: Kuglen push–pull hook, angled. (katalystsurgical.com).

Lens extraction hook: Lens extraction hook after Henning/Friedrich, Geuder 32,034.

Malyugin ring (6.25 mm) with injector: MST, (USA) MAL-0001.

Ocucoat ® (humidification of cornea): Bausch & Lomb.

Push Pull: Iris hook Dardenne (push–pull), Geuder 16,175.

Regular capsulotomy scissors. The instrument fits only through a main incision. Geuder 19,776.

Stiletto 23G. Indication: Lamellar sclerotomy. Beaver Visitec.

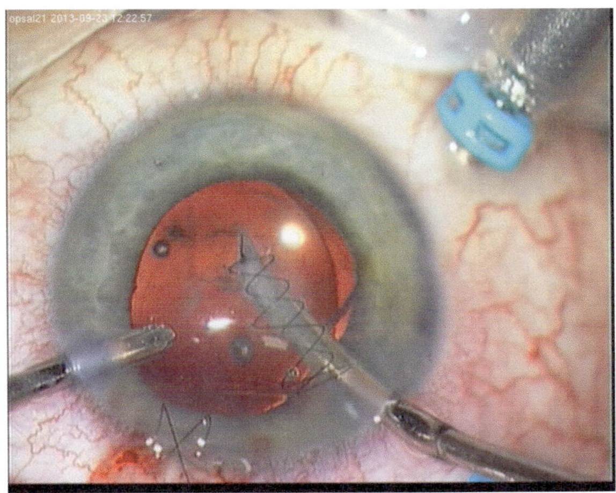

Fig. 36.12 Implantation of a 3-piece IOL into the sulcus

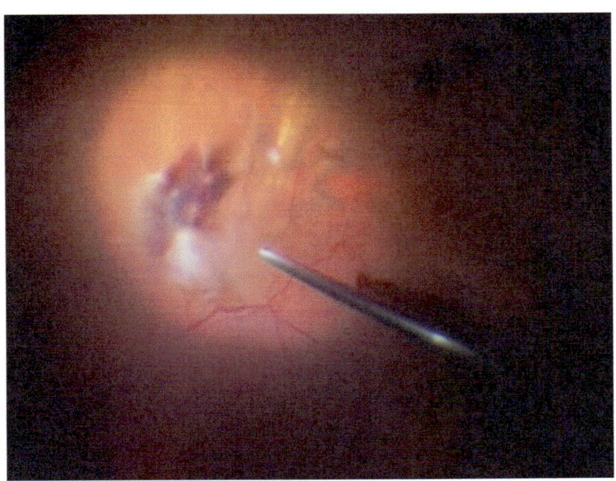

Fig. 36.13 A retinal perforation at 6 o'clock

Suture for scleral-fixated IOL: 2 curved needles. Alcon. Polypropylene, blue monofilament, double armed. 8,065,307,601th.

Suture for scleral-fixated IOL: 1 straight needle, 1 curved needle. Alcon. Polypropylene, blue monofilament, double armed. 8,065,304,901.

Sutures: Ethicon (www.ecatalog.ethicon.com/contact-us).

Suturing forceps. Castroviejo suturing forceps, Geuder, 19,023.

Triamcinolone acetonide (Volon A®): Pfizer.

Trocar forceps for removal of trocars. DORC No: 1278.

Tunnel incision knife, 2.4 mm wide. Indication: Main incision. Slit knife. Alcon. 8,065,992,445.

Tying forceps. Indication: Manipulation of suture or iris retractor. Tying forceps, Geuder, 19,032.

Fig. 36.14 Laser treatment around the impact edges

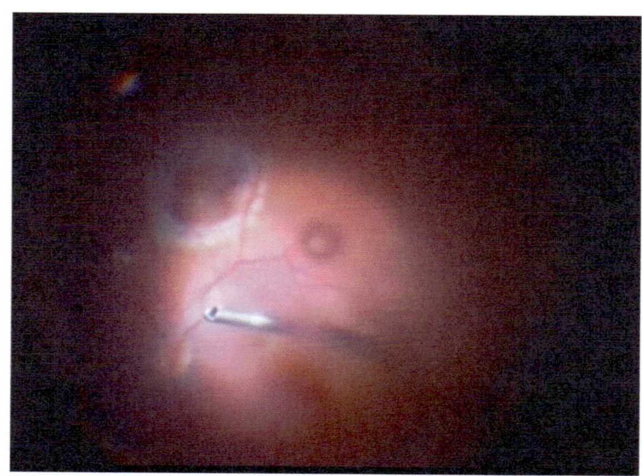

Fig. 36.15 At 12 o'clock a circular haemorrhage can be observed (1 month old). The retinal damage at 12 o'clock was treated with cryopexy

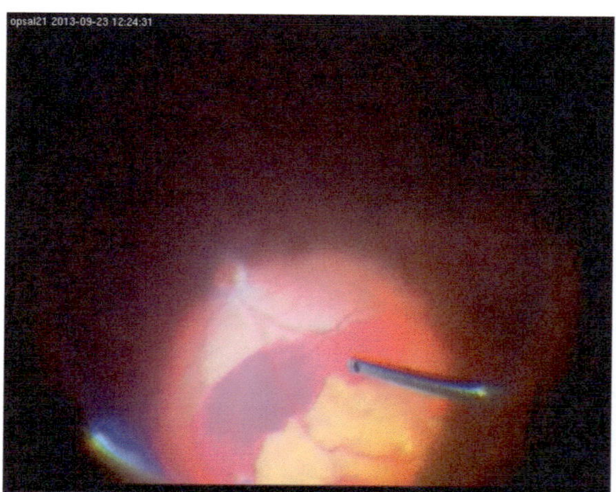

Fig. 36.16 3 Months postoperative. The corneal sutures are removed, and VA is 0,6

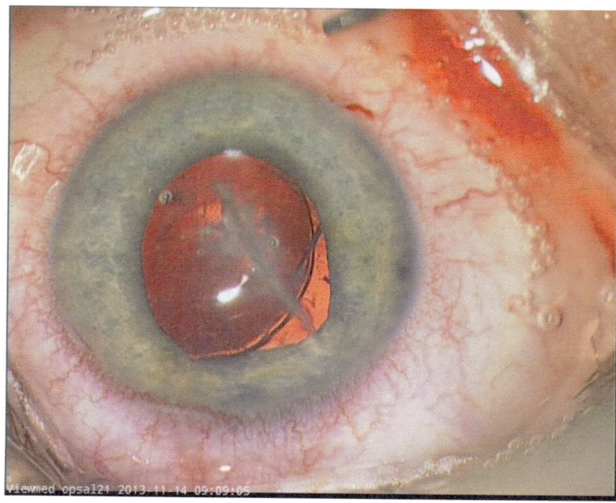

Trocars

(1)   Valved Trocar System by Alcon: 23G, 8,065,751,657;
(2)   Valved Trocar System by DORC: 23G, 1272.ED206

V-lance. 1.3 mm wide scleral and corneal diameter. Indication: Paracentesis and 20G sclerotomy. 20G V-lance. Alcon. 8,065,912,001.

Vannas scissors. Limbal peritomy. Geuder G-19760.

VisionBlue® (trypan blue): DORC.

Materials and Companies

Materials (in alphabetical order):

15° knife: Indication: Paracentesis. Alcon. 8,065,921,501

Acetylcholin, (Miochol®, Novartis). Indication: Pupil constriction

Backflush instrument: 23G disposable Eckardt backflush. DORC 1281.A5D06

Calipers, Castroviejo Geuder No.: 19135

Capsular tension ring with injector: CROMA, DORC, Morcher, Arcadophta

Capsule scissors after Kampik. The instrument fits through a paracentesis. Indication: Cutting of capsule or iris. Geuder 38,215

Capsulorhexis forceps. Geuder No.: 31299 or 31,308

Chandelier light of Synergetics: 25G Awh Chandelier 56.20.25; of ALCON: Constellation Chandelier Chandelier Accurus 8,065,751,574 or 8,065,751,577; DORC of: 27-gauge twin light of Eckardt 3269.MBD27;

Chopper: 1) Combined instrument with push–pull and chopper. Chopper by Neuhann, Geuder 32,162; 2) Chopper by Agarwal. Indication: Chopping of a hard nucleus. Geuder 32,282

Crescent bevel up blade. Indication: Dissection of a frown-incision. Crescent angled bevel up. Alcon. 8,065,990,002

Double-barreled cannula 23G for injecting PFCL: DORC. Eftiar Dual Bore Cannula
EFD.06

Fragmatome: Alcon (Accurus fragmentation Handpiece), DORC Fragmatome 3002.M and 20G or 23G Phaco Fragmentation cannula DORC 3005.F106

Fragment Forceps. Fragment forceps Gaskin. Geuder, No: 31624; Fragment forceps Kelman-McPherson, G-31623, Gaskin fragment forceps to Kansas. B & L. E-2030

Intravitreal scissors. 23G. Indication: Cutting of tissue in anterior or posterior chamber. DORC 1286.J06

Intravitreal serrated jaws forceps. 23G. Indication: Grasping of tissue in anterior or posterior chamber. DORC: 1286.C06

Iris prosthesis, foldable: Human Optics

Iris prosthesis, non foldable: Morcher, Opthec

Iris retractors: Alcon / Grieshaber: Flexible Iris Retractors REF 611.75

Kuglen hook: Katalyst: Kuglen push–pull hook, angled. (katalystsurgical.com)

© The Editor(s) (if applicable) and The Author(s), under exclusive license to Springer Nature Switzerland AG 2022

U. Spandau and G. B. Scharioth, *Complications During and After Cataract Surgery*, https://doi.org/10.1007/978-3-030-93531-3

Lens extraction hook: Lens extraction hook after Henning/Friedrich, Geuder 32,034
Malyugin ring (6.25 mm) with injector: MST, (USA) MAL-0001
Ocucoat ® (humidification of cornea): Bausch & Lomb
Push Pull: Iris hook Dardenne (push–pull), Geuder 16,175
Regular capsulotomy scissors. The instrument fits only through a main incision. Geuder 19,776
Stiletto 23G. Indication: Lamellar sclerotomy. Beaver Visitec
Suture for scleral fixated IOL: 2 curved needles. Alcon. Polypropylene, blue monofilament, double armed. 8,065,307,601th
Suture for scleral fixated IOL: 1 straight needle, 1 curved needle. Alcon. Polypropylene, blue monofilament, double armed. 8,065,304,901
Sutures: Ethicon (www.ecatalog.ethicon.com/contact-us)
Suturing forceps. Castroviejo suturing forceps, Geuder, 19,023
Triamcinolone acetonide (Volon A®): Pfizer
Trocar forceps for removal of trocars. DORC No: 1278
Tunnel incision knife, 2.4 mm wide. Indication: Main incision. Slit knife. Alcon. 8,065,992,445
Tying forceps. Indication: Manipulation of suture or iris retractor. Tying forceps, Geuder, 19,032

Trocars

(1) Valved Trocar System by Alcon: 23G, 8,065,751,657;
(2) Valved Trocar System by DORC: 23G, 1272.ED206

V-lance. 1.3 mm wide scleral and corneal diameter. Indication: Paracentesis and 20G sclerotomy. 20G V-lance. Alcon. 8,065,912,001
Vannas scissors. Limbal peritomy. Geuder G-19760
VisionBlue® (trypan blue): DORC

Companies' directory (in alphabetical order):

Alcon
Alcon Pharma GmbH
Blank Reute Address 1
79,108 Freiburg / Breisgau
Tel: 0049/761/13040
www.alcon-pharma.de

Arcadophta.
293, route de Seysses.
F-31100 Toulouse
Tel: 0033/561/405235
Fax: 0033/5617 408 466
info@arcadophta.com
www.arcadophta.com

Bausch & Lomb
Brunsbütteler Damm 165-173
13,581 Berlin
Tel: 030/330 935 702
Fax: 030/330 935 712
www.bausch-lomb.de

Beaver-Visitec International, Ltd.
Centurion Court
85c Milton Park
Abingdon, Oxfordshire
OX14 4RY
UK
www.Beaver-Visitec.com

CROMA GmbH
Industrial Line 6
2100 Leobendorf
Österrreich
Tel: + 43/2262/684680

DORC
D.O.R.C. Germany GmbH
Charlottenstr. 80
10,117 Berlin
Tel: 030/20188364
Fax: 030/20188365
Website: DORC.nl

Ethicon
Johnson & Johnson Medical GmbH
ETHICON Endo-Surgery Deutschland
Hummelsbütteler Steindamm 71
22,851 Norderstedt
Deutschland
www.ethicon.com

Eye Technology Ltd.
19 Totman Crescent
Brook Road Industrial Estate
Rayleigh
Essex SS6 7UY
United Kingdom
sales@eye-tech.co.uk

Fluoron GmbH
Magirus-Deutz-Straße 10
89,077 Ulm
Tel: 0731/20559970
Fax: 0731/205 599 728
info@fluoron.de
www.fluoron.de

Geuder
Hertzstr. 4
69,126 Heidelberg
Tel: 06,221/3066
Fax: 06,221/303122
info@geuder.de
www.geuder.de

Human Optics
Dr. Schmidt Intraocularlinsen GmbH
Westerwaldstraße 11–13
53,757 Sankt Augustin
Germany
e-mail: iris@humanoptics.com
www.artificial-iris.com

Katalyst Surgical Inc.
754 Goddard Avenue
Chesterfield, MO 63,005
USA
www.katalystsurgical.com

Medone Surgical Inc.
Sarasota, FL 34,243
USA
www.MedOne.com

Möller-Wedel GmbH
Rosengarten 10
22,880 Wedel
Germany
Phone: + 49 4103 709 01
Fax: + 49 4103 709 355
Email: sales@moeller-wedel.com
www.moeller-wedel.com

MorcherGmbH
Kapuzinerstrasse, 12
70,374 Stuttgart
Phone: + 49(0)711/95320–0
e-mail: info@morcher.com
www.morcher.com

MST (Microsurgical technology)
8415 154th Ave NE,
Redmond, WA 98,052
USA
www.microsurgical.com/

OASIS® Medical, Inc.
Sales & Marketing Office
OASIS Medical, Inc.
635 West Allen Avenue
San Dimas, CA 91,773
www.oasismedical.com

Oculus Optic device GmbH
Münchholzhäuser Strasse 29
D-35582 Wetzlar
Phone: 0641/20050
Fax: 0641/2005255
e-mail: sales@oculus.de
www.oculus.de

Opthec BV
Schweitzerlaan 15
9728 NR Groningen
Netherlands
Phone: + 31 050 5,251,944
www.opthec.com

Synergetics Germany GmbH
Körnerstraße 59
58,095 Hagen
Phone: 0641/20050
Fax: 0641/2005255
Email: blangohr@synergeticsusa.com
www.synergeticsusa.com

List of All Pits and Pearls

Pits & Pearls no. 1: Optics and constant irrigation during phaco and I/A.
Pits & Pearls no. 2: Soft nucleus.
Pits & Pearls no. 3: Epinucleus during phaco.
Pits & Pearls no. 4: Removal of phaco handpiece from anterior chamber.
Pits & Pearls no. 5: Unsuccessful quadrant removal.
Pits & Pearls no. 6: Unstable anterior chamber.
Pits & Pearls no. 7: Flat anterior chamber.
Pits & Pearls no. 8: Poor visualization of rhexis edge.
Pits & Pearls no. 9: Incomplete rhexis.
Pits & Pearls no. 10: Not round rhexis.
Pits & Pearls no. 11: Small pupil and white nucleus.
Pits & Pearls no. 12: Pressure from behind.
Pits & Pearls no. 13: Soft nucleus. pseudoexfoliation.
Pits & Pearls no. 14: Wound assisted IOL implantation.
Pits & Pearls no. 15: Both haptics inside the lens capsule.
Pits & Pearls no. 16: Incarcerated vitreous strand.
Pits & Pearls no. 17: IOL scaffolding.
Pits & Pearls no. 18: IOL capture.
Pits & Pearls no. 19: IOL extraction.
Pits & Pearls no. 20: Intrascleral IOL fixation.
Pits & Pearls no. 21: Combo iris-IOL prosthesis.
Pits & Pearls no. 22: Fixation of IOL-iris prosthesis with Scharioth method.

List of all videos

All videos can be found in a playlist of my YouTube channel:
https://www.youtube.com/playlist?list=PL0dKYclPD7yMJRuQAIt9Dr7pOtuI0
 Seex

Part II: Easy cataract: Divide and conquer.
Part II: Easy cataract, chop technique.
Part II: Malyugin ring
Part II: Sphincterectomy.

U. Spandau and G. B. Scharioth, *Complications During and After Cataract Surgery*,
https://doi.org/10.1007/978-3-030-93531-3

Part II: Difficult rhexis.
Part II: Special techniques for anterior chamber.
Part II: Simple technique for nucleus cracking.
Part II: Hard nucleus and small pupil.
Part II: Stuck IOL in main incision 1.
Part II: Stuck IOL in main incision 2.

Part III: Basis of anterior vitreous cutter.
Part III: Anterior vitrectomy from pars plana.
Part III: Would you call a vitreoretinal surgeon for this pathology.
Part III: Basics of management of PCR.
Part III: IOL scaffold.
Part III: PCR management with 1 trocar
Part III: Surgical management of a posterior capsular rent with 1 trocar
Part III: PCR with round capsular defect.
Part III: Removal of vitreous strands due to PCR.
Part III: Surgical management of positive vitreous pressure (PVP).
Part III: Removal of PCO from pars plana.

Part IV: SICS technique.
Part IV: Zonular lysisand phacoemulsification
Part IV: Traumatic cataract with inferior zonular lysis
Part IV: ICCE and iris claw IOL
Part IV: SICS and inferior zonular lysis
Part IV: Small pupil and phacodonesis.

Part V: IOL exchange.
Part V: IOL refolding.
Part V: IOL rolling.
Part V: Bi-section of silicone IOL.
Part V: Iris capture.

Part VI: Surgical management of anterior dislocated IOL from pars plana.
Part VI: Sulcus implantation for dummies.
Part VI: IOL extraction and iris claw IOL implantation.
Part VI: Subluxated IOL and Artisan IOL implantation, operated with one trocar
Part VI: Intrascleral PCIOL fixation (Scharioth).
Part VI: Intrascleral fixation with DORC forceps 1.
Part VI: Intrascleral fixation with DORC forceps 1.
Part VI: Yamane technique.
Part VI: Scleral fixation of IOL
Part VI: IOL refixation with Hoffmann technique
Part VI: Fixation of an IOL to iris with suture.
Part VI: Fixation of an IOL-in-the-bag with suture to iris, an elegant and simple technique.

Part VII: Insertion of trocar cannulas.
Part VII: Surgery of a dropped nucleus for dummies with phaco machine.
Part VII: Dropped nucleus with Infinity machine and phacoemulsification handpiece.
Part VII: Management of a dropped nucleus.
Part VII: Extraction of dropped nucleus with ICCE and retropupillar Artisan IOL.
Part VII: Combined phaco + PPV.
Part VII: Extraction of dropped nucleus with fragmatome and sulcus IOL.
Part VII: Posterior dislocated IOL retrieval and scleral fixation.

Part VIII: Corneal and scleral perforation with iris prolapse.
Part VIII: Traumatic cataract after paint ball trauma.
Part VIII: Traumatic cataract after blunt globe trauma_1.
Part VIII: Traumatic cataract after blunt globe trauma_2.
Part VIII: Iris claw IOL implantation and artificial pupil.
Part VIII: Iris suture and Artisan IOL for traumatic iris defect and aniridia.
Part VIII: Implantation of a foldable iris prosthesis

Bonus videos:

Bonus videos: Phaco nightmare and intrascleral fixation.
Bonus videos: Injection of Ozurdex pellet into a nucleus.
Bonus videos: Lens injury after intravitreal injection.
Bonus videos: Hyphema after complicated cataract surgery.
Bonus videos: IOL and capsular tension ring extraction and iris-claw IOL implantation.
Bonus videos: New technique for refixation of luxated IOL (Scharioth).
Bonus video: Subluxated nucleus and intrascleral IOL fixation (Scharioth).

Index

© The Editor(s) (if applicable) and The Author(s), under exclusive license to Springer Nature Switzerland AG 2022
U. Spandau and G. B. Scharioth, *Complications During and After Cataract Surgery*,
https://doi.org/10.1007/978-3-030-93531-3

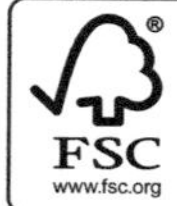

MIX
Papier aus verantwortungsvollen Quellen
Paper from responsible sources
FSC® C105338

If you have any concerns about our products,
you can contact us on
ProductSafety@springernature.com

In case Publisher is established outside the EU,
the EU authorized representative is:
Springer Nature Customer Service Center GmbH
Europaplatz 3, 69115 Heidelberg, Germany

Printed by Libri Plureos GmbH
in Hamburg, Germany